The Parasomnias

Editor

ALON Y. AVIDAN

SLEEP MEDICINE CLINICS

www.sleep.theclinics.com

March 2024 • Volume 19 • Number 1

ELSEVIER

1600 John F. Kennedy Boulevard • Suite 1800 • Philadelphia, Pennsylvania, 19103-2899

http://www.theclinics.com

SLEEP MEDICINE CLINICS Volume 19, Number 1
March 2024, ISSN 1556-407X, ISBN-13: 978-0-443-12925-4

Editor: Joanna Gascoine
Developmental Editor: Akshay Samson

Sleep Medicine Clinics (ISSN 1556-407X) is published quarterly by Elsevier Inc., 360 Park Avenue South, New York, NY 10010-1710. Months of issue are March, June, September and December. Business and Editorial Offices: 1600 John F. Kennedy Blvd., Ste. 1800, Philadelphia, PA 19103-2899. Customer Service Office: 3251 Riverport Lane, Maryland Heights, MO 63043. Periodicals postage paid at New York, NY and additional mailing offices. Subscription prices are $246.00 per year (US individuals), $100.00 (US and Canadian students), $283.00 (Canadian individuals), $292.00 (international individuals) $135.00 (International students). For institutional access pricing please contact Customer Service via the contact information below. Foreign air speed delivery is included in all *Clinics* subscription prices. All prices are subject to change without notice. **POSTMASTER:** Send change of address to *Sleep Medicine Clinics*, Elsevier Health Sciences Division, Subscription Customer Service, 3251 Riverport Lane, Maryland Heights, MO 63043. Customer Service: **Tel: 1-800-654-2452 (U.S. and Canada); 314-447-8871 (outside U.S. and Canada). Fax: 314-447-8029. E-mail: journalscustomerservice-usa@elsevier.com (for print support); journalsonlinesupport-usa@elsevier.com (for online support)**.

Reprints. For copies of 100 or more of articles in this publication, please contact the Commercial Reprints Department, Elsevier Inc., 360 Park Avenue South, New York, NY 10010-1710. Tel.: 212-633-3874; Fax: 212-633-3820; E-mail: reprints@elsevier.com.

Sleep Medicine Clinics is covered in *MEDLINE/PubMed (Index Medicus)*.

SLEEP MEDICINE CLINICS

SERIES OF RELATED INTEREST

Neurologic Clinics
https://www.neurologic.theclinics.com/

THE CLINICS ARE AVAILABLE ONLINE!
Access your subscription at:
www.theclinics.com

Contributors

CONSULTING EDITORS

TEOFILO LEE-CHIONG Jr, MD
Professor of Medicine, National Jewish Health,
Professor of Medicine, University of Colorado,
Denver, Colorado, USA; Chief Medical Liaison,
Philips Respironics, Murrysville, Pennsylvania,
USA

DIEGO GARCIA-BORREGUERO, MD, PhD
International Medical Director Instituto del
Sueño, Calle Padre Damián, Madrid, Spain

ANA C. KRIEGER, MD, MPH, FCCP, FAASM
Chief, Division of Sleep Neurology, Medical
Director, Weill Cornell Center for Sleep
Medicine, Professor of Clinical Medicine,
Professor of Medicine in Neurology and
Genetic Medicine, Weill Cornell Medical
College, Cornell University, New York, New
York, USA

EDITOR

ALON Y. AVIDAN, MD, MPH, FAAN, FAASM
Professor, Department of Neurology,
University of California, Los Angeles; Fellow,
American Academy of Sleep Medicine; Fellow,
American Academy of Neurology; Program

Director, University of California, Los Angeles
Sleep Medicine, Director, UCLA Sleep
Disorders Center, David Geffen School of
Medicine at University of California, Los
Angeles, Los Angeles, California, USA

AUTHORS

MONICA LEVY ANDERSEN, PhD
Associate Professor, Departamento de
Psicobiologia, Universidade Federal de São
Paulo (UNIFESP), Sleep Institute, São Paulo,
Brazil

R. ROBERT AUGER, MD
Psychiatrist, Sleep Medicine Specialist, Center
for Sleep Medicine, Mayo Clinic, Rochester,
Minnesota, USA

ALON Y. AVIDAN, MD, MPH, FAAN, FAASM
Professor, Department of Neurology,
University of California, Los Angeles; Fellow,
American Academy of Sleep Medicine; Fellow,
American Academy of Neurology; Program
Director, University of California, Los Angeles
Sleep Medicine, Director, UCLA Sleep
Disorders Center, David Geffen School of
Medicine at University of California, Los
Angeles, Los Angeles, California, USA

SOMAYYEH AZIMI, PhD
Research Officer, Clinical Research Centre,
Graylands Hospital, North Metropolitan Health
Service Mental Health, Perth, Western
Australia, Australia; Research Fellow, School of
Human Sciences, University of Western
Australia, Crawley, Western Australia, Australia

LUCIE BARATEAU, MD, PhD
Physician, Sleep-Wake Disorders Unit,
Department of Neurology, Gui-de-Chauliac
Hospital, CHU Montpellier, INSERM Institute of
Neurosciences of Montpellier, University of
Montpellier, Montpellier, France

DANIEL A. BARONE, MD, FAASM, FANA
Associate Medical Director, Weill Cornell
Center for Sleep Medicine, Associate
Professor of Clinical Neurology, Weill Cornell
Medicine, New York-Presbyterian, New York,
New York, USA

JAN DIRK BLOM, MD, PhD
Psychiatrist, Director of the Psychiatric Training Programme for Adult Psychiatry, Professor of Clinical Psychopathology, Parnassia Psychiatric Institute, The Hague, the Netherlands; Faculty of Social and Behavioural Sciences, Leiden University, Leiden, the Netherlands; Department of Psychiatry, University Medical Center Groningen, Groningen, the Netherlands

SOFIENE CHENINI, MD
Physician, Sleep-Wake Disorders Unit, Department of Neurology, Gui-de-Chauliac Hospital, CHU Montpellier, INSERM Institute of Neurosciences of Montpellier, University of Montpellier, Montpellier, France

RAMONA CORDANI, MD
Physician, Department of Neuroscience, Rehabilitation, Ophthalmology, Genetics, Maternal and Child Health, University of Genoa, Genoa, Italy

YVES DAUVILLIERS, MD, PhD
Director, Professor, Sleep-Wake Disorders Unit, Department of Neurology, Gui-de-Chauliac Hospital, CHU Montpellier, INSERM Institute of Neurosciences of Montpellier, University of Montpellier, Montpellier, France

DEEPALI M. DHRUVE, MS
Department of Psychology, Mississippi State University, Mississippi State, Mississippi, USA

ALAN S. EISER, PhD
Consultant, University of Michigan Sleep Disorders Center, Adjunct Clinical Assistant Professor, Department of Psychiatry, University of Michigan, Ann Arbor, Michigan, USA

DÓNAL G. FORTUNE, ClinPsyD, PhD
Chair of Clinical Psychology and Full Professor, Department of Psychology, University of Limerick; Health Service Executive, CHO 3 Mid West Region, Ireland; Health Research Institute, Univeristy of Limerick, Limerick, Ireland

VICTORIA R. GARRIQUES, MPS
Department of Psychology, Mississippi State University, Mississippi State, Mississippi, USA

BRIAN HOLOYDA, MD, MPH, MBA
Chief Psychiatrist, Contra Costa County Detention Health Services, Psychiatrist, Martinez Detention Facility, Martinez, California, USA; Adjunct Assistant Professor of Psychiatry, Department of Psychiatry and Behavioral Medicine, Medical College of Wisconsin, Milwaukee, Wisconsin, USA; Forensic Psychiatrist, Denver, Colorado, USA

MUNA IRFAN, MBBS
Associate Professor, Department of Neurology, University of Minnesota, Minneapolis Veterans Affairs Healthcare System, Eagan, Minnesota, USA

BRANDON M. JONES, MD, MS
Resident Physician, Department of Neurology, Mayo Clinic, Rochester, Minnesota, USA

FELICE DI LAUDO, MD
Neurology Resident, Department of Biomedical and NeuroMotor Sciences (DiBiNeM), University of Bologna, Bologna, Italy

IVAN LING, MBBS, FRACP
Respiratory and Sleep Physician, West Australian Sleep Disorders Research Institute, Perth, Western Australia, Australia; Department of Pulmonary Physiology and Sleep Medicine, Sir Charles Gairdner Hospital, Nedlands, Western Australia, Australia

MELISSA C. LIPFORD, MD
Neurologist, Sleep Medicine Specialist, Center for Sleep Medicine, Mayo Clinic, Rochester, Minnesota, USA

REGIS LOPEZ, MD, PhD
Physician, Sleep-Wake Disorders Unit, Department of Neurology, Gui-de-Chauliac Hospital, CHU Montpellier, INSERM Institute of Neurosciences of Montpellier, University of Montpellier, Montpellier, France

GRETA MAINIERI, MD
Neurologist, Department of Biomedical and NeuroMotor Sciences (DiBiNeM), University of Bologna, IRCCS Istituto delle Scienze Neurologiche di Bologna, Bologna, Italy

RONEIL MALKANI, MD, MS
Associate Professor, Department of
Neurology, Northwestern University
Feinberg School of Medicine, Neurology
Service, Jesse Brown Veterans Affairs
Medical Center, Chicago, Illinois,
USA

STUART J. McCARTER, MD
Assistant Professor, Department of
Neurology, Center for Sleep Medicine,
Mayo Clinic, Rochester, Minnesota,
USA

COURTNEY D. MOLINA, BS
Patient Education Liaison, Department of
Neurology, UCLA, David Geffen School of
Medicine at UCLA, Los Angeles, California,
USA

MICHAEL R. NADORFF, PhD
Professor, Department of Psychology,
Mississippi State University, Mississippi State,
Mississippi, USA

LINO NOBILI, MD, PhD
Director, Professor, Department of
Neuroscience, Rehabilitation, Ophthalmology,
Genetics, Maternal and Child Health, University
of Genoa, Genoa, Italy

FEDERICA PROVINI, MD, PhD
Professor, Neurologist, Department of
Biomedical and NeuroMotor Sciences
(DiBiNeM), University of Bologna, IRCCS
Istituto delle Scienze Neurologiche di Bologna,
Bologna, Italy

HELEN L. RICHARDS, ClinPsyD, PhD
Head of Department of Psychology, Mercy
University Hospital, Cork, Ireland; Adjunct Full
Professor, University of Limerick, Limerick,
Ireland

ADREANNE RIVERA, BS
Clinical Research Coordinator, UCLA Clinical
Translational Science Institute, Los Angeles,
California, USA

CARLOS H. SCHENCK, MD
Department of Psychiatry, Professor,
Minnesota Regional Sleep Disorders Center,
Hennepin County Medical Center, University of
Minnesota Medical School, Minneapolis,
Minnesota, USA

ROSALIA SILVESTRI, MD
Associate Professor, Sleep Medicine Center,
UOSD of Neurophysiopathology and Movement
Disorders, Department of Clinical and
Experimental Medicine, University of Messina,
Messina, Italy

AMBRA STEFANI, MD, PhD
Postdoctoral Clinical Research Fellow,
Neurological Clinical Research Institute,
Department of Neurology, Sleep Disorders
Clinic, Medical University of Innsbruck,
Innsbruck, Austria

QI TANG, MD
Department of Neurology, Sleep Disorders
Clinic, Medical University of Innsbruck,
Innsbruck, Austria

SERGIO TUFIK, MD, PhD
Professor, Departamento de Psicobiologia,
Universidade Federal de São Paulo (UNIFESP),
Sleep Institute, São Paulo, Brazil

FLAVIE WATERS, MSc, MPsych, PhD
Senior Research Fellow, Clinical Research
Centre, Graylands Hospital, North Metropolitan
Health Service Mental Health, Perth, Western
Australia, Australia; Research Professor,
School of Psychological Science, The
University of Western Australia, Crawley,
Western Australia, Australia

Contents

Parasomnias are defined as abnormal movements or behaviors that occur in sleep or during arousals from sleep. Parasomnias vary in frequency from episodic events that arise from incomplete sleep state transition. The framework by which parasomnias are categorized and diagnosed is based on the International Classification of Sleep Disorders–Third Edition, Text Revision (ICSD-3-TR), published by the American Academy of Sleep Medicine. The recent Third Edition, Text Revision (ICSD-3-TR) of the ICSD provides an expert consensus of the diagnostic requirements for sleep disorders, including parasomnias, based on an extensive review of the current literature.

Sexual behavior during sleep, known as sexual parasomnias, has captured the interest of researchers and clinicians. These parasomnias involve various sexual activities that occur unconsciously during sleep. Although relatively rare, they can profoundly affect well-being and relationships and can carry legal consequences. Understanding their nature, prevalence, and causes is crucial for advancing knowledge in this field. This article revisits the topic of sexsomnia, presenting new data and discussing cases published from 2007 to 2023. By analyzing these cases, we aim to enhance recognition, diagnosis, and management of sexsomnia, reducing stigma and providing better support for affected individuals.

Somnambulism, also called sleepwalking, classified as a non-rapid eye movement sleep parasomnia, encompasses a range of abnormal paroxysmal behaviors, leading to sleepwalking in dissociated sleep in an altered state of consciousness with impaired judgment and configuring a kind of hierarchical continuum with confusional arousal and night terror. Despite being generally regarded as a benign condition, its potential severity entails social, personal, and even forensic consequences. This comprehensive review provides an overview on the current state of knowledge, elucidating the phenomenon of somnambulism and encompassing its clinical manifestations and diagnostic approaches.

Sleep-related eating disorder is a non-rapid-eye movement parasomnia typified by recurrent episodes of eating/drinking following arousals, with associated partial/complete amnesia. Adverse health consequences and quality of life impairments are common. The condition can be idiopathic but most often accompanies unrecognized/untreated comorbid sleep disorders and/or is induced by psychoactive medications. As such, management consists of addressing comorbidities and removing potentially offending medications. While a thorough clinical history is often sufficient, additional sleep testing may help identify coexisting sleep disorders and/or other phenomena that may cause arousals. Limited data suggest benefit from topiramate and other medications in idiopathic or otherwise refractory cases.

 Video content accompanies this article at http://www.sleep.theclinics.com.

Sleep terrors, categorized under disorders of arousal, more prevalent in pediatric population, generally are self-limited but sometimes can persist or occur in adulthood. These are primed by factors enhancing homeostatic drive on backdrop of developmental predisposition and are precipitated by factors increasing sleep fragmentation resulting in dissociated state of sleep with some cerebral regions showing abnormal slow wave activity and others fast activity. This phenotypically evolves into abrupt partial arousal with individual arousing from N3 or N2 sleep with behaviors representing intense fear such as crying with autonomic hyperactivity. There is no recollection of the event, and lack of vivid dream mentation although fragmented imagery may be noted. Behavioral management is of prime importance including addressing precipitating factors, family reassurance, safety measures, and scheduled awakenings. Pharmacologic agents such as clonazepam and antidepressants are used infrequently in case of disruptive episodes.

Rapid eye movement (REM) sleep behavior disorder (RBD) classically presents with repetitive complex motor behavior during sleep with associated dream mentation. The diagnosis requires a history of repetitive complex motor behaviors and polysomnographic demonstration of REM sleep without atonia (RSWA) or capturing dream enactment behaviors. RSWA is best evaluated in the chin or flexor digitorum superficialis muscles. The anterior tibialis muscle is insufficiently accurate to be relied upon solely for RBD diagnosis. RBD may present with parkinsonism or cognitive impairment or may present in isolation. Patients should be monitored for parkinsonism, autonomic failure, or cognitive impairment.

Management of rapid eye movement sleep behavior disorder (RBD) includes reducing injurious dream-enactment behaviors, risk of injury to self and bedpartner, and vivid or disruptive dreams and improving sleep quality and bedpartner sleep disruption. Safety precautions should be reviewed at each visit. Medications to reduce RBD symptoms such as melatonin, clonazepam, pramipexole, and rivastigmine should be considered for most patients. Isolated RBD confers a high lifetime risk of neurodegenerative diseases with a latency often spanning many years. A patient-centered shared decision-making approach to risk disclosure is recommended. Knowledge of the risk allows for life planning and participation in research.

Trauma-associated sleep disorder (TASD) is a recently described parasomnia that develops following a traumatic event. It consists of trauma-related nightmares, disruptive nocturnal behaviors, and autonomic disturbances, and shares similarities with post-traumatic stress disorder and rapid eye movement behavior disorder. The underlying pathophysiology of TASD and how it relates to other parasomnias are still not entirely understood; proposed treatment is similarly nebulous, with prazosin at the forefront along with management of comorbid sleep disorders. The purpose of this article is to characterize and highlight the clinical features of this condition.

Recurrent isolated sleep paralysis has a 7.6% lifetime prevalence of at least one episode in the general population. Episodes resolve spontaneously and are benign. Sleep paralysis represents a dissociate state, with persistence of the rapid eye movement (REM)-sleep muscle atonia in the waking state. The intrusion of alpha electroencephalogram into REM sleep is followed by an arousal response and then by persistence of REM atonia into wakefulness. Predisposing factors include irregular sleep-wake schedules, sleep deprivation, and jetlag. No drug treatment is required. Patients should be informed about sleep hygiene. Cognitive behavioral therapy may be useful in cases accompanied by anxiety and frightening hallucinations.

This article presents a comprehensive review of nightmare disorder, covering diagnosis, treatment approaches, guidelines, and considerations. It begins with an introduction, defining the disorder and addressing its prevalence and psychosocial implications. The article explores assessment tools for diagnosis and then delves into psychological and pharmacologic treatment modalities, examining their efficacy and side effects. Considerations for optimizing therapeutic outcomes are highlighted, including medication versus psychotherapy, co-morbidities, cultural implications, and the use of technology and service animals. The review concludes by offering key recommendations for effective treatment and clinical care for individuals with nightmare disorder.

Exploding head syndrome (EHS) has historically been viewed as a disorder predominantly affecting older people and being more common in females. Through a comprehensive review of data since 2005, this scoping review provides updated evidence from 4082 participants reporting EHS across a variety of study designs on: how EHS presents; key information on comorbidity and correlates of EHS; how EHS is experienced in terms of symptoms and beliefs; causal theories arising from the research reviewed; and evidence-based information on how research has reported on the management of EHS. Since 2005, EHS has attracted increasing research interest; however, there are significant gaps in the research that are hindering a better understanding of EHS that might be helpful for clinicians.

The diagnostic category of sleep-related hallucinations (SRH) replaces the previous category of Terrifying Hypnagogic Hallucinations in the 2001 edition of International Classification of Sleep Disorders-R. Hypnagogic and hypnopompic hallucinations (HHH) that occur in the absence of other symptoms or disorder and, within the limits of normal sleep, are most likely non-pathological. By contrast, complex nocturnal visual hallucinations (CNVH) may reflect a dimension of psychopathology reflecting different combinations of etiologic influences. The identification and conceptualization of CNVH is relatively new, and more research is needed to clarify whether CNVH share common mechanisms with HHH.

In sleep-related dissociative disorders, phenomena of the psychiatrically defined dissociative disorders emerge during the sleep period. They occur during sustained wakefulness, either in the transition to sleep or following an awakening from sleep. Behaviors during episodes vary widely, and can result in injury to self or others. Daytime dissociative episodes and a background of trauma are almost always present; there is typically major co-existing psychopathology. Diagnosis is based on both clinical history and polysomnography; differential diagnosis primarily involves other parasomnias and nocturnal seizures. Information available about treatment is limited; in a few reported cases, psychological interventions have proven effective.

This article reports on the epidemiology, prevalence, and physiopathology of sleep-related urinary dysfunction, a new syndromic category proposed by the recently revised ICSD-3-TR classification. Sleep enuresis, whether primary or secondary, monosymptomatic or plurisymptomatic, will be reviewed in terms of risk factors, comorbidity, and diagnostic and therapeutic indications. A definition of nocturia and its impact on patients' health, quality of life, and mortality will follow. Finally, the impact of urge incontinence on various medical and neurologic disorders will be discussed. Special emphasis will be placed on the possible association of this parasomnia with several sleep disorders and poor, fragmented sleep.

COVID-19 had a massive impact on sleep, resulting in overall increase of sleep disturbances. During lockdown many factors contributed to sleep disturbances, in particular changes in sleep-wake habits and stress. This article will describe the frequency and features of the principal parasomnias and the impact of the pandemic and the government restriction measures on sleep. Among different pathophysiological hypotheses, we will discuss the role of stress, considered as an expression of the allostatic load. Finally, during the pandemic, parasomnias were mainly investigated by questionnaires, with controversial results; video-polysomnographic studies are crucial to obtain a definitive diagnosis, even in critical conditions.

Although many sleep-related behaviors are benign, others can result in physical or sexual aggression toward bed partners or others. Individuals who engage in sleep-related violence (SRV) and sexual behavior in sleep (SBS) may face legal sanctions for their behavior. Attorneys or legal decision-makers may call on an expert to evaluate a defendant and opine about the veracity of an alleged parasomnia diagnosis, the criminal responsibility of the defendant, and his risk of violence to others. This article reviews the phenomena of SRV and SBS and guides evaluators in the forensic considerations relevant to parasomnias.

This article serves to help reduce patient burden in searching for credible information about parasomnias—abnormal behaviors during sleep—including sleepwalking, night terrors, and rapid eye movement sleep behavior disorder. It exhibits a compiled list of accessible online resources about parasomnias as well as detailed descriptions about each resource. By increasing patient accessibility to clinically validated resources, patients are more empowered to take an active role in managing their conditions, collaborating with their health-care practitioners in clinical management, enrolling in registries, and joining newsletters sponsored by these resources.

Preface
The Parasomnias, "What Lies Beneath"

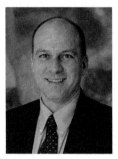

Alon Y. Avidan, MD, MPH, FAAN, FAASM
Editor

"In this stage, the sleep becomes much disturbed. The tremulous motion of the limbs occur during sleep, and augment until they awaken the patient, and frequently with much agitation and alarm...."
—*James Parkinson*

James Parkinson, Member of the Royal College of Surgeons

From "An Essay on the Shaking Palsy," London, 1817, one of the earliest descriptions of a Rapid Eye Movement sleep behavior disorder (RBD) parasomnia.

I am honored to serve as the guest editor for this issue of *Sleep Medicine Clinics* on "The Parasomnias." The parasomnias consist of some of the most fascinating and perplexing sleep disorders. While the diagnostic confirmation of most sleep disorders, requires objectively verifiable indicators, the parasomnias, with the exception of REM Sleep Behavior Disorder (RBD), lack formal assessment tools and remain allusive. Most sleep disorders rely on formal diagnostic polysomnography to assess patients for sleep-disordered breathing, central disorders of hypersomnia, and periodic leg movements disorder, and employ the use of actigraphy, sleep diaries, and wearable devices to shed light on insomnia and circadian rhythm disorders. Evaluation of parasomnias relies on key detailed historical and collateral data. The first step in the assessment of patients with complex behaviors is for the clinician to spend time with the patient to collect detailed and meticulous historically pertinent data. One might ask "What would Sherlock Holmes do if he encountered a patient with violent parasomnia?" One would need to reconstruct the "crime scene" and piece together a careful chronologic sequence of events, inquiring about any temporal associations with other conditions, medications, substances, and potential sleep/wake irregularities. The aspect of sleep medicine that is most rewarding for sleep medicine trainees confronted with complex nocturnal behaviors is the capacity to recreate these conditions and come up with a plausible explanation for these bizarre behaviors. While patients may disclose abnormal behaviors at night in the course of sleep medicine consultation, non–sleep clinicians may miss the red flags. I've encountered people who saw me for evaluation of RBD who were advised that it is "perfectly normal" to act out one's dream. One physician told a patient who punched a supposed intruder and experienced a subsequent wrist fracture that she may have a subconscious conflict with her spouse. She was referred to see a psychoanalyst to help uncover the origin of her "conflict" to control her aggressive behavior. Another physician advised a patient that her aggressive dream enactment was related to "eating too much pizza" the night before. Some physicians interpret RBD as sleep terrors or nightmares and tell patients that they will grow out of these episodes. One physician who read about RBD incorrectly advised a 22-year-old woman with narcolepsy type 1 that she now had "Parkinson's Disease". My intent in bringing up these scenarios is not to paint our non–sleep physician colleagues in a negative light, but to remind the readership that sleep medicine education continues to be lacking in medical school education curriculum. We need to do better in educating our colleagues about sleep. I try to use my sleep clinical consult note as an

Sleep Med Clin 19 (2024) xv–xvii
https://doi.org/10.1016/j.jsmc.2023.12.005
1556-407X/24/© 2023 Published by Elsevier Inc.

educational opportunity. I highlight key collateral clinical history that they may have forgotten to elicit. Over the years, I continue to illustrate to our trainees that clinical history gathered without a credible observer is partial and insufficient and may lead to unintended conclusions about the differential diagnosis. Our trainees are often baffled to hear reports of injurious nocturnal behaviors reported by bed partners that they may have dismissed if this attribute was not well corroborated by an observer.

Curating and developing this issue has been fulfilling because I've expanded on my education by reading the excellent reviews. I thank all the authors for the hours and weekends they spent contributing such exceptional articles. The issue is organized to mirror the parasomnia section of the international classification of sleep disorders, beginning with the non-REM parasomnias, progressing to REM parasomnias, other parasomnias, and concluding with special topics focusing on forensic complications of parasomnias, parasomnias in the setting of the COVID-19 Pandemic, and a unique article highlighting educational resources for patients who experience parasomnia.

I wrote the first article focusing on the clinical spectrum of parasomnias and have attempted to use high-impact visual tools to help reinforce the unique characteristics of the various parasomnias, highlighting their clinical semiologies and polysomnographic properties and utilizing high-impact diagrams and tables to help compare and contrast among the REM/NREM parasomnias while highlighting their differences from sleep-related epilepsy. The second article, "Understanding Sexual Parasomnias: A Review of the Current Literature on Their Nature, Diagnosis, Impacts, and Management," by Dr Monica Levy Andersen, Dr Carlos H. Schenck (a sleep medicine pioneer and the "father" of REM sleep behavior disorder), and Dr Sergio Tufik, summarize the sexsomnia, the first non-REM parasomnia, which is a unique subtype of confusional arousals. Many of these patients may not present to clinical attention until they experience marital or relation difficulties. I have taken care of several patients with sexsomnia who feel embarrassed and distressed by the nature of the episodes, highlighting the importance of providing reassurance and education for both patients and bed partners about the condition and acting as their advocates when they are subjected to legal actions. Drs Ramona Cordani, Regis Lopez, Lucie Barateau, Sofiene Chenini, Lino Nobili, and Yves Dauvilliers provided an elegant summary of somnambulism, highlighting the mechanism and differential diagnosis, and provided unique aspects about management.

Sleep-related eating disorder represents a unique subtype of somnambulism and is covered by Dr Melissa C. Lipford and Dr R. Robert Auger. The review of the most aggressive form of NREM parasomnias, sleep terrors, is concisely reviewed by Dr Muna Irfan. The review of REM sleep parasomnias begins with the most important in this category, RBD. "REM Sleep Behavior Disorder: Clinical Presentation and Diagnostic Criteria" is expertly reviewed by Dr Brandon M. Jones and Dr Stuart J. McCarter, while the management of RBD is detailed by Dr Roneil Malkani. Dr Ambra Stefani and Dr Qi Tang provide a nice summary of isolated sleep paralysis, which is rather common in the general population. Discussion of nightmare disorder is provided by Ms Victoria R. Garriques, Ms Deepali M. Dhruve, and Dr Michael R. Nadorff. The unique parasomnia, "Exploding Head Syndrome: a systematic scoping review," is discussed by Drs. Dónal G. Fortune and Helen L. Richards. The review of "Sleep-related Hallucinations" is expertly highlighted by Drs Flavie Waters, Ivan Ling, Somayyeh Azimi, and Jan Dirk Blom. An elegant review of "Sleep-Related Dissociative Disorders" is provided by Alan S. Eiser. Sleep-Related Urologic Dysfunction is nicely summarized by Dr Rosalia Silvestri. The unique spectrum of "Parasomnias during the COVID-19 Pandemic" is appraised by Drs Felice Di Laudo, Greta Mainieri, and Federica Provini. No review of parasomnias is complete without a discussion of its forensic implications, and this is expertly covered by Dr Brian Holoyda. The issue concludes with a helpful summary of "Educational Resources for Patients with Parasomnias" by Ms Courtney D. Molina and Ms Adreanne Rivera; both are premedical students with whom I have had the pleasure to work with in the capacity and during their support of our sleep clinic and RBD research. Courtney and Adreanne have a budding interest in a career in sleep medicine, which I hope they both pursue formally in the future.

I would like to conclude by thanking all the authors for their exceptional contributions. I have had the pleasure of working with many as colleagues and friends and their contribution is immensely appreciated. I would like to thank the editors of *Sleep Medicine Clinics*, Dr Ana C. Krieger and Teofilo Lee-Chiong Jr, for their gracious invitation to contribute to this work. I would also like to thank Ms Joanna Gascoine, *Sleep Medicine Clinics* Editor and editorial support, Mr Akshay Samson, Content Development Specialist and Jeyanthi Surendrakumar, Journal Manager. This work would not have been possible without their help, patience, and unwavering support in bringing this project to completion.

FUNDING STATEMENT

This work was funded by NIH-NIA National Institute on Aging, U19 AG071754, and the Karen Toffler Charitable Trust.

ACKNOWLEDGMENTS

The author would like to express his sincere appreciation and gratitude to the entire NAPS consortium, the Karen Toffler Charitable Trust (https://tofflertrust.org), and the Education Committee of the North American Prodromal Synucleinopathy Consortium for RBD, stage 2 (NAPS2, https://www.naps-rbd.org). Members of the RBD Education Committee include Carlos H. Schenck, MD, Emmanuel H. During, MD, Julie Flygare, JD (Ad hoc) Romy Hoque, MD, Joyce Lee-Iannotti, MD, Roneil Malkani, MD, MS, Jennifer McLeland, PhD, RPSGT, Ray Merrell, Adreanne Rivera, BS, Joshua P. Roland, MD, Erik K. St Louis, MD, MS, Leah Taylor, Aleksander Videnovic, MD, MSc, and Alon Y. Avidan, MD, MPH. This publication was supported in part by the National Institutes of Health grants R34AG056639 (NAPS) and U19-AG071754 (NAPS2). Its contents are solely the responsibility of the author and do not necessarily represent the official views of the NIH.

DISCLOSURE

Dr A.Y. Avidan has received consultant fees from Avadel, Merck, Takeda, AND Idorsia and speaker honoraria from Avadel and Idorsia.

Alon Y. Avidan, MD, MPH
Department of Neurology
David Geffen School of Medicine at UCLA
University of California, Los Angeles
RNRC, C153, Mail Code 176919
Los Angeles, CA, 90095-1769, USA

E-mail address:
Avidan@mednet.ucla.edu

The Clinical Spectrum of the Parasomnias

Alon Y. Avidan, MD, MPH

KEYWORDS

- Parasomnias • Non-REM parasomnias • Confusional arousal • Sleep walking • Sleep terror
- Sexsomnia • Sleep-related eating disorder • REM parasomnias
- REM Sleep Behavior Disorder (RBD)

KEY POINTS

- Parasomnias represent a spectrum of nocturnal behaviors ranging from mild nondisruptive confusion to aggressive and potentially injurious behaviors such as sleep terror, and dream-enactment behaviors.
- NREM-related parasomnias represent an incomplete transition from NREM deep sleep to wakefulness accompanied by partial or complete amnesia.
- Despite their peculiar clinical presentations, NREM parasomnias are readily explainable, diagnosable, and manageable. Comorbid sleep disorders, such as sleep apnea, may promote NREM-related parasomnia events.
- NREM parasomnias represent the activation of discrete neuronal networks. Aberrant physiology involving these regions gives rise to this incomplete transition culminating in complex behaviors.
- Parasomnias that emerge out of rapid eye movement (REM) sleep include REM sleep behavior disorder (RBD), REM nightmares, and isolated sleep paralysis. RBD may be prodromal to the future development of neurodegenerative conditions.

DEFINITION

Parasomnias are defined as undesirable and often abnormal motor or subjective phenomena that arise during arousals from sleep–wake transition and represent abnormal arousal as a universal phenomenon.[1–9] The episodes may include abnormal movements, behaviors, emotions, and autonomic activity, most of which are explainable, diagnosable, and manageable[5,7,10–13] These parasomnias may occur in response to internal factors, such as apneic episodes and fever, or may be triggered by external stimuli. The International Classification of Sleep Disorders–Third Edition, Text Revision (ICSD-3 TR)[14] defines non-rapid eye movement (NREM) parasomnias based on their disorders of arousal (DOAs) consisting of confusional arousals, sleep terrors, sleepwalking, and sleep-related eating disorder (SRED).[15–17] Sexsomnias are classified as a subtype of confusional arousals and

have an important impact on interpersonal relationships and forensic implications.[18]

CLASSIFICATION OF PARASOMNIAS

The ICSD- III Text Revision (TR) diagnostic criteria for the DOAs are outlined in **Box 1**.[19]

Box 1 illustrates the unique behavioral manifestation that may help differentiate between the three subtypes of NREM parasomnias. As a fundamental rule, the disorders are characterized by universal amnesia, beginning as partial arousals from slow wave sleep (SWS or stage N3 sleep), which are typically brief but may extend to about 30 minutes. Patients report dreamlike mentation, but not formed dreams. Arousals may emerge from any NREM sleep stage but primarily arise from stage N3 sleep with a propensity to occur during the first third of the night.[20]

Department of Neurology, UCLA Sleep Disorders Center, UCLA, David Geffen School of Medicine at UCLA, 710 Westwood Boulevard, RNRC, C153, Mail Code 176919, Los Angeles, CA 90095-1769, USA
E-mail address: avidan@mednet.ucla.edu

Sleep Med Clin 19 (2024) 1–19
https://doi.org/10.1016/j.jsmc.2023.12.003

Box 1
Classification of parasomnias

The ICSD-IIITR classifies parasomnias into three broad categories:

I. *Disorders of arousal (from NREM sleep)* consist of confusional arousals, sleepwalking, sleep terrors, and sleep-related eating disorder (SRED)

II. *Parasomnias emerging out of REM sleep* consisting of REM sleep behavior disorder (RBD), recurrent isolated sleep paralysis, and nightmare disorder

III. *Other parasomnias* consist of a relatively new category: sleep-related urologic dysfunction, exploding head syndrome, sleep-related hallucinations, and parasomnia due to drugs or substances, medical conditions, or unspecified

The universal behavioral manifestations of NREM parasomnias (DOA)[8,9,21–23] are shown in **Fig. 1**.

- *Diminished cognition:* Impairment or absence of higher cognitive functioning.
- *Confused demeanor and stare:* During an episode, the eyes are often wide-open, with a confused "glassy" stare.
- *Absence of or inappropriate response to external stimuli:* The patient may be very difficult to awaken and, even when the efforts succeed, the patient does not return to baseline function readily.

- *Sudden onset:* The patient typically experiences an abrupt to explosive onset associated with a variety of abnormal motor, behavioral, autonomic, or sensory symptoms.

INTRODUCTION AND NEUROPHYSIOLOGY

Parasomnias represent undesirable sensory, physical, or experiential phenomena that arise from sleep and may manifest in simple, complex, and dramatic behaviors. The pathophysiology for the parasomnias is believed to originate from disruption of sleep state stability. An overlap of the three different states of being—wakefulness, NREM sleep, and rapid eye movement (REM) sleep—gives rise to complex nocturnal behaviors (**Fig. 2**).[5]

Parasomnias may arise due to a disruption the traditionally well-orchestrated transition in and out of these states of being may give rise to an abnormal level of activity, whereas the individual remains asleep.[5] Another theory postulates that parasomnias arise from central pattern generators (CPGs) highlighted in **Fig. 3** are located along the neuroaxis (brain, brainstem, and spinal cord), responsible for involuntary motor behaviors such as oroalimentary automatisms, expression of fear, and complex involuntary motor events such as ambulatory behaviors.[24,25] Somnambulism is hypothesized to arise due to the deafferentation of the spinal and supraspinal locomotor neuronal network within the CPG. In addition to ambulatory behaviors, dissociation within the CPG likely promotes chewing, aggression, and sexual behavior

Diminished cognition: Impairment or absence of higher cognitive functioning.

Confused demeanor and stare: During an episode, the eyes are often wide-open, with a confused "glassy" stare.

Absence of or inappropriate response to external stimuli: The patient may be very difficult to awaken and, even when the efforts succeed, the patient does not return to baseline function readily.

Sudden onset: The patient typically experiences an abrupt to explosive onset associated with a variety of abnormal motor, behavioral, autonomic, or sensory symptoms.

Fig. 1. The universal behavioral manifestations of NREM parasomnias (DOA). (Image courtesy by Alon Y. Avidan, MD, MPH.)

Parasomnias: overlapping states

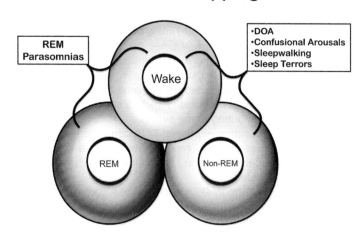

- •DOA
- •Confusional Arousals
- •Sleepwalking
- •Sleep Terrors

Fig. 2. Parasomnias as a state dissociation disorder. The abnormal admixture of the three states of being non-REM sleep, REM sleep, and wakefulness may overlap giving rise to parasomnias. Wakefulness and sleep are not mutually exclusive states and sleep-to-wake dissociation, incomplete transition, or oscillation from one sleep state to another leads to the parasomnias. Parasomnias are hypothesized to occur due to changes in brain organization across multiple states of being: incursion of wakefulness into non-rapid eye movement (REM) sleep leads to the disorder of arousal (DOA), and intrusion of wakefulness into REM sleep produces REM sleep parasomnias, REM sleep behavior disorder (RBD), being the most dramatic and important for sleep medicine providers. (*Modified after* Mahowald MW, Schenck CH. Non-rapid eye movement sleep parasomnias. Neurol Clin. Nov 2005;23(4):1077-1106, vii., and Avidan, A.Y. and N. Kaplish, The parasomnias: epidemiology, clinical features, and diagnostic approach. Clin Chest Med, 2010. 31(2): p. 353-70.)

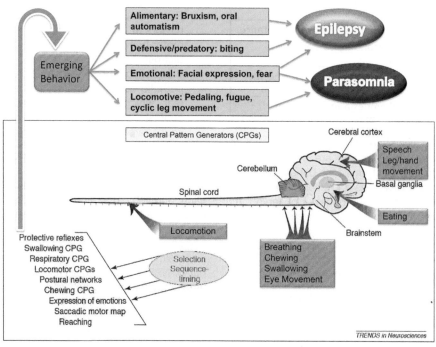

Fig. 3. Central pattern generators (CPGs). Several neuronal networks are found along all levels of the neuraxis stemming from the brain to the upper brainstem and spinal cord that when activated will produce different types of behavior (*upper panel*). The networks are collectively referred to as CPGs, depicted as the yellow regions in the bottom panel of the diagram. The spectrum of resulting behaviors may be simple and stereotyped such as rhythmic lip smacking and swallowing, to the more polymorphic and complex, such as those generating locomotion and search behaviors. The CPGs may be thought to lead to monomorphic spells which are stereotyped (automatisms) in which the possible etiology could be related to nocturnal seizures or highly complex (locomotive) polymorphic behavior in which the etiology may be a parasomnia. (*Modified from* Grillner S (2003) The motor infrastructure: from ion channels to neuronal networks. Nat Rev Neurosci 4:573–586, and *Tassinari, C.A., et al., Neuroethological approach to frontolimbic epileptic seizures and parasomnias: The same central pattern generators for the same behaviours. Rev Neurol (Paris), 2009.*)

disorders in the DOAs (NREM parasomnias). Some evidence for this admixture rests on studies showing that affected patients may have impaired awakening mechanisms.

Another recent theory implicates an abnormal timing of arousal-related slow-wave synchronization processes contributing to NREM parasomnias. This theory builds on the observation of specific electroencephalographic (EEG) changes previously reported during parasomnia episodes: "parasomnia awakenings" occur "inappropriately" when slow-wave activity (SWA) is high, implying a high "delta power," in contrast with normal awakenings seem to arise when certain levels of EEG activations have already been reached.[26]

CLINICAL FEATURES OF DISORDERS OF AROUSAL

The DOAs are classified as such based on the following common characteristics.

1. Underlying pathophysiology characterized by impaired arousal classically from stage N3 sleep
2. Genetic and familial patterns of inheritance
3. Predisposition secondary to sleep fragmentation
4. Impaired cognitive functioning during the event
5. Partial or total amnesia for the event[8,15,27–30]

The DOAs also share unique features based on the following attributes and are summarized in **Table 1**: clinical Spectrum of the behavioral manifestation of the DOAs, as a key for differentiating among them based on the behavior observed. All episodes are associated with universal amnesia as a rule.

Behavior/Semiology: Usually complex and variable clinical features. The patient's eyes are open, with little or no interaction with their environment.

- Confusional arousals: Arise from an abrupt awakening associated with confusion, disorientation, and, utterances of unintelligent speech.[8,29,31]
- Somnambulism: The occurrence of displacement out of bed would require reclassification as sleepwalking where the patient may engage in automatic non-goal-oriented behavior and less commonly would include complex, inappropriate, agitated behavior.[8,17]
- Sleep terrors: The hallmark of sleep terrors is a piercing scream signaling an abnormal arousal, associated with increased sympathetic activity and aggression.[32]

Age at Onset: Onset is common in childhood or the teens, generally after puberty, but may persist into young adulthood.

Frequency and Timing of Events: Events usually occur only a few times per month or week, but rarely with more than one event per night, and the arousals usually occur in the first half of the night. If episodes are frequent, the clinician should consider provocative factors such as sleep apnea contributing to the events.

Duration of Events: DOA can typically last from 20 seconds to minutes and may be protracted, especially when sleep inertia is prolonged[32] (**Table 2**).

Although DOA shares these common characteristics, the events are phenomenologically distinguished and differentiated by their unique semiology— "a fingerprint" of unique clinical presentations and behaviors.

- Confusional arousals usually consist of normal arousal behaviors, with abnormal duration rarely manifesting in explosive distress or motor behavior.[31–33]
- Somnambulism consists of normal arousal behaviors at onset, proceeding to non-agitated motor behavior including walking with lack of distress.[34,35]
- Sleep terrors begin with an explosion of sympathetic activity, distress, and expression of fear, which diminish over time. In contrast, confusional arousals and sleepwalking episodes rarely begin with distress.

Fig. 4 provides a graphic extrapolation of the spectrum of behavioral manifestations of the arousal disorders, illustrating the characteristic attributes for each: duration of the arousal episodes, the magnitude of displacement/ambulation, and the degree and intensity of distress as a function of time.[30] An admixture of multiple behavior types may wax and wane simultaneously.[30] All events usually emerge out of NREM sleep (most typically stage N3) and terminate either in wakefulness or transition into lighter NREM sleep. The episodes are typically brief but may occasionally be prolonged when an observer attempts to interrupt the behavior.[30]

CLINICAL EVALUATION OF PARASOMNIAS

The clinical evaluation of patients suspected to have parasomnias should focus on key clinical attributes and include collateral history, ideally from an observer—a family member/bed partner—to aid in establishing the diagnosis. These key attributes rely heavily on historical features provided by the patient and the observer, as well as a search for other associated features and priming factors.[27,29] The

Table 1
Clinical spectrum of the behavioral manifestation of the disorders of arousal, as a key for differentiating among them based on the behavior observed

Behavioral Semiology	DOA
Arousal progressing to sitting up in bed, verbal confusion, puzzled behaviour, and disorientation. If displacement occurs, then categorize as sleep walking.	Confusional arousal (CA)
Arousal followed by confusion, disorientation, automatic behavior, and displacement form the bed. May range from simple automatic non-goal-oriented behavior to more complex violent, inappropriate, agitated behavior.	Sleep walking (SW)
Eating behavior of edible and non-edible compounds	SRED (subtype of SW)
Sexual inappropriate behavior, out of character to typical behavior orientated toward bed partner or bystander next to patient	Sexomnia (subtype of CA)
Piercing scream, increased sympathetic response, and aggression. Attempts to interrupt behavior deepen confusion and aggression.	Sleep terror

All episodes are associated with universal amnesia as a rule.

Modified from American Academy of Sleep Medicine. The international classification of sleep disorders, revised: diagnostic and coding manual. 3rd edition. 3nd ed Revised. Darien, Ill.: American Academy of Sleep Medicine; 2023.

Table 2
The unique clinical attributes of non-rapid eye movement parasomnias

Attribute Category	Specific Features
Complex behavioral semiology	• Semiology refers to the clinically observed behavioral and motor events • In DOA, the semiology is complex with variable clinical features. • Although the patient's eyes are open, there is a universal lack of interaction between the patient and their environment and the observers.
Age at onset during early life	• Onset is common in childhood or teens, generally after puberty, but may persist into young adulthood.
Timing of events in the first half of the night	• Arousal usually occurs in the first half of the night.
Brief duration of episodes	• DOA typically lasts less than a minute, but episodes may be protracted when sleep inertia is prolonged

Courtesy by Alon Y. Avidan, MD, MPH.

key elements of the clinical semiology—age at onset, frequency, severity, complexity, and duration—are of fundamental importance in the initial evaluation.[2,32]

In general, patients with NREM parasomnias do not require in-laboratory investigation unless they are at risk for hurting themselves or others or are suspected of having another comorbid sleep or medical disorder, or if the events lead to insomnia, hypersomnia, or impairment in daytime functioning. People with dream-enactment behavior (DEB) must undergo polysomnography (PSG) with RBD montage to gain insight into the possibility of REM sleep-related atonia (RSWA). People who present with persistent nocturia, despite the appropriate medical management without clear signs of bladder outlet obstruction, should undergo formal sleep studies for evaluation of sleep-disordered breathing.[36]

Furthermore, signs of injury (as noted in **Fig. 4**) should be questioned and considered as to the potential for the patient to have injurious behaviors during events. These findings reinforce the need for PSG.[37]

Although most patients with parasomnias have normal findings on examination, the clinician should include a formal upper airway examination including a Modified Mallampati examination, tonsillar size, and include a movement may suggest the need for further evaluation. Patients who present with DEB and parkinsonism symptoms such as bradykinesia, rest tremor, rigidity, and postural and gait impairment may benefit from a formal evaluation by a movement disorders specialist.

Predisposing Conditions Responsible for the Non-Rapid Eye Movement Parasomnias

Predisposing factors, such as obstructive sleep apnea in this case, lead to fragmentation of sleep

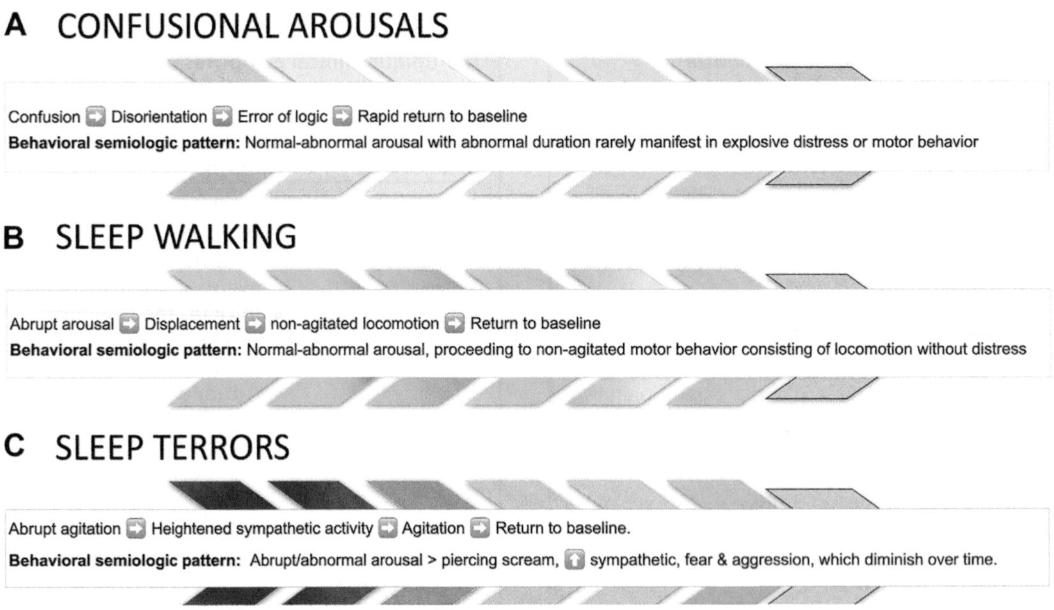

A CONFUSIONAL AROUSALS

Confusion ➡ Disorientation ➡ Error of logic ➡ Rapid return to baseline

Behavioral semiologic pattern: Normal-abnormal arousal with abnormal duration rarely manifest in explosive distress or motor behavior

B SLEEP WALKING

Abrupt arousal ➡ Displacement ➡ non-agitated locomotion ➡ Return to baseline

Behavioral semiologic pattern: Normal-abnormal arousal, proceeding to non-agitated motor behavior consisting of locomotion without distress

C SLEEP TERRORS

Abrupt agitation ➡ Heightened sympathetic activity ➡ Agitation ➡ Return to baseline.

Behavioral semiologic pattern: Abrupt/abnormal arousal > piercing scream, ⬆ sympathetic, fear & aggression, which diminish over time.

Fig. 4. Semiology of DOA as a function of time. Diagrammatic representation of the common behavioral semiologic pattern as a function of time depicting the key disorders of arousals (non-REM parasomnias). Here, the clinical semiology represented as hierarchical combinations of the 3 l behavior states on the vertical axis (Arousal→ non-agitated motor → distressed state as a function of time (1–10 min) on the horizontal axis). (A) *Confusional Arousals:* confusional arousal spells consists of normal arousal behaviors but of abnormal duration only. (B) *Sleep Walking:* somnambulistic events comprising of normal arousal behaviors at onset, proceeding to non-agitated motor behavior. (C) *Sleep Terror:* beginning with a distressed, predominantly negative emotional behavior typically of sudden onset motor and normal arousal behaviors are usually also seen during these events, either at onset or offset. *Parasomnia Overlap:* an admixture of two arousal disorders, comprising waxing and waning of the multiple behavior types. All events usually start in stage N3 NREM sleep and terminate either in wakefulness or lighter NREM sleep. (Image courtesy Alon Y. Avidan, MD, MPH; Modified after: C. P. Derry, A. S. Harvey, M. C. Walker, J. S. Duncan, and S. F. Berkovic. 2009. Nrem arousal parasomnias and their distinction from nocturnal frontal lobe epilepsy: A video eeg analysis. *Sleep* 32, no. 12: 1637-44.)

architecture as exemplified by the hypnogram highlighting apneic spells (bottom blue bars), arousals (top blue bars), and oxygen desaturations (red tracing) (**Fig. 5**). In susceptible individuals (ie, with a family history of non-REM parasomnias), the precipitating factor triggers EEG arousals which lower the threshold for the arousal disorder (**Table 3**).

SPECIFIC DISORDERS OF AROUSAL
Confusional Arousals

Confusional arousal (**Fig. 6**), also referred to as "*sleep drunkenness,*" consists of a brief period of confusion and disorientation following an arousal from SWS.[38,39] The episodes emerge during the first half of the night, in keeping with the higher propensity for arousal out of stage N3 sleep.[37] Polysomnographic recordings during the episodes demonstrate arousals from deep slow wave associated with brief episodes of delta activity, stage N1 theta patterns, with repeated micro-sleeps, or a diffuse and poorly reactive alpha rhythm (**Fig. 7**).[37]

Sexsomnias

Sexsomnias are considered a subtype of confusional arousals and consist of inappropriate amnestic sexual behaviors, sometimes triggered by primary sleep disorders.[40–43] Sexsomnias consist of abrupt and inappropriate sexual behaviors occurring with limited awareness during the act, unresponsiveness to the external environment, and amnesia for the event.[43]

Somnambulism

Somnambulism, or sleepwalking, consists of complex behaviors that are initiated during SWS and result in walking during sleep (**Fig. 8**). The episodes range from sitting up in bed, simple walking to agitated walking, and rarely, in extreme cases, frantic efforts to escape a perceived threatening situation, sometimes accompanied by inappropriate behavior such as urinating.[44] Precipitating factors include acute sleep deprivation, untreated sleep apnea, and the use of selective serotonin reuptake,[45,46] bupropion,[47] mirtazapine,[48] paroxetine,[49]

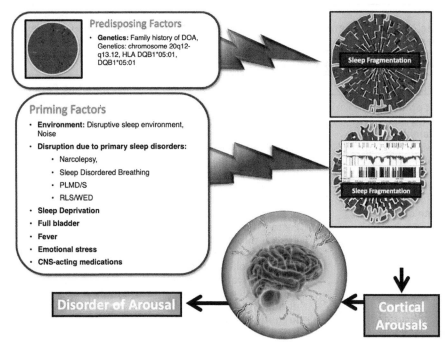

Fig. 5. Predisposing conditions responsible for the disorders of arousals. Predisposing factors, such as obstructive sleep apnea in this case, lead to fragmentation of sleep architecture as exemplified by the hypnogram highlighting apneic spells (*bottom blue bars*), arousals (*top blue bars*), and oxygen desaturations (*red tracing*). In susceptible individuals (ie, with a family history of non-REM parasomnias), the precipitating factor triggers EEG arousals which lower the threshold for the arousal disorder. CNS, central nervous system; DOAs, disorders of arousal; OSA, obstructive sleep apnea; PLMD, period limb movement disorder; WED, Willis–Ekbom disease. (Image courtesy Alon Y. Avidan, MD, MPH; Howell, M.J., Schenck, C.H/ .NREM Sleep Parasomnias in Adults: Confusional Arousals, Sleepwalking, Sleep Terrors and Sleep Related Eating Disorder" In: Barkoukis, T.J., Matheson, J.K., Ferber, R.F. Doghramji, K.,Eds. Therapy in Sleep Medicine. Philadelphia, Pennsylvania: Elsevier Press 2011, Guilleminault C, Palombini L, Pelayo R, Chervin RD. Sleepwalking and sleep terrors in prepubertal children: what triggers them? Pediatrics 2003;111:e17-25.)

and norepinephrine reuptake inhibitors.[50] Polysomnographic findings in patients with sleepwalking episodes usually show frequent arousals from SWS, the emergence of hypersynchronous slow-wave EEG just before and during arousals, and diminished delta activity.

Sleep-Related Eating Disorder

These events of amnestic eating occur after partial arousal from sleep, consumption of unusual food items, such as inedible substances (eg, a bar of soap) or unusual/odd food choices/combination (eg, eating mayonnaise out of a jar, consuming a frozen pizza, or preparing a cat food–dish soap sandwich). PSG during amnestic SRED is depicted in **Fig. 9**. This is a recording during non-REM sleep in a patient with known SRED. **Fig. 9** shows the patient having an arousal and chewing popcorn, his favorite sleep-related eating food item, which he was instructed to bring with him to the sleep laboratory. The patient had no recollection of this awakening and eating behavior in the morning. The patient has repetitive chewing movements rhythmic masticatory muscle activity (RMMA), as noted in the bracket, associated with arousals during non-REM sleep.

The main concerns with SRED are related to the safety and welfare of the patient during the preparation of food (ie, cutting and cooking) and the potential metabolic consequences (obesity, poor glucose control). Injurious behaviors may occur and require special attention to safety assessment and management (**Figs. 10** and **11**).

SLEEP TERRORS

Sleep terrors, also known as night terrors (*pavor nocturnus*), consist of a sudden arousal from deep sleep manifested by a piercing scream accompanied by heightened autonomic arousal and behavioral manifestations of extreme fear (**Fig. 12**). Sleep terrors represent the most dramatic of the DOA and is

Table 3
Predisposing, priming, and precipitating factors responsible for the non-rapid eye movement parasomnias

NREM Parasomnias: Etiologic Factors		
Predisposing Factors	**Priming Factors**	**Precipitating Factors**
Factors that promote susceptibility • Genetic/familial predisposition (HLA gene DQB1*05:01 and *04 alleles, chromosomes 20q12-q13.12) • NREM sleep instability, impaired arousal from N3 sleep, state dissociation;	Factors that promote sleep state stability • Factors that increase the proportion or depth of N3 NREM sleep per night, example: CNS medications (benzodiazepine receptor agonists, antipsychotics, antidepressants) • Factors that increase the arousal threshold • Acute sleep deprivation • Recovery following acute sleep deprivation, example: Stage N3 sleep rebound during PAP titration. • Irregular sleep/wake schedules, shift or night work, circadian rhythm disorders • Emotional stress	Trigger that interacts with the predisposing and priming factors to set off the parasomnia • Fragmented or insufficient sleep due to sleep apnea or sleep deprivation • Untreated/unrecognized primary sleep disorders (sleep apnea, narcolepsy, restless legs) • Environmental factors such as noise and touch. • Forced awakenings, noise, light, pain, enuresis, itch, dyspnea, fever, or apnea

Abbreviations: PAP, positive airway pressure.
  * The WHO HLA Nomenclature Committee for Factors of the HLA System establishes that if the sequence for the HLA alleles is unknown at any point in the alignment, it is represented by an asterisk.
  Courtesy by Alon Y. Avidan, MD, MPH.

characterized further by extreme panic, and confusion, associated with heightened sympathetic activity and a state of cerebral hyperresponsiveness manifested by extreme agitation, escape behavior, marked confusion amnesia, and disorientation.[3,51]

Polysomnographic features reveal high-voltage, symmetric, hypersynchronous SWA followed by a sudden and incomplete arousal accompanied by a marked increase in muscle tone and change in respiratory and heart rates, inconsolable crying along with

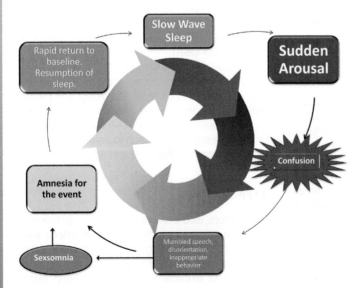

Fig. 6. Characteristic pattern of confusional arousal. Confusional arousals are sudden and abrupt arousals from deep sleep with demarcated by confusion mentation, inappropriate behavior, minimal motor, or autonomic activity, but typically terminating in rapider return to baseline with amnesia to the preceding event. Sexsomnias are classified by the ICSD-III as a subtype of confusional arousals manifested by inappropriate sexual behaviors typically oriented at the bed partners followed with complete amnesia for the behavior. (Image courtesy Alon Y. Avidan, MD, MPH.)

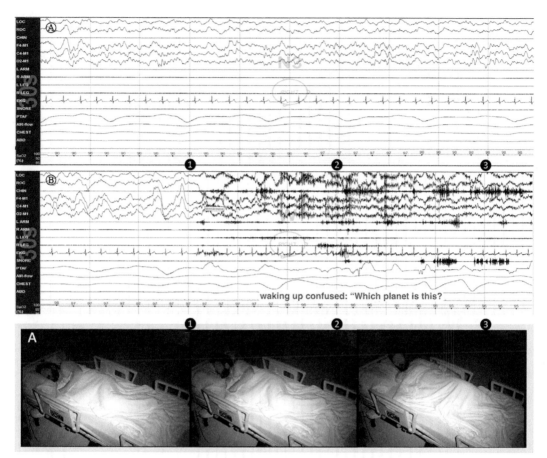

Fig. 7. Characteristic pattern of sleep walking. The evolution of a confusional arousal out of stage N3 sleep. The PSG recording is from a patient with recurrent nocturnal confusion. The episode is highly representative of the patient's abnormal arousal out of N3 sleep. The spell was remarkable for abrupt arousal accompanied by the eye-opening facial expression of confusion and perplexed vocalization (asking "Where am I?" and "Which planet is this?"). The event was not preceded by a respiratory event, and the EEG showed no epileptiform abnormalities (A and B). (C) The demeanor of his behavior during the spell, from the abrupt arousal (1) to the expression of confusion (2) and return to baseline (3). The patient reported no recall of the event on awakening in the morning. (A) A 30-s epoch just before an episode of confusion arousal experienced by the patient highlighting normal stage N3 sleep. (B) A 30-s epoch illustrating hypersynchronous delta activity preceding episode of confusional arousal experienced by the patient, who woke up saying, "which planet is this?" Electrooculogram LOC and ROC left and, respectively, right outer cantus electrooculography (EOG) electrodes, CHIN, Chin electromyogram (EMG). Electroencephalogram [(EEG), M1: Left mastoid electrode location. F3, C4, O2, right frontal, central, and respectively, occipital electroencephalography electrodes. Limb EMG (L, left LEG/ARM; R, right LEG/ARM)]. LEG limb placement: Tibialis anterior, ARM limb placement: Biceps. AIR-flow, nasal-oral airflow; CHEST and ABD, chest and abdominal wall motion effort; EKG, electrocardiogram; PTAF, pressure transducer airflow; SNORE, snore sensor sound; SpO2, percent oxygen saturation by pulse oximetry by finger probe. (Image courtesy by Alon Y. Avidan, MD, MPH.)

screaming, and sympathetic hyperactivation **(Fig. 13)**.[52]

Rapid Eye Movement Sleep Behavior Disorder

REM stage sleep behavior disorder (RBD) is characterized by an abnormal loss of muscle atonia during REM sleep and REM sleep without atonia (RSWA as illustrated in **Fig. 14**) observed on PSG. Observed complex DEBs consist of complex nocturnal motor behaviors and vocalizations during sleep. DEBs are not unique to RBD and may occur in other conditions highlighting the importance of careful history taking and PSG (**Table 4**). RBD confers an important prognostic implication for future progression to neurodegenerative alpha-synucleinopathies including Parkinson's disease, dementia with Lewy bodies, and multiple system atrophy. RBD can arise in the setting of serotonergic antidepressants. RBD manifests as

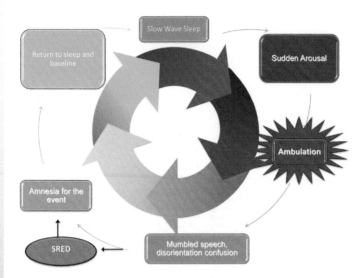

Fig. 8. Characteristic pattern of sleep walking. Somnambulism consists of a sudden arousal followed by bizarre motor activity, typically walking, but occasionally with other semipurposeful tasks such as moving objects, expression of unintelligent speech with minimal aggressive, autonomic or affective involvement. When eating or drinking occurs, then sleep-related eating disorders (SREDs) are diagnosed. (Image courtesy by Alon Y. Avidan, MD, MPH.)

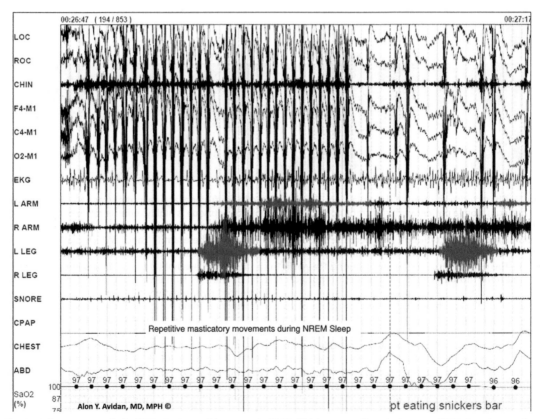

Fig. 9. Polysomnography in SRED. Patient with amnestic SRED. This is a recording during non-REM sleep in a patient with known sleep-related eating disorder (SRED). The patient having an arousal and chewing popcorn, his favorite sleep-related eating food item, which he was instructed to bring with him to the sleep laboratory. The patient had no recollection of this awakening and eating behavior in the morning. The patient has repetitive chewing movements rhythmic masticatory muscle activity (RMMA), as noted in the bracket, associated with arousals during non-REM sleep. A 30-s epoch depicting sleep-related eating disorder. Related muscle activity was identified by repetitive masticatory movements during NREM sleep as the patient was eating a snicker bar. There was no recollection of eating in the morning. Electrooculogram LOC and ROC left and, respectively, right outer cantus electrooculography (EOG) electrodes, F3, C4, O2, right frontal, central, and respectively, occipital electroencephalography electrodes. Limb EMG (L, left LEG/ARM; R, right LEG/ARM). LEG limb placement: Tibialis anterior, ARM limb placement: Biceps. AIR-flow, nasal-oral airflow; CHEST and ABD, chest and abdominal wall motion effort; EKG, electrocardiogram; PTAF, pressure transducer airflow; SNORE, snore sensor sound; SpO₂, percent oxygen saturation by pulse oximetry by finger probe. (Image courtesy by Alon Y. Avidan, MD, MPH.)

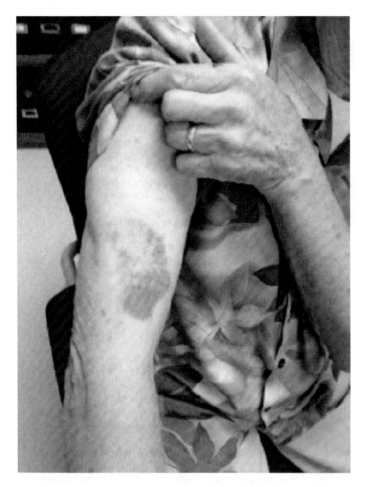

Fig. 10. Injury sustained during sleep walking event in a patient with SRED. A 68-year-old gentleman presented with ecchymosis and bruising over his arms first noted after being treated with a hypnotic agent to "help improve an urge to move the legs and restlessness." He was witnessed by his wife to get up at night and prepare raspberry jam and mustard sandwiches. The photograph was taken during a recent clinic visit with the author, highlighting right arm ecchymosis following a night in which he experienced a typical episode. The patient was diagnosed with Willis–Ekbom disease (WED) and was managed with a dopaminergic agent. The hypnotic agent was discontinued and his spells terminated shortly thereafter. (Image courtesy by Alon Y. Avidan, MD, MPH.)

repeated events of complex motor phenomena or vocalizations during sleep. The associated symptoms put both patients and bed partners at risk for physical injury as movements potentially corresponding to dream content become able to be enacted. The condition is one of the few parasomnias where in-laboratory PSG is recommended for diagnosis outside of just ruling out concomitant sleep pathology. Treatment goals typically target improving patient and bed partner safety and

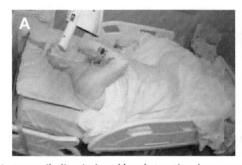
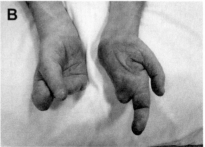

Fig. 11. Autocannibalism induced by obstructive sleep apnea. (*A*) The photograph on the left side is from the patient's video polysomnogram capturing the actual behavior. This example is provided to illustrate the bizarre, perplexing, and dramatic nature of the severe injury that may be seen in severe cases. The video example is highlighted in (https://doi.org/10.1016/j.sleep.2017.01.017) the article "Autocannibalism induced by obstructive sleep apnea, Sleep Medicine, Volume 37, 2017, Pages 72-73." (*B*) The right side of this figure illustrate the hands of a patient with untreated sleep apnea who experienced cervical spinal cord damage and consequent tetraplegia. The photograph illustrates the resulting injury after the autocannibalism which left the patient with only the thumb and index finger on each hand.

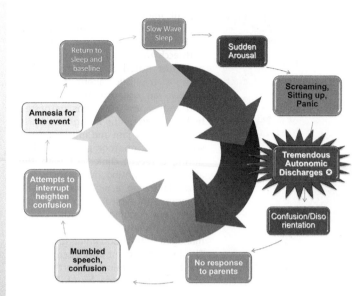

Fig. 12. Clinical course of sleep terrors. Sleep terrors (pavor nocturnus) are dramatic events are characterized by a sudden and abrupt arousal associated with a panicky scream, agitation, intense anxiety, and heighted autonomic activity☉. The general duration is about a minute, but they can last for up to 10 minutes. Inconsolability is almost universal and the patient is unresponsive to the efforts of others to console him. The child is incoherent and has altered perception of the environment appearing confused. This behavior may potentially be dangerous and could result in injury. (*Modified after* Avidan, A.Y. and N. Kaplish, The parasomnias: epidemiology, clinical features, and diagnostic approach. Clin Chest Med, 2010. 31(2): p. 353-70.)

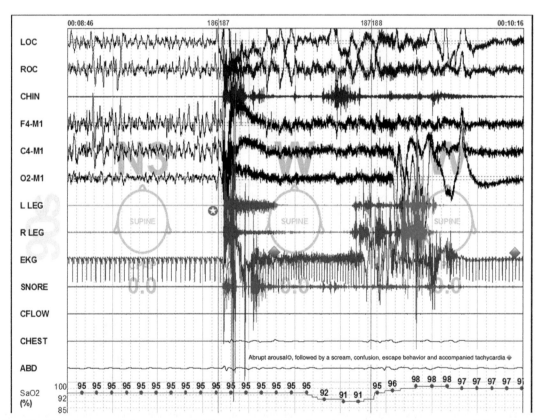

Fig. 13. Clinical course of sleep terrors. A 90-s epoch depicting sleep terror. The recording captured the patient's representative spells: an abrupt arousal out of slow-wave sleep demarcated by the star, accompanied by screaming, tachycardia, and amnesia for the event in the morning. The abrupt arousal is demarcated by ☉, followed by, a scream, confusion, escape behavior, and accompanied tachycardia◆. Channels are as follows: electrooculogram (left: E1-M2, right: E2-M1), chin EMG (Chin1-chin2), EEG (right: frontal-F4, central-C4, occipital-O2, right mastoid-M2), two ECG, two-limb EMG (LAT, RAT), snore, nasal-oral airflow-N/O, nasal pressure signal-NPRE, respiratory effort (thoracic, abdominal), and oxygen saturation (SaO₂). ECG, electrocardiogram; EEG, electroencephalogram; EMG, electromyogram; LAT, left anterior tibialis; RAT, right anterior tibialis. (Image courtesy by Alon Y. Avidan, MD, MPH.)

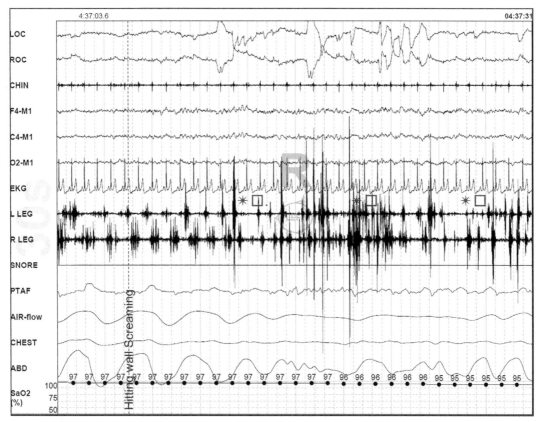

Fig. 14. Polysomnography in RBD illustrating RSWA. A 30-s polysomnograph epoch a patient with dream enactment behavior. Note the elevated EMG activity in the lower extremities (LAT1-LAT2 in *brown*) characteristic of "REM sleep without atonia," (*) with simultaneous REMs in the electrooculogram (LOC-A2 and ROC-A1 in *blue*), and EEG appearance of REM sleep (low amplitude, mixed frequency).

frequently require a combination of environmental and pharmacotherapy, often through the usage of clonazepam or melatonin. Some patient may use home remedies to protect themselves from injurious dream enactment, as illustrated in **Fig. 15**.

RECURRENT ISOLATED SLEEP PARALYSIS

Sleep paralysis (SP) describes an inability to initiate any voluntary movement or to vocalize on awakening. The episodes can last a few seconds to a few minutes. This distressing phenomenon can start at sleep onset or sleep offset and relates to an overlap of REM-related atonia and despite the patient's wakefulness. The presence of daytime somnolence, sleep attacks, and cataplexy should always be sought through a careful interview to differentiate these episodes from narcolepsy.[53]

NIGHTMARES

Nightmares affect up to 10% to 50% of children and up to 75% of the population can remember at least one or a few nightmares in the course of their childhood. Half of all adults admit to having an occasional nightmare, whereas 1% report more than a single nightmare a week. Nightmares consist of vivid and prolonged dream pattern that tends to become progressively more complicated and frightening terminating in an arousal and recall. Episodes may increase during times of stress, particularly following traumatic events.[54] PSG depicts an abrupt awakening from REM sleep associated with an increased REM-seep density and variability in heart and respiratory rates. **Table 5** highlights the differences between sleep terrors and nightmares.

DIFFERENTIAL DIAGNOSIS OF PARASOMNIAS

Parasomnias must be differentiated from other parasomnias and nocturnal events.

DOA or NREM parasomnias are characterized by abrupt arousal and amnesia, without dream recollection.

REM Parasomnias: The differential diagnosis should include REM nightmares, nocturnal anxiety attack related to obstructive sleep apnea, nocturnal cardiac ischemia, and sleep-related

Table 4
Differential diagnosis of dream-enacted behaviors

Disorder	NREM N3 Parasomnia	RBD	Acute PTSD	Sleep-Related Epilepsy
Sleep stage	N3	R	N2, R	N1, N2
Behaviors during the episode				
Eyes	Open	Closed	Open	Open
Ambulation	Frequent	Exceptional	Rarely jumping out of bed and walking	Rare running and nocturnal wandering
Interaction with environment	Frequent	Less frequent	Frequent	Frequent
Motor behavior and movements	Similar to wake movements; confusional arousals with orientation behavior or complex, purposeful, prolonged behaviors	Various varying from jerky simple movements to complex, usually brief purposeful behavior. Absent tremor and absent bradykinesia	Frequent, explosive, violent movements, thrashing, shaking, startling	Stereotyped paroxysmal arousals, tonic posturing, focal cloning activity, gestures, semi-purposeful automatism; bicycling, hand rubbing
Vocalizations	Moaning, sentences, swearing interrogative tone	Moaning, sentences, insults, imperative tone	Frequent vocalizations, grunting, yelling, screaming	Moaning, palilalia speech comprehensible words
Subject experiences and dreams associated with the behavior				
Recall of associated mentation	Infrequent recall (occasion in 70%)	Frequent recall	Frequent recall (but startling may occur in absence of dream recall except fear)	Frequent recall of the seizure, but no associated dreams
Complexity	Brief visual scenes	More complex dreams and nightmares	Complex nightmares	No dreams
Content	Misfortune or aggression	Threat or aggression, rarely related to personal history	Replays of prior combat or traumatic experiences	No dreams
Response of the dreamer	Tends to flies from danger, rarely attacks the bed partner	Tends to fight back, may attack the bed partner	Defensive or offensive behaviors may attack the bed partner	No dreams
Emotions	Frequently fear, apprehension	More variable, can laugh too	Intense fear	Possible fear

Differential diagnosis of dream-enacted behaviors illustrating the key features of NREM parasomnia, REM sleep behavior disorder, post-traumatic stress disorder, and sleep-related frontal lobe epilepsy.

Abbreviations: NREM, non-rapid eye movement sleep; PTSD, post-traumatic stress disorder; RBD, rapid eye movement sleep behavior disorder.
From Rocha AL, Arnulf I. NREM parasomnia as a dream enacting behavior. *Sleep Medicine.* 2020;75:103-105. doi: https://doi.org/10.1016/j.sleep.2020.02.024.

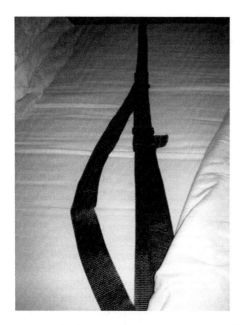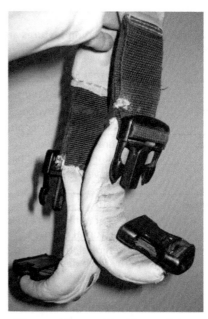

Fig. 15. A set of handcuffs and mattress belts constructed by a 65-year-old man with a history of dream enactment episodes to prevent himself from moving and hurting himself and his wife. The nocturnal episodes became extremely dangerous in the months before his initial presentation at the author's sleep disorder clinic in 2008. His neurologic examination then was completely normal. When the patient was seen in November 2023, he pheno-converted and his neurologic examination revealed hypomimia, decreased blinking, a resting tremor, and increased tone in the upper extremities, specifically cogwheel rigidity, bradykinesia, slow gate, reduced arm swing, resting tremor, and gait apraxia consistent with Parkinson's disease. (*From* Avidan, A.Y., 2009. Parasomnias and movement disorders of sleep. Semin. Neurol. 29, 372–392.)

epilepsy (SRE). Differentiation from nightmares is most important, however. Nightmares are distinguishable from sleep terrors in that the former often are associated with a vivid recall of the dream event during REM sleep, the clinical presentation is less dramatic, and many patients do not experience the typical autonomic hyperarousal that characterizes the latter.[2,27,35]

RBD will be differentiated based on the polysomnographic signature of RSWA, which is required for diagnosis as well as DEB.[55,56] RBD is typically more common in older individuals and associated with

Table 5
Differences between sleep terrors and nightmares

Characteristic	Sleep Terror	Nightmare
Timing during the night	First third (deep slow wave sleep)	Last third (REM Sleep)
EEG characteristics	Stage N3 sleep	Stage REM
Movements	Common	Rare
Anxiety level	High (difficult to control)	Minimum
Severity	Severe	Mild
Vocalizations	Common	Rare
Autonomic discharge	Severe and intense	Mild
Recollection	No (amnestic, occasional fragmentary recall of frightening images)	Yes (good recollection)
State on walking	Vague, confused, disoriented	Function well, vivid, and clear
Injuries	Common	Rare
Violence	Common	Rare
Displacement from bed	Common	Very rare

Table 6
Key similarities and differentiating features among the non-rapid eye movement parasomnias and nocturnal seizures

	Nocturnal Seizures	Non-REM Parasomnias
Length of event	Typically brief (<1 min)	Longer in duration (5–15 min)
Motor activity	Generally stereotyped	More likely to be complex, variable
Onset	Within 30 min of sleep onset	Within 2 h of sleep onset
Frequency	Generally more likely to occur nightly and multiple times per a night	Usually <3 times per a month, more than several times per week.
Recall	Can have lucid recall	Amnestic of event. Partial recall with complex partial seizures
Age of onset	14 ± 10	<10 y
Family history	39% more likely in especially in Nocturnal frontal lobe epilepsy	Frequently positive 62%–96%
Triggering factors	Not typical, but may be precipitated by sleep deprivation.	Yes: sleep deprivation, febrile illness, anxiety, stress, sleep apnea, moto disorders of sleep
Other	Presence of aura, dystonic or tonic posturing, abrupt offset	Interaction with environment, wander outside bedroom, slow offset or ending of event
Common features of both	Commonly start in childhood, may have vocalizations, motor artifact seen on EEG	

dream mentation and reasonable recollection.[57] The eyes are closed during REM parasomnias and the behaviors vary with the dream in contrast with NREM parasomnias, where the eyes are open and dream mentation is absent. NREM parasomnias are common in the first third of the night and may occur as multiple events throughout the night in contrast with REM parasomnias which generally take place when the propensity for REM sleep is greater. Displacement is less common in patients with RBD but sleepwalking in RBD may represent a greater predilection to develop Parkinson's disease. The differential diagnosis of DEB includes obstructive sleep apnoea (OSA) pseudo-RBD, periodic limb movement disorder pseudo-RBD, NREM parasomnia (such as sleepwalking and sleep terrors), sleep-related epilepsy (SRE), nocturnal panic attacks and post-traumatic stress disorder (PTSD) summarized in **Table 4**.[58]

SREs also may occur multiple times during the night but are stereotypic in behavior. Amnesia is not always universal as the seizure must involve both medial temporal lobe structures to produce amnesia.[59] SRE emerges between the ages of 10 and 20 years but occurrence later in life is not uncommon.[60,61] In contrast with SRE, parasomnias are infrequent and have more complex and polymorphic semiology, as opposed to the stereotypical semiology and higher frequency of events.[62] Key similarities and differentiating features among

the non-REM and nocturnal seizures are depicted in **Table 6**.

Table 6 shows that differentiating between sleep terrors and SRE is occasionally difficult and the use of electroencephalography is helpful in patients in whom the episodes are atypical, unusually frequent, or less responsive to management.[62,63] Nocturnal seizures, especially complex partial seizures of temporal and frontal origin, may have a major fear component and manifest with many of the characteristics found in sleep terrors including screaming, panic, fear, tachycardia, and vague frightening perceptions.

For this reason, history and clinical semiology alone are not sufficient to conclusively differentiate sleep terrors from seizures. In these challenging cases, video polysomnographic recording with a full set of EEG electrodes is essential when the spells are frequent, repetitive, or refractory to conventional therapy or have atypical features.[64] Videopolysomnographic recordings capturing multiple events may be helpful in demonstrating stereotypic behaviors suggestive of an epileptic origin, even in the face of no EEG change.[65,66]

SUMMARY

Sleep clinicians are often enlisted to help diagnose, evaluate, and manage complex nocturnal behaviors and differentiation from parasomnias is paramount. Parasomnias are undesirable emotional or physical events that accompany sleep that span across our lifespan and may be age-appropriate but can contribute to severe injury and might be a harbinger of future neurodegenerative conditions. Parasomnias are hypothesized to be due to changes in brain organization across multiple states of being and are particularly apt to occur during the incomplete transition or oscillation from one sleep state to another. Parasomnias are often explained on the basis that wakefulness and sleep are not mutually exclusive states; abnormal intrusion of wakefulness into NREM sleep produces arousal disorders; and intrusion of wakefulness into REM sleep produces REM sleep parasomnias, RBD, the most dramatic and important parasomnia. The DOAs are a unique group of sleep disorders that share similar characteristics and have a common underlying pathophysiology. Successful amelioration of the parasomnias is critically important and depends on a detailed, concise, and accurate diagnosis and requires time and dedication to the clinical history. The videos 1-5 have been included as supplementary resources at the end of this article which has been already published.

CLINICS CARE POINTS

- Parasomnias are enigmatic nocturnal behaviors comprising of emotional experiences, movements, behaviors, perceptions, and hallucinatory or autonomic nervous system phenomena.

- While they are universal and generally benign during childhood, they can persist and emerge during adulthood with substantial quality-of-life, prognostic, and potentially forensic implications for patients and their bed-partners Non-REM Parasomnias represent a unique group of sleep disorders that share similar characteristics and have a common underlying pathophysiology.

- Successful amelioration of these nocturnal behaviors is contingent on establishing an accurate diagnosis, based on distinguishing features and differentiation from other complex events.

- Management typically includes patient education and reassurance, while attending to proper sleep duration and regularity because these disorders can be exacerbated by sleep deprivation, sleep-wake circadian irregularities, substances, and untreated sleep apnea.

- It is well recognized that these comorbid sleep disorders promote the risk of parasomnias by facilitating sleep instability and frequency of arousals from sleep which lower the threshold for parasomnias.

- When parasomnias are frequent or involve aggressive or dramatic behaviors, pharmacotherapy with a benzodiazepine, particularly clonazepam, at night is the preferred approach with most of the disorders of arousal.

- Other therapy relies on the use of short-acting benzodiazepines, such as diazepam and alprazolam, or tricyclic antidepressants in the case of sleep terrors.

- Relaxation training and guided imagery may be helpful strategies for some patients, especially those with disorders of arousal.

- RBD is a fascinating parasomnia that is prodromal of neurodegenerative disease, specifically α-synucleinopathies such as pure autonomic failure, multiple system atrophy, dementia with Lewy bodies, and Parkinson's disease.

- The finding of REM sleep without atonia (RSWA) and dream enactment behavior requires careful assessment as these findings may be heralding symptoms of neurodegenerative pathology.

- People suffering from RBD should be assessed longitudinally for early signs of neurodegenerative diseases and prognostic counseling should be deployed based on the ethical principles for disclosure exercising a shared decision-making approach.

- An appropriate and timely referral to a sleep specialist trained in the application of polysomnographic techniques in evaluating complex nocturnal behaviors is necessary to optimize patient and bed-partner safety

ACKNOWLEDGMENTS

The author would like to express his sincere appreciation and gratitude to the entire NAPS consortium, the Karen Toffler Charitable Trust (https://tofflertrust.org), and the Education Committee of the North American Prodromal Synucleinopathy Consortium for RBD, Stage 2 (NAPS2, https://www.naps-rbd.org). This publication was supported in part by the National Institutes of Health, United States grants R34AG056639 (NAPS) and U19-AG071754 (NAPS2). Its contents are solely the responsibility of the author and do not necessarily represent the official views of the NIH, United States.

DISCLOSURE

Dr A.Y. Avidan has received consultant fees from Avadel, Merck, Takeda, and Idorsia and speaker honoraria from Avadel and Idorsia. This work was funded by NIH-NIA National Institute on Aging, United States, U19 AG071754 and the Karen Toffler Charitable Trust, United States.

SUPPLEMENTARY DATA

Video 1: NREM parasomnia, Confusional Arousal, Loud Vocalization.

Video 2: Supplementary video 1 - REM behavior disorder and neurodegenerative diseases.

Video 3: Video 21-41. REM Sleep Behavior Disorder with Obstructive Sleep Apnea.

Video 4: Video 1 - NREM parasomnia as a dream-enacting behavior.

Video 5: Parasomnias and Nocturnal Frontal Lobe Epilepsy (NFLE): Lights and shadows - Controversial Points in the Differential Diagnosis.

REFERENCES

1. Baldini T, Loddo G, Sessagesimi E, et al. Clinical features and pathophysiology of disorders of arousal in adults: a window into the sleeping brain. Front Neurol 2019;10:526.
2. Brooks S, Kushida CA. Behavioral parasomnias. Curr Psychiatr Rep 2002;4:363–8.
3. Schenck CH. REM sleep behavior disorder as a complex condition with heterogeneous underlying disorders: clinical management and prognostic implications [Commentary]. Sleep Breath 2022;26: 1289–98.
4. Irfan M, Schenck CH, Howell MJ. NonREM disorders of arousal and related parasomnias: an updated review. Neurotherapeutics 2021;18:124–39.
5. Mahowald MW, Bornemann MC, Schenck CH. Parasomnias. Semin Neurol 2004;24:283–92.
6. Hu MT. REM sleep behavior disorder (RBD). Neurobiol Dis 2020;143:104996.
7. Broughton R. Behavioral parasomnias. Boston, MA: Butterworth-Heinemann; 1998.
8. Fleetham JA, Fleming JA. Parasomnias. CMAJ (Can Med Assoc J) 2014;186:E273–80.
9. Mahowald MW, Ettinger MG. Things that go bump in the night: the parasomnias revisited. J Clin Neurophysiol 1990;7:119–43.
10. Kowey PR, Mainchak RA, Rials SJ. Things that go bang in the night. N Engl J Med 1992;327:1884.
11. Parkes JD. The parasomnias. Lancet 1986;2: 1021–5.
12. Stores G. Dramatic parasomnias. Journal of the Roayal Society of Medicine 2001;94:173–6.
13. Thorpy MJ, Glovinsky PB. Parasomnias. Psychiatric Clinics of North American 1987;10:623–39.
14. Medicine AAoS. International classification of sleep disorders. 3rd Edition. Darien, IL: American Academy of Sleep Medicine; 2023. Text Revision (ICSD-3-TR).
15. Irfan M, Schenck CH, Howell MJ. Non-rapid eye movement sleep and overlap parasomnias. Continuum 2017;23:1035–50.
16. Howell MJ. Parasomnias: an updated review Neurotherapeutics. Journal of the American Society for Experimental NeuroTherapeutics 2012;9:753–75.
17. Kotagal S. Sleep-wake disorders of childhood. Continuum 2017;23:1132–50.
18. Arino H, Iranzo A, Gaig C, et al. Sexsomnia: parasomnia associated with sexual behaviour during sleep. Neurologia 2014;29:146–52.
19. American Academy of Sleep Medicine. The international classification of sleep disorders, revised: diagnostic and coding manual. 3rd edition. 2nd ed. Darien, Ill: American Academy of Sleep Medicine; 2014.
20. Pressman MR. Hypersynchronous delta sleep EEG activity and sudden arousals from slow-wave sleep in adults without a history of parasomnias: clinical and forensic implications. Sleep 2004;27: 706–10.
21. Mahowald MW, Schenck CH. NREM sleep parasomnias. Neurol Clin 1996;14:675–96.
22. Mahowald MW. Parasomnias. Med Clin North Am 2004;88:669–678 ix.
23. Mahowald MW, Bornemann MC, Schenck CH. Parasomnias. Semin Neurol. 2004;24(3):283–92.
24. Tassinari CA, Rubboli G, Gardella E, et al. Central pattern generators for a common semiology in fronto-limbic seizures and in parasomnias. A neuroethologic approach. Neurol Sci 2005;26(Suppl 3): s225–32.
25. Tassinari CA, Cantalupo G, Hogl B, et al. Neuroethological approach to frontolimbic epileptic seizures and parasomnias: the same central pattern generators for the same behaviours. Rev Neurol (Paris) 2009;S0035-3787(09):00370–1 [pii].
26. Cataldi J, Stephan AM, Marchi NA, et al. Abnormal timing of slow wave synchronization processes in non-rapid eye movement sleep parasomnias. Sleep 2022;45. https://doi.org/10.1093/sleep/zsac111.
27. Avidan AY, Kaplish N. The parasomnias: epidemiology, clinical features, and diagnostic approach. Clin Chest Med 2010;31:353–70.
28. Mahowald MW, Schenck CH. Non-rapid eye movement sleep parasomnias. Neurol Clin 2005;23: 1077–106.
29. Ekambaram V, Maski K. Non-rapid eye movement arousal parasomnias in children. Pediatr Ann 2017; 46:e327–31.

30. Derry CP, Harvey AS, Walker MC, et al. NREM arousal parasomnias and their distinction from nocturnal frontal lobe epilepsy: a video EEG analysis. Sleep 2009;32:1637–44.

31. Ohayon MM, Priest RG, Zulley J, et al. The place of confusional arousals in sleep and mental disorders: findings in a general population sample of 13,057 subjects. J Nerv Ment Dis 2000;188:340–8.

32. Zadra A, Pilon M. NREM parasomnias. Handb Clin Neurol 2011;99:851–68.

33. Ohayon MM, Mahowald MW, Leger D. Are confusional arousals pathological? Neurology 2014;83:834–41.

34. Zergham AS, Chauhan Z. Somnambulism (sleep walking). Treasure island (FL): StatPearls; 2020.

35. Arnulf I. Sleepwalking. Curr Biol 2018;28:R1288–9. https://doi.org/10.1016/j.cub.2018.09.062.

36. Di Bello F, Napolitano L, Abate M, et al. Nocturia and obstructive sleep apnea syndrome: a systematic review". Sleep Med Rev 2023;69:101787.

37. Lopez R, Shen Y, Chenini S, et al. Diagnostic criteria for disorders of arousal: a video-polysomnographic assessment. Ann Neurol 2018;83:341–51.

38. Hilditch CJ, McHill AW. Sleep inertia: current insights. Nat Sci Sleep 2019;11:155–65.

39. Tassi P, Muzet A. Sleep inertia. Sleep Med Rev 2000;4:341–53.

40. Bejot Y, Juenet N, Garrouty R, et al. Sexsomnia: an uncommon variety of parasomnia. Clin Neurol Neurosurg 2010;112:72–5.

41. Underwood A. It's called 'sexsomnia'. Newsweek 2007;149:53.

42. Andersen ML, Poyares D, Alves RS, et al. Sexsomnia: abnormal sexual behavior during sleep. Brain Res Rev 2007;56:271–82.

43. Shapiro CM, Trajanovic NN, Fedoroff JP. Sexsomnia–a new parasomnia? Canadian Journal of Psychiatry Revue Canadienne de Psychiatrie 2003;48:311–7.

44. Frank NC, Spirito A, Stark L, et al. The use of scheduled awakenings to eliminate childhood sleepwalking. J Pediatr Psychol 1997;22:345–53.

45. Lam SP, Fong SY, Ho CK, et al. Parasomnia among psychiatric outpatients: a clinical, epidemiologic, cross-sectional study. J Clin Psychiatry 2008;69:1374–82.

46. Ott GE, Rao U, Lin KM, et al. Effect of treatment with bupropion on EEG sleep: relationship to antidepressant response. Int J Neuropsychopharmacol 2004;7:275–81.

47. Oulis P, Kokras N, Papadimitriou GN, et al. Bupropion-induced sleepwalking. J Clin Psychopharmacol 2010;30:83–4.

48. Yeh YW, Chen CH, Feng HM, et al. New onset somnambulism associated with different dosage of mirtazapine: a case report. Clin Neuropharmacol 2009;32:232–3.

49. Kawashima T, Yamada S. Paroxetine-induced somnambulism. J Clin Psychiatry 2003;64:483.

50. Kunzel HE, Schuld A, Pollmacher T. Sleepwalking associated with reboxetine in a young female patient with major depression–a case report. Pharmacopsychiatry 2004;37:307–8.

51. Basyuni S, Quinnell T. Autocannibalism induced by obstructive sleep apnea. Sleep Med 2017;37:72–3.

52. Leung AKC, Leung AAM, Wong AHC, Hon KL. Sleep Terrors: An Updated Review. Curr Pediatr Rev 2020;16(3):176–82.

53. Rauf B, Sharpless BA, Denis D, et al. Isolated sleep paralysis: clinical features, perception of aetiology, prevention and disruption strategies in a large international sample. Sleep Med 2023;104:105–12.

54. El Sabbagh E, Johns AN, Mather CE, et al. A systematic review of Nightmare prevalence in children. Sleep Med Rev 2023;71:101834.

55. Porter VR, Avidan AY. Clinical overview of REM Sleep behavior disorder. Semin Neurol 2017;37:461–70.

56. Schenck CH, Hurwitz TD, Mahowald MW. REM sleep behavior disorder. Am J Psychiatr 1988;145:652.

57. Boeve BF. REM sleep behavior disorder: updated review of the core features, the REM sleep behavior disorder-neurodegenerative disease association, evolving concepts, controversies, and future directions. Ann N Y Acad Sci 2010;1184:15–54.

58. Rocha AL, Arnulf I. NREM parasomnia as a dream enacting behavior. Sleep Med 2020;75:103–5.

59. Boursoulian LJ, Schenck CH, Mahowald MW, et al. Differentiating parasomnias from nocturnal seizures. J Clin Sleep Med : JCSM 2012;8:108–12.

60. Somboon T, Grigg-Damberger MM, Foldvary-Schaefer N. Epilepsy and sleep-related breathing disturbances. Chest 2019;156:172–81.

61. Carreno M, Fernandez S. Sleep-related epilepsy. Curr Treat Options Neurol 2016;18:23.

62. Tinuper P, Bisulli F, Cross JH, et al. Definition and diagnostic criteria of sleep-related hypermotor epilepsy. Neurology 2016;86:1834–42.

63. Jain SV, Dye T, Kedia P. Value of combined video EEG and polysomnography in clinical management of children with epilepsy and daytime or nocturnal spells. Seizure. Journal of the British Epilepsy Association 2019;65:1–5.

64. Zucconi M. Sleep-related epilepsy. Handb Clin Neurol 2011;99:1109–37.

65. Derry CP, Davey M, Johns M, et al. Distinguishing sleep disorders from seizures: diagnosing bumps in the night. Arch Neurol 2006;63(5):705–9.

66. El Youssef N, Marchi A, Bartolomei F, et al. Sleep and epilepsy: A clinical and pathophysiological overview. Revue Neurologique 2023. https://doi.org/10.1001/archneur.63.5.705.

Understanding Sexual Parasomnias

A Review of the Current Literature on Their Nature, Diagnosis, Impacts, and Management

Monica Levy Andersen, PhD[a,b,]*, Carlos H. Schenck, MD[c],
Sergio Tufik, MD, PhD[a,b]

KEYWORDS

- Sleep • Sexsomnia • Parasomnia • Sleepsex • Sexuality • Sleepwalking • Confusional arousals
- Obstructive sleep apnea

KEY POINTS

- Sleep is essential for physiologic and cognitive functions, supporting physical restoration, memory consolidation, emotional regulation, and overall brain health. Sufficient sleep is linked to improved mental health, cognitive performance, and quality of life, whereas inadequate or disrupted sleep can cause a range of health issues and impairments.
- Sexual parasomnias, including sexsomnia, involve atypically-timed sexual behaviors and experiences during sleep, occurring outside of conscious awareness.
- Despite being relatively rare, sexual parasomnias have a significant influence on well-being and interpersonal relationships and can carry legal consequences.
- Increased awareness and improved support and care for individuals with sexsomnia can help reduce stigma and provide better outcomes for affected individuals.

INTRODUCTION

Sleep plays a vital role in various physiologic and cognitive functions, promoting physical restoration, memory consolidation, emotional regulation, and overall brain health. It is crucial for maintaining immune function, metabolic balance, cardiovascular health, and hormonal regulation.[1] Adequate sleep is also correlated with improved mental health, cognitive performance, and overall quality of life. Insufficient or disrupted sleep, however, can lead to a wide range of health problems and impairments.[1]

Sleep is a complex process characterized by distinct stages and cycles. These stages include non-rapid eye movement (NREM) sleep, which further consists of 3 stages (N1, N2, and N3 or slow-wave sleep), and rapid eye movement (REM) sleep.[2] Each stage has unique physiologic and electroencephalographic characteristics. NREM sleep is marked by slow brain waves, reduced muscle activity, and vital functions working to restore the body. REM sleep, often associated with dreaming, involves REMs, activated brain activity, and temporary paralysis of skeletal muscles.[2]

[a] Departamento de Psicobiologia, Universidade Federal de São Paulo (UNIFESP), São Paulo, Brazil; [b] Sleep Institute, São Paulo, Brazil; [c] Department of Psychiatry, Minnesota Regional Sleep Disorders Center, Hennepin County Medical Center and University of Minnesota Medical School, R7701 Park Avenue, Minneapolis, MN 55415, USA
* Corresponding author. Rua Napoleão de Barros, 925, Vila Clementino, São Paulo, São Paulo 04024-002, Brazil.
E-mail address: ml.andersen12@gmail.com

Sleep Med Clin 19 (2024) 21–41
https://doi.org/10.1016/j.jsmc.2023.10.002
1556-407X/24/© 2023 Elsevier Inc. All rights reserved.

Sleep disorders encompass a range of conditions that can significantly disrupt the quality and quantity of sleep. The latest edition of the International Classification of Sleep Disorders, that is, ICSD-3, by the American Academy of Sleep Medicine (AASM) published in 2014 provides a comprehensive taxonomy for categorizing sleep disorders,[3] now updated with the ICSD-3 Text Revision.[4] The classification system includes several main categories of sleep disorders, each with its distinct set of characteristics and diagnostic criteria. These categories involve a broad spectrum of conditions and provide a structure for accurate diagnosis and appropriate treatment planning. Some of the major categories of sleep disorders include insomnias, sleep-related breathing disorders, hypersomnias, circadian rhythm sleep–wake disorders, sleep-related movement disorders, and parasomnias. Parasomnias comprise various abnormal behaviors, movements, emotions, or experiences during sleep, including REM sleep behavior disorder (RBD), and also the NREM parasomnias involving sleepwalking (SW), sleep terrors (ST), sleep-related eating disorder, and sleep-related sexsomnia that are classified as a variant of confusional arousals.[3] Identifying these sleep disorders is essential for an accurate diagnosis and effective treatment, ultimately improving individuals' sleep quality and overall well-being (**Table 1**).

Within the realm of sleep disorders, sexual parasomnias have emerged as a captivating and distinct phenomenon, engaging the attention of researchers and clinicians alike, along with the general public.[5] These complex conditions cover a full spectrum of sexual behaviors and experiences that occur during sleep, frequently manifesting outside the space of conscious awareness.[6] Despite their relatively low prevalence, sexual parasomnias can significantly affect an individual's overall well-being and interpersonal relationships. Therefore, comprehensively grasping the nature, prevalence, underlying mechanisms, personal and interpersonal consequences, and available treatment approaches for sexual parasomnias is of the utmost importance.

In 2007, we published a comprehensive review that delved into the key aspects of sexsomnia, examining the available published cases up to that point.[7] Since our previous review, significant advancements have been made in the field of sleep disorders and sexual behaviors during sleep (SBS). Researchers worldwide have reported and documented new cases, and Editorials have been written,[8,9] contributing to our growing knowledge of sexsomnia. One of the authors (CHS) has investigated and reported on the clinical and forensic aspects of sexsomnia for the past 3 decades, with additional updates provided in this review. With the goal of revisiting this intriguing topic, our current aim is to present new findings and discuss the latest cases published between 2007 and 2023. By analyzing and synthesizing these recent cases, we gain an updated insight into sexsomnia's prevalence, clinical presentation,

Table 1
Differential diagnosis

Condition/Disorder	Similar Symptoms	Key Differences
Sexsomnia	Involuntary sexual behaviors, including at times aggressive/violent sexual contact with the bed partner	Typically occurs during deep NREM sleep; involves sexual behaviors (that can be aggressive/violent)
Rapid eye movement sleep behavior disorder (RBD)	Violent or potentially harmful physical acts during sleep, such as kicking, punching, or other vigorous movements	Occurs during REM sleep; involves aggressive physical actions
KLS	Recurrent episodes of prolonged sleep, with hypersexuality/peculiar sexuality during wake during the episodes, hyperphagia (excessive eating), and at times child-like behavior	Involves episodes of excessive sleep and altered wakeful sexuality during the episodes, and at times child-like behavior
Persistent sexual arousal syndrome	Intense and persistent spontaneous sexual arousal during sleep and/or wake without apparent sexual stimulation	Can be associated with sleep and/or wake

underlying mechanisms, associated comorbidities, and potential treatments. By presenting new data and discussing the latest cases, we hope to contribute to increased recognition, accurate diagnosis, and appropriate management of sexsomnia. Exploring the topic of sexsomnia enhances our understanding of the complex interplay between sleep, sexuality, and consciousness, ultimately leading to improved support and care for affected individuals. Moreover, it helps dispel misconceptions, reduce stigma, and promote empathy and support for individuals experiencing sexsomnia and their partners.

DATA SOURCES AND SEARCH STRATEGIES

In May 2023, we undertook a comprehensive search of the PubMed database for articles published between 2007 and 2023. Only articles written in English were considered. We used the following search terms: "sexsomnia," "parasomnia sexual," "sleepsex." The database was searched using Boolean operators "AND" and "OR" in a similar sequence. The inclusion criteria were applied all throughout the selection and screening process, and the entire process of the literature search was well documented using text analysis tools. All resulting citations were moved into EndNoteWeb, and any duplicates found were removed manually. A total of 55 articles were retrieved from the searches, with 3 being excluded because they were not written in English. The remaining citations were then screened using the content of the title and abstract, as well as through characterization of the data of the full-text articles.

SEXSOMNIA

Sexsomnia, also described as "sexual sleepwalking" or "sleepsex," belongs to the group of parasomnias, more precisely those that occur during the NREM sleep phase, where an abnormal arousal leads to the execution of atypically timed sexual acts while still in a nonawake state.[3] These behaviors can range from being harmless, such as masturbation, sexual vocalizations, and spontaneous orgasms, to being aggressive and violent, with attempts at nonconsensual penetration of a bed partner. However, sexual vocalizations during sleep masturbation at times can result in serious negative marital consequences, as illustrated by 2 reported cases from Paris[10] and Sao Paulo[11] of married women who uttered the names of men—who were not their husbands—while engaging in sleep masturbation during many nights, with their husbands sleeping alongside them in bed. Understandably, this caused great personal and marital distress, despite the lack of any evidence suggesting an extramarital affair. Despite the gradual demystification of human sexuality during the twentieth century, becoming a subject of medical and scientific interest—notably through the studies of Sigmund Freud, which still elicited indignant reactions from some sections of society at the time—sexual confusional arousals and SW remain a topic that is inadequately addressed and still insufficiently studied[12] but there is a recent growing momentum in published case series and case reports across the world that is raising more awareness of sexsomnia, its causes, consequences, and treatment. A recent literature review (that is complementary to the review contained herein), which included reports published in languages other than English (eg, Turkish, Dutch, and Spanish), and also published abstracts, identified 220 sexsomnia cases (from 15 countries and 5 continents), with most of these cases reported in 4 large case series and 2 comprehensive reviews.[9,13] Notable findings included male predominance (84%), with an age range of 14 to 77 years, indicating that sexsomnia can emerge throughout the postpuberty life span. Nevertheless, the typical age of onset is in early adulthood (26–33 years old in one series).[6] A study using an online questionnaire concluded that symptomatic onset may occur earlier in patients with a prior history of SW.[14] Moreover, besides a strong comorbidity with other NREM parasomnias (eg, SW, ST, sleep-related eating disorder, and so forth), obstructive sleep apnea (OSA) was found to be a known trigger for sexsomnia, with control of the OSA by continuous positive airway pressure (CPAP)[15,16] or by mandibular advancement device[17,18] also controlling the sexsomnia in most cases.

Despite the growing literature that was just mentioned, the prevalence of sexsomnia remains underestimated. This may be due to the undervaluation of symptoms by patients and health-care professionals, or even due to the discomfort of both parties in reporting or tracking them, respectively, thus hindering their recognition.[19] The underestimation of the disorder is possibly due to feelings of shame and humiliation experienced by patients and their partners, leading them to conceal the situation from health-care professionals.[7] Additionally, the association of amnesia with episodes of sexsomnia, as reported in several cases, may contribute to the underrecognition of the disorder. These arguments support the hypothesis of underdiagnosis rather than the epidemiologic rarity of sexsomnia. However, there has been an increasing interest in sexsomnia recently, due to the serious psychological, social, and legal implications it can entail.[10,11,13,15]

Sexsomnia episodes mostly occur in the first half of the night, with a highly variable frequency, ranging from a single episode in a lifetime to several episodes per week. Similar to other subtypes of NREM sleep-related parasomnias, the pathophysiology is unknown, and it is only speculated that it may stem from a disturbance in the awakening mechanisms, manifesting as disordered arousals from (usually) deep NREM sleep. Several studies using electroencephalography (EEG) and polysomnography (PSG) have observed frequent arousals concurrent with slow and fast electroencephalographic activities, suggesting the occurrence of partial arousals, particularly during the N3 sleep stage characterized by slow-wave activity. To date, there have been 18 published cases of sexual behaviors documented during video-polysomnography (vPSG) that involved masturbation from N3 arousals in 17 of these cases.[20]

In 2007, Trajanovic and colleagues executed a study aiming to expand the knowledge about sexsomnia.[14] Previous research primarily focused on a specific group of middle-aged men with extensive medico-legal exposure. However, anecdotal evidence suggested that a younger population might be more affected, with a gender distribution similar to other NREM sleep parasomnias. Unfortunately, there was a lack of epidemiologic information regarding this condition. To overcome the challenges of reaching this elusive population, the researchers implemented a 28-item Internet survey, which was posted on a sexsomnia reference site and distributed to prospective respondents, mostly registered visitors to the site.[14] Respondents had the option to complete the survey anonymously, necessitating the screening of fraudulent and duplicate submissions. Ultimately, 219 validated responses were collected and analyzed. The findings revealed a higher representation of women, accounting for 31% of the total number of respondents, and a wider age distribution with a mean age of 30.4 years. Most respondents reported experiencing multiple episodes of sexsomnia, often triggered by body contact, stress, and fatigue. A relatively small proportion of participants reported the involvement of legal authorities (8.6% of men and 3% of women) from their sexsomnia episodes, including involvement of minors in 6% of the total sample. Although it is important to acknowledge the limitations inherent in survey-based research, this study significantly contributed to the understanding of this complex nocturnal behavior. It corroborated the subjective evidence regarding gender and age distribution while providing insights into key aspects such as precipitating factors, types of behavior, medication usage, personal medical history, and medico-legal implications.

The most commonly documented sexual behaviors in patients with sexsomnia include attempts to initiate sexual intercourse, attempted penetration, fondling of the bed partner, masturbation, vocalization of orgasms, and even sexual assault, understood as submission to nonconsensual sexual acts during sleep.[7] In reported cases involving women experiencing sexsomnia episodes, masturbation, and spontaneous orgasms are the most frequent and almost exclusive manifestations during sleep.[21] The sexual behavior exhibited by individuals with sexsomnia during sleep can sometimes differ from their waking behavior. Some individuals become more tender and affectionate with their partners, whereas others become more direct, aggressive, and even violent, engaging in sexual acts that differ from their usual practices.[5] Typically, during wakefulness, patients have a normal sexual life without a history of sexual abuse, trauma, paraphilias, or psychiatric disorders. It is characteristic for partners to feel perplexed when confronted in the middle of the night, and in most cases, they reject these sexual behaviors on understanding that they are not voluntary acts by their partners.[5] One peculiar aspect of this sexual behavior during sleep is that individuals engage in these behaviors only when alone or when with their bed partner. It is uncommon for individuals with sexsomnia to leave the bed and seek out their partner, suggesting that physical contact may trigger an episode. In general, almost all patients wake up with complete amnesia of the events that occurred during the previous night and are questioned by their bed partners.[8] Sexsomnia episodes do not seem to be associated with erotic (or any) dream content.

SLEEP ARCHITECTURE AND SLEEP DISRUPTIONS

Sleep architecture and disruptions are critical factors in the development and manifestation of sleep disorders, including sexsomnia. Sleep architecture refers to the cyclical progression of different sleep stages, including NREM sleep and REM sleep.[22] Disruptions in sleep architecture can occur due to various factors, such as external stimuli, physiologic changes, or underlying sleep disorders. For instance, frequent arousals or awakenings can significantly affect sleep architecture and increase the likelihood of sleep-related behaviors, including sexsomnia.[19] Fragmented sleep, characterized by interrupted or fragmented sleep stages, may disrupt the normal sleep–wake cycle and contribute to the occurrence of sexsomnia episodes.

In sexsomnia, these sleep disruptions may lead to the initiation of SBS. The transitions between sleep stages, particularly the NREM sleep stages, have been implicated in the occurrence of sexsomnia episodes.[22] During NREM sleep, arousal thresholds are generally higher, and the individual is less responsive to external stimuli. However, disruptions in the transitions between NREM sleep stages, such as from deep sleep (N3) to lighter sleep stages, may lower arousal thresholds and increase the probability of engaging in sleep-related sexual behaviors.[22]

Sleep pattern can be influenced by various factors. Coexisting sleep disorders, for example, OSA, restless legs syndrome (RLS), or sleep-related movement disorders, can contribute to sleep fragmentation and increase the risk of sexsomnia episodes.[19] These conditions often involve repetitive movements or arousals during sleep, leading to disturbances in sleep architecture and potentially triggering sexsomnia behaviors.

Medications and substances can influence sleep architecture and arousal thresholds, thereby influencing the occurrence of sleep-related sexual behaviors. Certain medications, including sedatives, hypnotics, and antidepressants, may alter sleep stages and increase the possibility of sleep disruptions.[23] The use of substances, such as alcohol, illicit drugs, or specific prescription medications, can lower inhibitions, disrupt normal sleep patterns, and contribute to the manifestation of sexsomnia. The role of alcohol has been controversial: recently, with the ICSD-3-Text Revision a lack of firm correlation of alcohol use with arousal disorders was noted, and also alcohol intoxication was stated to be an exclusion criterion.[4] The diagnostic and statistical manual of psychiatric disorders, 5th edition (DSM-5) also supports this idea by excluding alcohol from the list of potential precipitants of SW.[24] Understanding the role of sleep architecture and disruptions in relation to sexsomnia is essential for accurate diagnosis and tailored treatment approaches. PSG, a comprehensive sleep study that includes the monitoring of brain waves, muscle activity, and other physiologic parameters during sleep, can provide valuable insights into sleep architecture and help identify disruptions linked with sexsomnia.

Sleep Disorders and Comorbidities

Coexisting sleep disorders, including OSA, RLS, and sleep-related movement disorders, have been suggested as potential precipitating factors for sexsomnia.[23] These conditions may contribute to sleep fragmentation and increase the likelihood of sexsomnia episodes.

OSA, a prevalent sleep disorder[25] characterized by recurrent pauses in breathing during sleep, has shown a triggering association with sexsomnia.[15–18] The fragmented sleep patterns resulting from sleep apnea can disrupt the normal sleep architecture and increase the risk of sleep-related sexual behaviors—in predisposed individuals, with male gender being a major predisposing factor. The intermittent hypoxia and arousals related with sleep apnea may further contribute to the occurrence of sexsomnia episodes. A study was conducted to examine the prevalence of parasomnias in relation to the presence and severity of OSA.[26] The study included 4372 patients referred to a Norwegian university hospital for suspected OSA, with an average age of 49.1 years and 69.8% being men. OSA diagnosis was confirmed using standard respiratory polygraphy, and participants completed a comprehensive questionnaire regarding their experiences with parasomnias during the previous 3 months. The findings revealed that among the participants, 34.7% had no OSA, 32.5% had mild OSA, 17.4% had moderate OSA, and 15.3% had severe OSA. The overall prevalence of parasomnias was as follows: 3.3% for SW, 2.5% for sleep-related violence (SRV), 3.1% for sexual acts during sleep, 1.7% for sleep-related eating, and 43.8% for nightmares. Adjusted logistic regression analysis indicated that the odds of SW were significantly higher in individuals with severe OSA compared with those with mild OSA.[26]

RLS, a neurologic disorder characterized by uncomfortable sensations and an irresistible urge to move the legs, has also been linked to sexsomnia. The disrupted sleep continuity caused by RLS symptoms can heighten the risk of sleep-related sexual behaviors. The motor restlessness and sleep disturbances connected with RLS may contribute to the manifestation of sexsomnia episodes.[27]

Sleep-related movement disorders, such as periodic limb movement disorder (PLMD), have also been implicated as comorbidities in sexsomnia cases. PLMD involves repetitive limb movements during sleep, which can lead to sleep fragmentation and arousal. These disruptions in sleep architecture increase the susceptibility to sleep-related sexual behaviors observed in sexsomnia.[19]

Della Marca and colleagues (2009) investigated the characteristics of abnormal nocturnal sexual behaviors in 3 male patients who sought evaluation at a sleep laboratory due to others sleep-related problems (**Table 2**).[28] The clinical and PSG findings were carefully examined to gain

Table 2
Case summaries for individuals with episodes of sexsomnia since 2007

Gender	Age	Family History of Parasomnia	Personal History of Parasomnia	Precipitating Factors	PSG	Epworth	Abnormal Behavior During Sleep	Frequency	Respiratory Events	Medico-legal Issues	Refs
MAN	42	No	No	Sleep disorder (OSAS)	Yes	U	Sexual intercourse with his wife	2–3/wk	OSA	No	Marca et al.[28] 2009
MAN	32	Yes	Yes	Sleep disorder (somnambulism)	Yes	U	Sexual intercourse with his wife	2–3/wk	No	No	Marca et al.[28] 2009
MAN	46	No	No	Sleep disorder (rapid eye movement behavior disorder—RBD)	Yes	U	Sexual intercourse with his wife	3–4/wk	OSA	No	Marca et al.[28] 2009
WOMAN	36	No	No	SW and alcohol	Yes	U	Sexual intercourse with her husband	4–5/y	No	No	Béjot et al.[45] 2010
WOMAN	40	No	No	Marijuana and heroin	Yes	U	Violent masturbation, insertion of objects into her vagina and anus, inflicting pain on her husband's genitals, moaning and sexually provocative phrases	1/mo	No	No	Béjot et al.[45] 2010
WOMAN	61	No	Yes	SW and sleeptalking	Yes	5	Masturbation	2–3/wk	OSA	No	Cicolin et al.[29] 2010
MAN	41	Yes	Yes	SW and sleeptalking	Yes	3	Sexually touching his daughter (remove her clothing and fondle)	3–5/wk	No	Yes	Cicolin et al.[29] 2010
MAN	31	No	No	NA	Yes	U	Masturbation, unintelligible talk, moving around, and hallucinations	3–4/night	No	No	Pelin[56] 2012
MAN	29	No	Yes	Sleeptalking	Yes	U	Sexual intercourse	2–3/wk	OSA	No	Ariño et al.[31] 2014

WOMAN 40	No	Yes	SW	Yes	U	Masturbation	2–3/wk	No	No	Ariño et al.[31] 2014
MAN 42	No	Yes	Confusional arousals	Yes	U	Sexual intercourse	2–3/wk	OSA	No	Ariño et al.[31] 2014
MAN 25	No	Yes	Confusional arousals	Yes	U	Sexual intercourse and masturbation	2–3/wk	No	No	Ariño et al.[31] 2014
WOMAN 41	No	No	Narcolepsy and mild cataplexy	Yes	U	Sexually assaulted her husband	Lasted for 3 wk	No	No	Devesa et al.[38] 2016
MAN 20	No	U	Sleep deprivation	Yes	U	Masturbation	Every night	No	No	Yeh et al.[39] 2016
MAN 27	No	Yes	SW	Yes	U	Sexual intercourse and disrobing his wife	1–2/mo	OSA	No	Meira e Cruz et al.[18] 2016
MAN 42	NA	No	No	Yes	U	Masturbation and talking sexual connotations	4–5/wk	OSA	No	Soca et al.[30] 2016
MAN 33	No	Yes	Hypnagogic hallucinations, sleep paralysis, night terrors, and SW	Yes	U	Sexual behaviors	4/y	No	No	Mioč et al.[57] 2017
MAN 37	U	U	Sleep deprivation	Yes	12	Sexual intercourse with his wife	1–2/wk	OSA	No	Khawaja et al.[17] 2017
WOMAN 57	U	U	Narcotic use	Yes	U	Masturbation and sleep-related orgasms	Several times weekly to every 6 mo	OSA	No	Irfan et al.[61] 2018
MAN 49	No	Yes	Bruxism	Yes	11	Masturbation without ejaculation	Every night	OSA	No	Martynowicz et al.[32] 2018
MAN 38	U	Yes	Smoker and bruxism	Yes	16	Masturbation	Every night	OSA	No	Martynowicz et al.[32] 2018
MAN 16	No	No	Attention deficit hyperactivity disorder, mood disorder, and anxiety; pineoblastoma resection; chemotherapy, and panhypopituitarism	Yes	U	Masturbation		OSA	No	Contreras et al.[41] 2019

(continued on next page)

Table 2
(continued)

Gender	Age	Family History of Parasomnia	Personal History of Parasomnia	Precipitating Factors	PSG	Epworth	Abnormal Behavior During Sleep	Frequency	Respiratory Events	Medico-legal Issues	Refs
MAN	44	No	ST, somniloquy	No	Yes	8	Masturbation	1–3/night	No	No	Pirzada et al.[43] 2019
MAN	26	Somnambulism	Somnambulism	Exertion and exhaustion	Yes	10	Sexual intercourse	2–3/night	No	No	Pirzada et al.[43] 2019
MAN	38	Somnambulism	Somnambulism	No	Yes	10	Sexual intercourse	3/wk	OSA	No	Pirzada et al.[43] 2019
WOMAN	47	No	Nightmare disorder and somniloquy	Menstruation	Yes	10	Sexual dream enactment	1–2/wk	No	No	Pirzada et al.[43] 2019
MAN	40	No	Yes, SW and talking	Alcohol	Yes	U	Sexual intercourse	2–6/mo	No	No	Kumar et al.[62] 2020
WOMAN	42	U	Yes	Stress	Yes	13	Moaning, sexual phrases, "dirty talk," masturbation and sexual intercourse	U	OSA	No	Toscanini et al.[11] 2021
MAN	40	Yes, SW	No	Anxiety and depression	Yes	U	Masturbation, partial coherence, ejaculation, and cleaning hands after masturbation	U	OSA	No	Kim et al.[48] 2021
WOMAN	44	No	No	KLS, childhood sexual trauma, cluster headaches, major depressive disorder, anxiety, and restless leg syndrome.	No	No	Masturbation, partnered stimulation, and orgasm	Everyday	U	No	Zwerling et al.[33] 2021

Sex	Age			Sleep-related head jerks			Masturbation, sexual intercourse/attempted intercourse, and sexual vocalizations				Reference
MAN	33	No	Yes, SW	No	Yes	U	Masturbation, sexual intercourse/attempted intercourse, and sexual vocalizations	1/mo to several nights a week	No	No	Bušková et al.[63] 2022
MAN	41	No	No	No	Yes	U	Sexual intercourse with his wife	10/life	No	No	Fernandez et al.[47] 2023
MAN	27	No	No	No	Yes	U	Sexual intercourse with his wife	U	No	No	Fernandez et al.[47] 2023
MAN	25	No	No	No	Yes	U	Sexual intercourse with his wife	5/wk	OSA	No	Fernandez et al. (2023)[47]
MAN	50	No	No	No	Yes	U	Sexual intercourse with his wife; aggressive movements and struggling	50% of the nights for the past 5 y	OSA	No	Fernandez et al.[47] 2023

English language articles.
Abbreviations: OSA, obstructive sleep apnea; PSG, polysomnography; U, unspecified.

insights into the nature of their behaviors and their underlying sleep disorders. The patients exhibited different sleep disorders: one had severe obstructive sleep apnea syndrome (OSAS), another had NREM sleep parasomnia in the form of somnambulism (SW), and the third displayed rapid eye movement sleep behavior disorder (RBD). This diversity suggests that sleep-related sexual behaviors can manifest in connection with various sleep disorders, each with its own distinct mechanisms and treatment approaches.[28] The utilization of PSG played a crucial role in examining these behaviors. By monitoring and recording various physiologic parameters during sleep, PSG provided valuable information regarding the pathophysiology of the abnormal sexual behaviors. This knowledge, in turn, guided the development of appropriate treatment strategies for each patient. The 3 male patients included in this study were aged 32, 42, and 46 years, respectively.[28]

In 2011, Cicolin and coworkers (see **Table 2**) conducted a study that shed light on the coexistence of RBD and NREM sleep parasomnias[29] in a phenomenon known as parasomnia overlap disorder (POD).[3] Specifically, the study focused on SBS, which are categorized as confusional arousals and SW under the ICSD-2 classification of parasomnias. The study presented 2 cases of patients with documented SBS associated with POD, confirmed through PSG. In one case, a 60-year-old female patient exhibited SBS during slow-wave sleep (SWS). Video-PSG recordings captured a brief episode of masturbation, preceded by the specific EEG pattern of deep slow-wave sleep. Importantly, the patient had no awareness of the behavior and did not recall any related dreams. The second case involved a 41-year-old male patient with a history of SW and RBD. He faced legal charges for sexually fondling a young girl during the night. PSG confirmed the presence of POD in this patient. The court accepted the defense of parasomnia, including sleepsex, and the patient was acquitted. This report holds significant importance because it provides evidence of SBS occurring in patients with PSG-confirmed POD.[29] It should be noted that these 2 patients each had a total of 5 NREM/REM motor parasomnias, calling attention to the inappropriate and excessive activation of "central pattern [motor] generators" in the brainstem.[8] Thus, the Cicolin and colleagues report highlights the utility of video-PSG in documenting SBS, enabling a more comprehensive understanding of the behaviors linked with this complex POD.[29] Indeed, POD seems to be strongly connected with cases of sexsomnia. Soca and colleagues described a case of a 42-year-old man who exhibited a history of abnormal nighttime behaviors (see **Table 2**).[30] For 7 to 10 years, he had been SW and consuming food. Additionally, he started talking during sleep, initially with inappropriate content and later with sexual connotations. According to his bed partner, he made attempts to engage in sexual activities during sleep. Concurrently, the patient was diagnosed with severe OSA and prescribed CPAP therapy, which improved his SW and sleep eating but had no effect on the sexual behaviors. During evaluation at the sleep clinic, the patient reported experiencing sexual episodes 4 to 5 nights per week, primarily involving masturbation (see **Table 2**). He did not recall having any sexual dreams and could easily go back to sleep after becoming aware of an episode. The patient had a medical history of generalized anxiety disorder, resolved alcohol abuse, irritable bowel syndrome, esophageal reflux, type 2 diabetes, gout, and hypertension. His medications at the time included multiple drugs for these conditions. Physical examination yielded no significant findings, and video-PSG showed no respiratory events during the night.[30] Noteworthy observations during video-PSG included arousal from stage N3 sleep accompanied by violent leg movements and increased muscle tone during REM sleep, accompanied by episodes of yelling profanities and leg kicking. The patient was prescribed clonazepam 0.5 mg at bedtime, which reduced the frequency of sexual episodes to 1 to 2 nights per week but the nature of the episodes remained the same. There was one instance of SW after initiating treatment, and a higher dose of clonazepam led to excessive daytime sleepiness.[30]

Ariño and colleagues (2014) performed a study describing 4 cases of sexsomnia. The patients, aged between 28 and 43 years, reported engaging in these behaviors for varying durations, including masturbation, and attempted sexual intercourse.[31] They had no recollection of these events, and their partners provided accounts of their behavior. Medical histories revealed correlations with SW, confusional arousals, OSA, and periodic leg movements. Treatment with clonazepam resulted in a reduction in the frequency of both confusional arousals and sexsomnia episodes. Overall, sexsomnia commonly affects young adults and can be associated with other sleep disorders, mainly OSA and PLMD. Additionally, 2 new cases link sleep bruxism to recurrent episodes of sexsomnia, as depicted in **Table 2**.[32] These findings emphasize the need for further exploration of the relationship between sexsomnia and a wide range of sleep-related disorders, including bruxism, which could lead to improved management strategies for both conditions.

The accurate diagnosis and effective management of sexsomnia require consideration of coexisting sleep disorders. In individuals with sexsomnia, evaluating and treating OSA, RLS, and sleep-related movement disorders are essential to improve sleep quality and reduce the occurrence of sleep-related sexual behaviors. A comprehensive approach that combines both sleep disorder treatment and sexsomnia management strategies can yield favorable outcomes.

Kleine-Levin syndrome (KLS) is a rare sleep disorder that has gained attention due to its association with concurrent sexual dysfunction. This disorder has prompted a review of existing literature to explore the relationship between sleep disorders and women's sexual health. In this review, a notable case study involving a patient named J.C. with KLS and persistent genital arousal disorder was presented.[33] J.C., a 44-year-old woman, sought help at a sexual medicine clinic because she experienced persistent and distressing sexual arousal. Despite trying various forms of stimulation, her symptoms persisted, leading to multiple self-stimulations throughout the day. This condition affected her social life and relationships. J.C.'s recent diagnosis of KLS revealed cycles of hyperphagia, intense clitoral arousal, and hypersomnia lasting between 2 and 28 days. Her medical history included childhood sexual trauma, cluster headaches, major depressive disorder, anxiety, and RLS. Previous treatments, including medications and physical therapy, had not yielded significant results. During the examination, mild pelvic floor hypertonus was observed but J.C.'s vaginal tissues seemed normal. Hormone evaluations fell within the normal range. To address her symptoms, a multimodal treatment approach was adopted. J.C. was prescribed intravaginal diazepam suppositories, topical lidocaine ointment, and an increased dose of duloxetine. After 3 months of treatment, her symptoms improved, and the frequency of self-stimulation decreased. Her other KLS symptoms were being managed separately by a sleep specialist. These findings underscore the importance of considering sleep quality and potential sleep disorders when addressing sexual health concerns (see **Table 2**). It highlights the importance of the awareness of health-care professionals of the need to evaluate sleep patterns and disorders in patients with sexual health complaints. By adopting a comprehensive approach, incorporating both sleep and sexual health evaluations, health-care providers can provide more effective and holistic care to patients.

Future research should focus on elucidating the underlying mechanisms linking sleep apnea, RLS, sleep-related movement disorders, and sexsomnia. Longitudinal studies with larger sample sizes can provide insights into the prevalence and causal relationships between these comorbidities. Developing targeted interventions and treatment guidelines specific to individuals with sexsomnia and coexisting sleep disorders will enhance clinical care and improve patient outcomes.

Confusional Arousals

Confusional arousals are classified as an NREM parasomnia within the ICSD-3.[3] It is also known as Elpenor syndrome and is often casually referred to as "sleep drunkenness" due to its resemblance to the mental fog experienced on waking from a deep sleep. The condition predominantly occurs during deep NREM sleep and is characterized by partial awakening, leading to confusion and cognitive impairment.

Confusional arousals typically presents as sudden awakening accompanied by symptoms, such as confusion, decreased responsiveness, slowed speech, and impaired cognitive function. Individuals affected by confusional arousal may also display automatic behaviors, repetitive movements, or complex motor acts. The episodes are usually brief, lasting from a few minutes to an hour but they can recur and be distressing for both the individual and their bed partner. The prevalence of confusional arousal varies across different age groups, with higher rates reported in children and adolescents compared with adults. According to one study conducted in the United Kingdom, approximately 4.2% of adults experience confusional arousals.[34] Other studies have indicated that up to 15.2% of adults may experience confusional arousals within a year.[35] The AASM has noted a higher prevalence of the disorder among children, with around 17%, whereas the prevalence in individuals aged older than 15 years is approximately 3% to 4%.[36] It is worth mentioning that children diagnosed with confusional arousal disorder may later develop SW during their later childhood or adolescence.

Confusional arousals and sexsomnia are 2 distinct but overlapping parasomnias that have been found to exhibit a relationship, potentially due to shared underlying factors. In fact, the official term for sexsomnia in the ICSD-3 is "sleep-related abnormal sexual behaviors" as a recognized variant of confusional arousals.[3] Research suggests that individuals with confusional arousal may have an increased susceptibility to experiencing sexsomnia episodes.[37] This correlation could be attributed to disruptions in the arousal systems during sleep, contributing to the occurrence of both conditions.

Numerous cases reported in the literature have documented the co-occurrence of confusional arousals in episodes of sexsomnia, further supporting their association.[11,19,22,23,29,31,32,38–40] Several factors have been identified as potential risk factors for confusional arousals, namely the use of certain medications, drugs, and alcohol. These substances can disrupt the normal sleep architecture and contribute to the occurrence of confusional arousals. Furthermore, certain medical conditions, sleep deprivation, and high levels of stress have also been recognized as potential risk factors for confusional arousals. Understanding these risk factors is crucial in the identification and management of confusional arousals, underscoring the importance of addressing substance use, promoting healthy sleep practices, and addressing underlying medical conditions to mitigate their occurrence.

MEDICATIONS, SUBSTANCES, AND SEXSOMNIA: AN INTRIGUING RELATIONSHIP

Certain medications have been implicated in the occurrence of sexsomnia episodes. Sedative-hypnotics, commonly prescribed for sleep disorders or anxiety, may alter sleep architecture, and increase the risk of sleep-related sexual behaviors. These medications can affect arousal thresholds, impair inhibitory control mechanisms, and disrupt the normal sleep–wake cycle, potentially contributing to the manifestation of sexsomnia.[8] Antidepressants, particularly those with serotonergic effects, have also been correlated with sexsomnia.[6] The precise mechanisms underlying these connections remain to be fully elucidated.

Muza and colleagues (2016) conducted a review with the aim of enhancing our understanding of the clinical characteristics of patients with sexsomnia and exploring the diverse range of clinical manifestations associated with this condition.[6] Their review encompassed the literature published in the past decade (2008–2014) as well as their own clinical experience with patients with sexsomnia identified retrospectively during a 6-year period at a tertiary sleep clinic.[6] The findings indicated that the prevalence of SBS remains uncertain, but it seems to primarily affect younger adult men who frequently exhibit other NREM parasomnias. Instances of sexsomnia induced by medication have also been documented, and there is a significant variability in the approach to treatment. Within their study group of 41 individuals with sexsomnia, with a mean age of 32 years (including 37 men), the manifestations of sexsomnia varied. Overall, sexual

intercourse was the most commonly reported behavior, although a majority of the 4 women engaged in masturbation. Incidents of violence and aggression were described in 11 cases. All patients had no recollection of the events, and 73% had a history of other parasomnias.[6]

The use of substances, such as alcohol, illicit drugs, and specific prescription medications, has been linked to an increased risk of sexsomnia. Alcohol, a central nervous system depressant, can suppress inhibitory mechanisms and lead to disinhibition during sleep. This disinhibition can result in the initiation of sleep-related sexual behaviors in individuals predisposed to sexsomnia.[41,42] Illicit drugs, such as cannabis and stimulants, can also disrupt sleep architecture and increase the likelihood of sleep-related sexual activities.[41,42] Nevertheless, the ICSD-3 Text Revision clearly states that an NREM parasomnia (including sexsomnia) cannot be diagnosed (in both clinical and legal settings) in the context of alcohol intoxication or other drug intoxication.[4] Certain prescription medications, including those used for the treatment of Parkinson disease or erectile dysfunction, have also been related with sexsomnia episodes, although further research is needed to establish the causal relationship.[43]

A research study was conducted to investigate the occurrence of parasomnias in individuals with addictions and during addiction treatment.[44] The study involved a systematic search of published articles to gather information on parasomnias that occur during both REM and non-REM sleep in individuals using substances or during abstinence. The study identified 17 articles, and several associations were found between specific substances and the occurrence of parasomnias.[44] Alcohol consumption was linked to arousal disorders, such as sexsomnia and sleep-related eating disorder. Additionally, RBD was reported during alcohol withdrawal. Cocaine abuse was connected with RBD featuring drug-related dream content.[44] These findings open an important avenue of research in respect of the prevalence of parasomnias among individuals with addictions.

The exact mechanisms through which medications and substances contribute to the development of sexsomnia are still not fully understood and remain highly controversial. Future research should focus broadly on predisposing, triggering, and perpetuating factors for sexsomnia that could facilitate the most appropriate interventions. However, it is thought that alterations in sleep architecture, arousal thresholds, inhibitory control mechanisms, and neurotransmitter modulation play significant roles.

In one report, a patient, a 41-year-old woman with narcolepsy and mild cataplexy, initially received modafinil treatment without a response.[38] Subsequently, the patient was switched to sodium oxybate, which led to a positive response and significant improvement in symptoms. However, after taking a high dose of sodium oxybate in a single administration, the patient experienced a confusional arousal episode accompanied by sexsomnia and sleep-related eating disorder. During these episodes, she sexually assaulted her husband and engaged in unintelligible sleep talking of an obscene nature. She displayed excessive eating, particularly of carbohydrates. The symptoms persisted for 3 weeks but on temporary discontinuation of sodium oxybate, they immediately ceased. Gradual reintroduction of sodium oxybate did not trigger a recurrence of the symptoms. Confusional arousal disorders occurring during non-REM sleep can result in the disinhibition of primitive behaviors such as eating, sexual activities, or aggression. It is hypothesized that a central pattern generator may be involved in these disorders, with the prefrontal cortex normally inhibiting such behaviors during wakefulness. Dissociation of brain regions, activation of the central pattern generator, sleep inertia, and sleep-state instability are thought to contribute to confusional arousal disorders. The case report suggested that the observed side effects of confusional arousals, including sexsomnia, in the patient may be attributed to the increase in SWS induced by sodium oxybate treatment.[38]

When evaluating individuals with sexsomnia, it is crucial to assess their medication history and substance use patterns. Identifying medications or substances that may contribute to sleep-related sexual behaviors is essential for comprehensive diagnosis and management. Health-care professionals should consider alternative medication options and educate patients about the potential risks associated with certain pharmacologic agents and substances. Collaborative efforts between sleep specialists, psychiatrists, and addiction specialists may be beneficial in managing sexsomnia in individuals with coexisting substance use disorders.

PSYCHOLOGICAL AND EMOTIONAL FACTORS

Psychological and emotional factors, such as stress, anxiety, trauma, and relationship issues, have been suggested as potential triggers for sexsomnia. Emotional distress and unresolved psychological conflicts may manifest during sleep as sexual behaviors, possibly influenced by altered dream content or emotional processing during sleep.

In 2010, Béjot and colleagues presented 2 cases demonstrating the influence of psychological factors on sexsomnia (see **Table 2**).[45] In the first case, a 36-year-old married woman with a history of SW and alcohol consumption exhibited abnormal behavior during sleep. Her husband reported instances where she sexually assaulted him while he was asleep, typically between 2 and 6 AM. These episodes occurred around 4 to 5 times per year and persisted until sexual intercourse was completed. Interestingly, the woman had no memory of these events afterward. Further psychological evaluation revealed social difficulties during her childhood, as well as a history of being placed in a children's home and experiencing sexual abuse. A psychiatric assessment indicated an obsessive-compulsive personality but no major depressive or dissociative disorders were identified. Physical examination, brain MRI, and EEG results were all within normal ranges. PSG indicated spontaneous arousals from SWS, suggesting a parasomnia condition. Although video recordings did not capture any sexual activity, the patient was prescribed an antidepressant (escitalopram), which resulted in a decrease in the frequency of SW episodes. Within the first year of treatment, 3 episodes of abnormal sexual behavior were reported but they were limited to vocalization and dirty talk. Eventually, the abnormal behavior ceased completely.[45] In the second case, a 40-year-old woman with a history of substance abuse (marijuana and heroin) during adolescence displayed episodes of abnormal sexual behavior during sleep. The first episode occurred at the age of 35 years, where she violently assaulted her husband while appearing to be "not present" and confused. Subsequent episodes occurred irregularly but at least once a month, typically between 1 and 3 AM, with the patient having no memory of these events. The episodes involved various forms of sexual assault, including violent masturbation, insertion of objects into her vagina and anus, and inflicting pain on her husband's genitals. The patient also experienced episodes of vocalization during sleep, involving moaning and sexually provocative phrases. These behaviors caused feelings of shame and guilt for the patient, as well as concern for her husband. Psychological assessment revealed emotional deprivation during childhood, witnessing her mother's rape, and a history of depressive symptoms. Borderline personality traits and moderate-severity major depressive disorder were diagnosed. PSG indicated spontaneous arousals from SWS but did not record any sexual activity, and brain MRI results were normal. The patient was prescribed a serotonin reuptake inhibitor (escitalopram), resulting in a significant reduction in abnormal sexual behavior and a recovery from major depressive disorder. Treatment was continued based on these positive outcomes.[45]

Psychological factors seem to be a trigger for sexsomnia. A study examined 335 patients with NREM parasomnias during 15 years, identifying 65 with SBS.[46] The SBS cohort consisted of 58 men and 7 women, representing 19.4% of the overall cohort. SBS onset was more common in adulthood, associated with psychiatric diagnoses, and triggered by alcohol consumption, relationship difficulties, and sleep deprivation. SBS patients often reported concurrent SW. Men were accompanied by bed partners, whereas women presented alone. Individuals in the armed forces or police had a higher prevalence of SBS.[46]

The military environment poses significant challenges for service members, including sleep deprivation, shift work, and heightened psychosocial stress. These factors can potentially increase the risk of experiencing various NREM parasomnias, including sexsomnia. Considering that sexsomnia has been invoked in military sexual assault lawsuits, it is crucial for the military community to have a clear understanding of how this condition typically presents itself to address its medicolegal implications more effectively. In this context, Fernandez and coworkers[47] demonstrated the largest case series of sexsomnia in active duty military service members to date (see **Table 2**). The patients ranged in age from 25 to 50 years old. They did not have a history of parasomnias, regular consumption of alcohol or stimulants, or the use of sleep aids. Some cases revealed evidence of OSA based on overnight PSG results, whereas others did not. REM atonia was intact in all cases where it was assessed. In case 1, a 50-year-old man with loud snoring, possible OSA, presented episodes of sexsomnia. CPAP therapy effectively resolved the sleep-related behaviors. Case 2 involved a 25-year-old man with sexsomnia episodes primarily occurring within the first hour of sleep. The patient had mild OSA. In case 3, a 27-year-old man reported sleep-related sexual activity and difficulties waking up in the morning. The PSG showed no evidence of OSA, and the diagnosis was insufficient sleep syndrome. Case 4 featured a 41-year-old man with occasional sleep-related sexual activity, vivid dreams, and confusion on waking. No evidence of OSA was observed in the PSG findings.[47] Overall, these cases illustrate the occurrence of sexsomnia in male active-duty military service members in different age groups.[47,48] The importance of evaluating and addressing sleep-related issues to promote well-being and ensure safety in this population is highlighted.

In addition to the cases mentioned earlier, Yeh and Schenck[39] documented another case of sexsomnia in a military setting. The patient was a 20-year-old Taiwanese man serving mandatory military duty. He presented to a sleep clinic with a history of SW and sleep masturbation episodes on his military base. The SW episodes had initially occurred between the ages of 6 and 11 years but resurfaced when he started his military service, which involved irregular sleep–wake schedules and sleep deprivation. During the episodes, the patient engaged in sleep masturbation, and these behaviors were witnessed by other military personnel. Medical history, physical and neurologic examinations, and brain MRI were all unremarkable. Video-PSG monitoring conducted at the hospital captured one episode of sleep talking during N3 sleep and 2 episodes of sleep masturbation (one from N2 and the other from N3). The patient remained in a supine position and a light sleep stage during these episodes. Snoring was observed but did not trigger the sleep masturbation, and the patient had no recollection of the events on awakening. The final diagnoses included SW, sexsomnia during confusional arousals as a non-REM parasomnia, and sleep talking. Clonazepam was prescribed to address the SW but it did not suppress the sleep masturbation. After completing military service, the patient planned to discontinue clonazepam therapy and anticipated that both sleep masturbation and SW would cease once he returned home and resumed a normal sleep–wake schedule. During the most recent follow-up, the patient was living at home, maintaining a regular sleep–wake cycle, and had not experienced any SW episodes according to his mother. The status of sleep masturbation in relation to the cessation of SW remains unknown because the patient sleeps alone and does not have a girlfriend.[39]

These cases emphasize the occurrence of sexsomnia in military service members. The relationship between sleep disturbances, military duties, and the resurfacing of parasomnia episodes underscores the impact of irregular sleep patterns and sleep deprivation on sleep-related behaviors.

Understanding the unique challenges faced by service members and the potential influence of sleep disorders such as sexsomnia is essential for ensuring the well-being of military personnel. By addressing these issues, appropriate measures can be implemented to support their health, promote safety, and facilitate effective forensic investigations when necessary. Importantly, none of the cases in this series was involved in legal issues. Recognizing the legal aspects surrounding parasomnias is crucial, given the general lack of laws addressing this topic. SW and sexsomnia are being increasingly used as defenses in criminal cases, raising concerns about their validity and the heavy reliance on expert opinions in forensic sleep disorders.[49] It is essential to establish evidence-based guidelines, conduct more research, and initiate legal reforms to ensure fair outcomes in SRV cases. Taking a multidisciplinary approach is vital to address these complex issues and enhance our comprehension of parasomnias within the legal framework.

NAVIGATING THE COMPLEXITIES: MEDICAL-LEGAL CASES AND SEXSOMNIA

Medical legal cases involving sexsomnia pose unique challenges due to the complex nature of the condition. Sexsomnia can lead to legal issues and potential accusations of sexual assault or misconduct.[50] These cases require careful evaluation to differentiate between consensual sexual activity and sexsomnia episodes because individuals experiencing sexsomnia are typically unaware of their actions and have no recollection of the events.[51] Legal authorities and medical professionals need to consider comprehensive medical assessments, including PSG and psychiatric evaluations, to establish the presence of sexsomnia and its impact on the individual's behavior. This approach is crucial in ensuring a fair and accurate understanding of sexsomnia-related incidents in the legal context.

Ingravallo and colleagues carried out a systematic review to examine medical-legal cases involving SRV and SBS.[52] A comprehensive search was performed on the PubMed and PsychINFO databases, covering the period from 1980 to 2012, supplemented by a review of reference lists. Case reports were included if they presented a sleep disorder as a defense during criminal trials and provided information about the forensic evaluation of the defendant. Qualitative analysis was performed to extract data on legal issues, defendant and victim characteristics, circumstantial factors, and forensic evaluations. The review identified a total of 18 cases, consisting of 9 SRV and 9 SBS cases, encompassing charges ranging from murder to sexual assault. SW was the predominant defense strategy used, and favorable trial outcomes were observed in most instances. The defendants were primarily young men, whereas victims were often adult relatives or unrelated young girls/adolescents. Criminal events typically occurred within 1 to 2 hours after sleep onset, with various triggering factors reported. Forensic evaluations exhibited considerable heterogeneity across cases.[52] This study emphasizes the pressing need for an international multidisciplinary consensus on the forensic evaluation of SRV and SBS as a critical priority.

Mohebbi and colleagues demonstrated a series of legal cases involving sexsomnia and the subsequent forensic evaluation.[51] In these cases, the defendants were predominantly men, and the victims were generally female minors who were known to the defendant. Forensic evaluators play a crucial role in educating judges and juries about sleep-related sexual behaviors, including sexsomnia. However, sleep studies are not routinely conducted in these evaluations because they are not always considered conclusive evidence. In some cases where sleep studies were performed, they did not show aberrant SBS, yet the forensic experts still offered a diagnosis based on other factors.[50] Sleep medicine experts emphasize that sleep evaluations have limited utility in assessing sexsomnia, and the absence of sexsomnia on PSG does not rule out its occurrence during the alleged incidents. Despite these limitations, guidelines have been developed for forensic sleep assessments, including assessing for malingering and considering collateral reports. Observation in a clinical setting or correctional facility can also provide supporting evidence.

Sleep experts play a crucial role in legal proceedings by providing their expertise to help determine the mental state of the accused during alleged criminal behavior. However, this task is challenging due to the limited scientific literature on sleep disorders, particularly SW and other parasomnias, which primarily consists of case and series reports. The evidentiary value of much of this literature is unclear. Presenting sleep behavior evidence in court poses various difficulties, highlighting the dilemmas faced by expert witnesses when dealing with ambiguous data and uncertain interpretive principles.[53] Moreover, there are significant policy considerations at stake that are not always adequately addressed in expert testimony.

In regards to violence in relation to sleep, Bornemann, in a review, presented the 3 most prevalent criminal allegations among 351 consecutive referrals related to sleep forensic issues received by a single sleep medicine center during the previous 11 years (2006–2017).[54] These allegations were sexual assault, homicide/manslaughter or attempted murder, and driving under the influence. Among these cases, sexsomnia was the most commonly implicated possible sleep disorder, accounting for 41% or 145 out of 351 cases. Out of the 351 referrals, 111 were accepted after a thorough case review. Cases that were not accepted were typically deemed to have little or no merit or were influenced by alcohol intoxication. Among the accepted cases, around 50% supported the initial claim that a sleep phenomenon was involved, with most being NREM disorders of arousal. There were no cases attributed to RBD. The medical-legal topic of sexsomnia and sexsomnia assault has recently been comprehensively addressed.[13]

In 2020, Munro analyzed the use of sleepsex as a defense in cases of alleged sexual assault.[42] The ICSD-3 states that disorders of arousal should not be diagnosed when alcohol intoxication is present,[3] favoring the prosecution hypothesis. Bayesian methodology was used, using the likelihood ratio (LR) to assess the impact of alcohol intoxication on guilt odds. Cross-sectional and longitudinal studies on sexual assault, alcohol use, and parasomnias informed the LR (alcohol). The analysis contradicted the ICSD-3, suggesting strong support for the prosecution hypothesis with an LR of approximately 1,000,000. ICSD-3's statistical reasoning is unclear, potentially involving Bayesian conditional inversion and neglecting to consider alcohol intoxication in the defense hypothesis.[42] The study recommends that the AASM review ICSD-3's statistical methodology in order to improve its accuracy and validity. However, the key issue in this context is not statistical but rather phenomenological: intoxicated behavior cannot be reliably distinguished from sleep-related behavior, and so sexsomnia cannot be diagnosed (or established in a legal setting) in the context of alcohol intoxication, which is the basis for the ICSD-3-TR statement.[4] The other pertinent issue is that an individual must be held legally responsible for the consequences of voluntary alcohol intoxication.

UNRAVELING THE MYSTERY: DIAGNOSTIC CHALLENGES IN SEXSOMNIA

The diagnostic challenge remains a hallmark of sexsomnia, whether due to patients' reluctance to report their condition or the lack of suitable tools to ensure accurate diagnosis. In 2014, a scale was developed to assess the severity of arousal disorders (Paris Arousal Disorders Severity Scale [PADSS]).[55] This controlled study, conducted at a university hospital, included consecutive patients aged 15 years and older with SW and/or ST, individuals with previous SW/ST, normal controls, and patients with RBD. The self-rated PADSS scale consisted of 3 parts: PADSS-A listed 17 parasomnia behaviors, PADSS-B assessed their frequency, and PADSS-C evaluated the consequences. The scale demonstrated high sensitivity, specificity,

internal consistency, and test–retest reliability. The total PADSS score ranged from 0 to 50 and varied significantly between different groups. The scale's complexity factors correlated with scores for the total PADSS, highlighting its potential use for screening, stratifying patients, and evaluating treatment effects.[55]

Sexsomnia is often prone to be confused with other conditions, or vice versa. The differential diagnosis of nocturnal attacks poses challenges for neurologists, particularly when distinguishing between sleep disorders, psychiatric disturbances, and epileptic seizures.[56] These attacks may exhibit various behavioral patterns, including abnormal motor behavior, autonomic activation, or unconventional SBS. The complexity originates from the broad spectrum of sexual behaviors observed, encompassing diverse activities that deviate from typical circumstances. It is crucial to note that misinterpretation of results can occur, leading to potential diagnostic errors.[57] This highlights the need for comprehensive clinical and neurophysiological evaluations to ensure accurate diagnoses and appropriate management strategies. In this context, Pelin and coworkers (2012) presented a case that exemplifies the challenges in diagnosis and the potential for misinterpretation.[56] A 31-year-old man exhibited abnormal behaviors during sleep, including muscle contractions, incoherent speech, disrobing, and unconventional sexual behaviors. These symptoms persisted for several years and were initially characterized by laughter, banging on walls, and clapping hands during sleep. However, the episodes evolved and occurred frequently, involving masturbation, unintelligible speech, movement, and hallucinations. Despite having no recollection of these events and being unrecognizable to others during episodes, the patient experienced significant behavioral and personality changes, including increased libido, inappropriate sexual advances, social isolation, and occupational impairment. Initial treatment with ziprasidone showed no improvement, leading to the diagnosis of psychomotor epilepsy. Subsequent evaluations, including video-EEG monitoring and cranial MRI, revealed specific findings supporting the diagnosis of psychomotor epilepsy. However, challenges developed during treatment, necessitating adjustments and additional medications to manage symptoms effectively.[56] This case underscores the importance of meticulous evaluation and the potential risks associated with misdiagnosis or misinterpretation, highlighting the need for a comprehensive approach to accurately diagnose and manage sleep-related disorders involving abnormal sexual behaviors.

A recent study aimed to assess the applicability of recent EEG and behavioral criteria for arousal disorders in the diagnosis of sexsomnia.[20] The researchers conducted a retrospective analysis, comparing EEG and behavioral markers during N3 sleep interruptions in video-PSG among 3 groups: 24 participants with sexsomnia, 41 participants with arousal disorders, and 40 healthy controls. The study aimed to evaluate the specificity and sensitivity of previously suggested EEG and behavioral cutoffs for diagnosing arousal disorders in the sexsomnia group compared with the control group. The results revealed that both participants with sexsomnia and those with arousal disorders displayed higher N3 fragmentation index, slow/mixed N3 arousal index, and number of eye openings during N3 interruptions compared with the healthy controls. Notably, 41% of participants with sexsomnia exhibited sexual behaviors during N3 arousal, including masturbation, sexual vocalization, and pelvic thrusting. The study identified specific criteria that were highly specific (95%) but had low sensitivity (46% and 42%) for diagnosing sexsomnia, such as an N3 sleep fragmentation index 6.8/h or greater of N3 sleep and 2 or more N3 arousals associated with eye opening. An index of slow/mixed N3 arousals 2.5/h or greater of N3 sleep showed 73% specificity and 67% sensitivity. Additionally, an N3 arousal characterized by trunk raising, sitting, speaking, displaying fear/surprise, shouting, or exhibiting sexual behavior was 100% specific for diagnosing sexsomnia. In conclusion, this study demonstrated that video-PSG-based markers of arousal disorders in individuals with sexsomnia fall between those of healthy individuals and patients with other arousal disorders.[20] These findings support the idea that previously validated criteria for arousal disorders partially apply to individuals with sexsomnia. The results contribute to a better understanding of the diagnostic methods and characteristics of sexsomnia, aiding in the development of more accurate diagnostic criteria for this specific parasomnia.[20]

AWAKENING SOLUTIONS: TREATMENT APPROACHES FOR SEXSOMNIA

Treatment options for patients with sexsomnia can vary depending on the severity and frequency of symptoms, as well as the underlying causes. Sleep hygiene and lifestyle modifications, such as maintaining a regular sleep schedule and avoiding sleep deprivation, can help reduce the occurrence of sexsomnia episodes.[7] Medications, such as benzodiazepines or selective serotonin reuptake inhibitors, may be prescribed to manage symptoms. Cognitive-behavioral therapy techniques, for example, relaxation exercises and imagery rehearsal therapy, can also be used to address underlying psychological factors contributing to sexsomnia.[11] In some cases, a combination of these approaches may be recommended to effectively treat sexsomnia and improve overall sleep quality. It is important for individuals experiencing sexsomnia to consult with a health-care professional to determine the most appropriate treatment plan based on their specific needs and circumstances.

Mioč and colleagues unveiled a successful case of alternative therapy for sexsomnia treatment.[57] The patient, a 33-year-old man, had a history of hypnagogic hallucinations, sleep paralysis, night terrors, and SW since childhood. In his adolescence, he began experiencing more frequent nocturnal motor events accompanied by vivid dream content. At 18 years of age, he started engaging in SBS involving his girlfriend and a female friend, occurring about 4 times per year and lasting less than a minute. These episodes could easily be interrupted by his girlfriend. Video-PSG at age 22 revealed sudden arousals from NREM sleep with actions such as raising his head and trunk, jumping out of bed, and screaming. Clonazepam treatment was ineffective. A second PSG at age 31 showed stereotyped motor behaviors with autonomic activation and immediate awareness at the end of the episodes. Despite normal EEG and brain MRI results, the episodes' characteristics led to a diagnosis of "clinical SHE" (sleep-related hypermotor epilepsy). Antiepileptic treatment exacerbated the episodes and caused self-injuries. Subsequent psychotherapy, focusing on stress management and hypnotic age regression, conducted once a week, significantly reduced the frequency of episodes, as confirmed in a follow-up PSG.

The use of devices other than CPAP for treating OSA is also highly effective in ceasing episodes of sexsomnia.[17,18] In this regard, the case of a 37-year-old man is noteworthy.[17] He exhibited a history of loud snoring and witnessed apneas, indicating moderate-to-severe sleep apnea. The Epworth Sleepiness Scale indicated daytime sleepiness (see **Table 2**). During the clinic visit, it was discovered that the patient and his wife had been engaging in sexual activity during sleep for many years, with the patient initiating it but having no recollection of it. Video-PSG confirmed the OSA and demonstrated that CPAP effectively treated it. The patient later tried a mandibular advancement device (MAD) but experienced jaw pain and reverted to CPAP. The patient became aware of his sleep-related sexual behaviors and expressed embarrassment and remorse. With the initial use of MAD, the sexsomnia ceased, and it continued to be absent during CPAP therapy during the follow-up period.

FUTURE PERSPECTIVES

Sexsomnia, a complex sleep disorder characterized by SBS, has garnered increasing attention in recent years. The research conducted on sexsomnia has provided valuable insights into its prevalence, clinical presentation, diagnostic criteria, triggers, and associated factors. However, there are still several areas within the field that warrant further exploration and investigation. One promising avenue for future research is the neurobiological underpinnings of sexsomnia. Although the exact mechanisms remain unclear, studying the neural correlates and brain activity during sexsomnia episodes could shed light on the neurologic basis of this disorder. Advanced neuroimaging techniques, such as functional MRI and EEG, especially high-density EEG during vPSG[9,58] could offer valuable insights into the brain regions and networks involved in sexsomnia as a form of NREM parasomnia. More comprehensive studies are needed to better understand the prevalence and incidence of sexsomnia, as well as its relationship with other sleep disorders, including POD,[3] and psychiatric conditions. For example, the NREM parasomnia component of POD now also includes appetitive behaviors (feeding with sleep-related eating disorder and sex with sexsomnia) and rhythmic movement disorders (including sleep bruxism).[4] Longitudinal studies could provide valuable information about the natural course of sexsomnia, its risk factors, and potential comorbidities. Moreover, research focusing on the impact of sexsomnia on individuals' quality of life, relationships, and overall well-being could help guide therapeutic interventions and support strategies. This point is illustrated by a recent novel case report of sexsomnia in an adolescent woman (a rare clinical scenario) with complex psychosocial and medical issues.[59] In addition, the complexity of the neurophysiological underpinnings for SBS has recently been expanded by a series of 5 cases in which the nondominant hand was repeatedly used for sleep masturbation, raising questions about disturbed brainstem functioning during sleep in these sexsomnia cases.[60] The data presented in a recent publication on hand dominance in sexsomnia offer intriguing insights that may support an underlying mechanism involving central pattern generators (CPGs) in the pathophysiology of sexsomnias.[60] In this case series, a distinct pattern of adult sleep masturbatory behavior was reported to primarily involve the nondominant (left) hand in 4 out of 5 cases, with one ambidextrous patient also predominantly using the left hand. Interestingly, there was no evidence of gender predilection, suggesting that hand dominance, rather than gender, plays a significant role in these sexsomnias.[60] Our speculation is that sexsomnia may originate from CPGs located in the brainstem and spinal cord (**Fig. 1**). This hypothesis is based on the observed preference for the nondominant hand in these cases. If the cerebral cortex were primarily responsible for these behaviors, one might expect a more even distribution between dominant and nondominant hands. The fact that individuals with sexsomnia exhibit amnesia for these events further supports the notion that cerebral motor control is not the primary driver. CPGs in the brainstem and spinal cord are responsible for generating rhythmic motor patterns, often without the need for higher cortical input. These generators are involved in various motor behaviors, and their involvement in sexsomnia could explain the involuntary nature of these actions during sleep. Although this case series provides valuable insights, further research is needed to validate these hypotheses and explore the exact mechanisms involved in sexsomnias. Understanding the role of CPGs and their interplay with sleep physiology could offer crucial insights into the pathophysiology of sexsomnias and potentially lead to more effective diagnostic and therapeutic approaches in the future.

In terms of diagnosis and assessment, the development of standardized protocols and diagnostic criteria specific to sexsomnia would be beneficial. Currently, sexsomnia is often diagnosed based on clinical history, PSG findings, and the exclusion of other sleep disorders. Refining the diagnostic criteria and establishing more reliable and valid assessment tools would enhance the accuracy and consistency of sexsomnia diagnosis. Furthermore, therapeutic interventions for sexsomnia could be explored further. Currently, treatment options primarily involve addressing underlying sleep disorders, modifying sleep environments, and implementing behavioral interventions. Investigating the efficacy of pharmacologic interventions, such as medications targeting specific neurotransmitter systems or hormones, could open up new possibilities for managing sexsomnia symptoms.

Finally, raising awareness and reducing the stigma surrounding sexsomnia as a *bona fide* sleep disorder that is classified in the official sleep nosology[3] are crucial for supporting affected individuals and fostering a supportive environment. Education campaigns targeting health-care professionals, the general public, and military

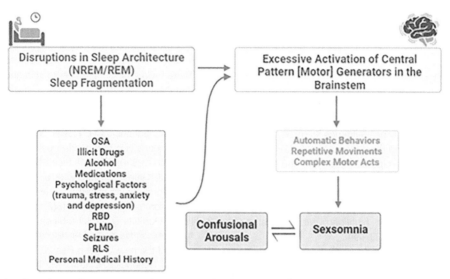

Fig. 1. Pathophysiology of sexsomnias. The exact pathophysiology of sexsomnia is not fully understood but it is thought to involve disruptions in the normal sleep cycle and the transition between sleep stages. Sexsomnia typically occurs during NREM sleep, specifically during deep NREM stages. These stages are associated with SWS, and disruptions in SWS can lead to abnormal behaviors. Sleep fragmentation and disruptions in sleep architecture, often caused by factors such as OSA, illicit drug use, alcohol, medications, RBD, RLS, and psychological factors, can substantially contribute to the development of sexsomnia. These conditions lead to an excessive activation of central pattern [motor] generators in the brainstem, resulting in automatic behaviors, repetitive movements, and complex motor acts associated with sexsomnia. Confusional arousals may also be interconnected with episodes of sexsomnia and vice versa. NREM, non-REM; OSA, obstructive sleep apnea; PLMD, periodic limb movement disorder; RBD, REM sleep behavior disorder; REM, rapid eye movement; RLS, restless legs syndrome. (Created with BioRender.com.)

personnel could help promote understanding and empathy toward sexsomnia as a legitimate sleep disorder.

In conclusion, although significant progress has been made in the research on sexsomnia, there are still numerous avenues for future exploration. Advancements in neurobiology, epidemiology, diagnosis, treatment, and awareness are essential to further our understanding of sexsomnia and improve the lives of those affected by this complex sleep disorder. By continuing to invest in research and collaboration, we can strive toward better recognition, management, and support for individuals with sexsomnia.

CLINICS CARE POINTS

- Sexsomnia is usually a NREM sleep parasomnia that is associated with a current and/or past history of other NREM sleep parasomnias.

- Sexsomnia can also be associated with RBD, as a manifestation of the "Parasomnia Overlap Disorder" together with other NREM sleep parasomnias.

- The second most common cause of Sexsomnia is Obstructive Sleep Apnea (OSA), with OSA-induced arousals triggering the Sexsomnia episodes.

- Treatment of OSA comorbid with Sexsomnia, either with CPAP or with MAD (mandibular advancement device) usually controls both the OSA and the Sexsomnia.

- Treatment of Sexsomnia as a NREM parasomnia with bedtime clonazepam, paroxetine, and various other medications, is usually effective.

- Presumed Sexsomnia emerging for the first time that results in legal consequences should be viewed with extreme skepticism as a valid diagnosis.

ACKNOWLEDGMENTS

Our studies were supported by the Associação Fundo de Incentivo à Pesquisa, São Paulo, Brazil. MLA is a fellowship recipient from Conselho Nacional de Desenvolvimento Científico e Tecnológico. This article was written with the assistance of Mariana Toricelli.

DISCLOSURE

The authors have no conflict of interest to disclose.

REFERENCES

1. Tufik S, Andersen ML, Bittencourt LR, et al. Paradoxical sleep deprivation: neurochemical, hormonal and behavioral alterations. Evidence from 30 years of research. An Acad Bras Cienc 2009;81(3):521–38.
2. Bon OL. Relationships between REM and NREM in the NREM-REM sleep cycle: a review on competing concepts. Sleep Med 2020;70:6–16.
3. Sateia MJ. International classification of sleep disorders-third edition: highlights and modifications. Chest 2014;146(5):1387–94.
4. American Academy of Sleep Medicine. International classification of sleep disorders. 3rd edition. Darien, IL: American Academy of Sleep Medicine; 2023. text revision.
5. Underwood A. It's called 'sexsomnia'. Newsweek 2007;149(24):53.
6. Muza R, Lawrence M, Drakatos P. The reality of sexsomnia. Curr Opin Pulm Med 2016;22(6):576–82.
7. Andersen ML, Poyares D, Alves RS, et al. Sexsomnia: abnormal sexual behavior during sleep. Brain Res Rev 2007;56(2):271–82.
8. Schenck CH. RBD, sexsomnia, sleepwalking, and sleep paralysis comorbidities: relevance to pulmonary, dental, and behavioral sleep medicine. Sleep Sci 2021;14(2):87–91.
9. Schenck CH. New insights into the neurophysiology of sleep-related abnormal sexual behaviors [Editorial]. Sleep 2023. https://doi.org/10.1093/sleep/zsad078.
10. Dubessy AL, Leu-Semenescu S, Attali V, et al. Sexsomnia: a specialized non-REM parasomnia? Sleep 2017;40(2). https://doi.org/10.1093/sleep/zsw043.
11. Toscanini AC, Marques JH, Hasan R, et al. Sexsomnia: case based classification and discussion of psychosocial implications. Sleep Sci 2021;14(2):175–80.
12. McRae L. Blaming rape on sleep: a psychoanalytic intervention. Int J Law Psychiatr 2019;62:135–47.
13. Cramer Bornemann MA SC. Sexsomnia and sexual assault: the role of the sleep forensics investigator in court. 2nd edition. Oxford University; 2023 (in press).
14. Trajanovic NN, Mangan M, Shapiro CM. Sexual behaviour in sleep: an internet survey. Soc Psychiatr Psychiatr Epidemiol 2007;42(12):1024–31.
15. Schenck CH, Arnulf I, Mahowald MW. Sleep and sex: what can go wrong? A review of the literature on sleep related disorders and abnormal sexual behaviors and experiences. Sleep 2007;30(6):683–702.
16. Schenck C. Update on sexsomnia, sleep related sexual seizures, and forensic implications. NeuroQuantology 2015;13(4):518–41.
17. Khawaja IS, Hurwitz TD, Schenck CH. Sleep-related abnormal sexual behaviors (sexsomnia) successfully treated with a mandibular advancement device: a case report. J Clin Sleep Med 2017;13(4):627–8.
18. Meira E Cruz M, Soca R. Sexsomnia and REM- predominant obstructive sleep apnea effectively treated with a mandibular advancement device. Sleep Science 2016;9(3):140–1.
19. Irfan M, Schenck CH, Howell MJ. Non-rapid eye movement sleep and overlap parasomnias. Continuum 2017;23(4):1035–50. Sleep Neurology.
20. Rossi J, Gales A, Attali V, et al. Do the EEG and behavioral criteria of NREM arousal disorders apply to sexsomnia? Sleep 2023;46(7):zsad056.
21. Idir Y, Oudiette D, Arnulf I. Sleepwalking, sleep terrors, sexsomnia and other disorders of arousal: the old and the new. J Sleep Res 2022;31(4):e13596.
22. Irfan M, Schenck CH, Howell MJ. NonREM disorders of arousal and related parasomnias: an updated review. Neurotherapeutics 2021;18(1):124–39.
23. Longe O, Omodan A, Leschziner G, et al. Non-REM parasomnias: a scoping review of dreams and dream-like mentation. Croat Med J 2022;63(6):525–35.
24. Reynolds CF, O'Hara R. DSM-5 sleep-wake disorders classification: overview for use in clinical practice. Am J Psychiatr 2013;170(10):1099–101.
25. Tufik S, Santos-Silva R, Taddei JA, et al. Obstructive sleep apnea syndrome in the Sao Paulo epidemiologic sleep study. Sleep Med 2010;11(5):441–6.
26. Lundetræ RS, Saxvig IW, Pallesen S, et al. Prevalence of parasomnias in patients with obstructive sleep apnea. a registry-based cross-sectional study. Front Psychol 2018;9:1140.
27. Gossard TR, Trotti LM, Videnovic A, et al. Restless legs syndrome: contemporary diagnosis and treatment. Neurotherapeutics 2021;18(1):140–55.
28. Della Marca G, Dittoni S, Frusciante R, et al. Abnormal sexual behavior during sleep. J Sex Med 2009;6(12):3490–5.
29. Cicolin A, Tribolo A, Giordano A, et al. Sexual behaviors during sleep associated with polysomnographically confirmed parasomnia overlap disorder. Sleep Med 2011;12(5):523–8.
30. Soca R, Keenan JC, Schenck CH. Parasomnia overlap disorder with sexual behaviors during sleep in a patient with obstructive sleep apnea. J Clin Sleep Med 2016;12(8):1189–91.
31. Ariño H, Iranzo A, Gaig C, et al. Sexsomnia: parasomnia associated with sexual behaviour during sleep. Neurologia 2014;29(3):146–52.
32. Martynowicz H, Smardz J, Wieczorek T, et al. The co-occurrence of sexsomnia, sleep bruxism and other sleep disorders. J Clin Med 2018;7(9):233.
33. Zwerling B, Keymeulen S, Krychman ML. Sleep and sex: a review of the interrelationship of sleep and sexuality disorders in the female population, through

the lens of sleeping beauty syndrome. Sex Med Rev 2021;9(2):221–9.

34. Ohayon MM, Guilleminault C, Priest RG. Night terrors, sleepwalking, and confusional arousals in the general population: their frequency and relationship to other sleep and mental disorders. J Clin Psychiatry 1999;60(4):268–76. quiz 77.

35. Ohayon MM, Mahowald MW, Leger D. Are confusional arousals pathological? Neurology 2014; 83(9):834–41.

36. Westchester I. AASM. International classification of sleep disorders Diagnostic and coding manual. American Academy of Sleep Medicine. Available at: https://www.scirp.org/(S(351jmbntvnsjt1aadkposz je))/reference/ReferencesPapers.aspx?Reference ID=408248. Accessed May, 2023.

37. Bjorvatn B, Grønli J, Pallesen S. Prevalence of different parasomnias in the general population. Sleep Med 2010;11(10):1031–4.

38. Gomis Devesa AJ, Ortega Albás JJ, Denisa Ghinea A, et al. Sexsomnia and sleep eating secondary to sodium oxybate consumption. Neurologia 2016;31(5):355–6.

39. Yeh SB, Schenck CH. Sexsomnia: a case of sleep masturbation documented by video-polysomnography in a young adult male with sleepwalking. Sleep Sci 2016;9(2):65–8.

40. Drakatos P, Marples L, Muza R, et al. Video polysomnographic findings in non-rapid eye movement parasomnia. J Sleep Res 2019;28(2):e12772.

41. Contreras JB, Richardson J, Kotagal S. Sexsomnia in an adolescent. J Clin Sleep Med 2019;15(3): 505–7.

42. Munro NA. Alcohol and Parasomnias: the statistical evaluation of the parasomnia defense in sexual assault, where alcohol is involved. J Forensic Sci 2020;65(4):1235–41.

43. Pirzada A, Almeneessier AS, BaHammam AS. Abnormal sexual behavior during sleep: sexsomnia and more. Sleep and Vigilance 2019;3(1):81–9.

44. Jiménez-Correa U, Santana-Miranda R, Barrera-Medina A, et al. Parasomnias in patients with addictions-a systematic review. CNS Spectr 2022; 27(1):58–65.

45. Béjot Y, Juenet N, Garrouty R, et al. Sexsomnia: an uncommon variety of parasomnia. Clin Neurol Neurosurg 2010;112(1):72–5.

46. Riha RL, Dodds S, Kotoulas SC, et al. A case-control study of sexualised behaviour in sleep: a strong association with psychiatric comorbidity and relationship difficulties. Sleep Med 2023;103:33–40.

47. Fernandez JD, Soca R. Sexsomnia in active duty military: a series of four cases. Mil Med 2023; 188(1–2):e436–9.

48. Kim DS, Foster BE, Scott JA, et al. A rare presentation of sexsomnia in a military service member. J Clin Sleep Med 2021;17(1):107–9.

49. Morrison I, Rumbold JM, Riha RL. Medicolegal aspects of complex behaviours arising from the sleep period: a review and guide for the practising sleep physician. Sleep Med Rev 2014;18(3):249–60.

50. Mohebbi A, Holoyda BJ, Newman WJ. Sexsomnia as a defense in repeated sex crimes. J Am Acad Psychiatry Law 2018;46(1):78–85.

51. Holoyda BJ, Sorrentino RM, Mohebbi A, et al. Forensic evaluation of sexsomnia. J Am Acad Psychiatry Law 2021;49(2):202–10.

52. Ingravallo F, Poli F, Gilmore EV, et al. Sleep-related violence and sexual behavior in sleep: a systematic review of medical-legal case reports. J Clin Sleep Med 2014;10(8):927–35.

53. Idzikowski C, Rumbold J. Sleep in a legal context: the role of the expert witness. Med Sci Law 2015; 55(3):176–82.

54. Cramer Bornemann MA, Schenck CH, Mahowald MW. A review of sleep-related violence: the demographics of sleep forensics referrals to a single center. Chest 2019;155(5):1059–66.

55. Arnulf I, Zhang B, Uguccioni G, et al. A scale for assessing the severity of arousal disorders. Sleep 2014;37(1):127–36.

56. Pelin Z, Yazla E. Abnormal sexual behavior during sleep in temporal lobe epilepsy: a case report. Balkan Med J 2012;29(2):211–3.

57. Mioč M, Antelmi E, Filardi M, et al. Sexsomnia: a diagnostic challenge, a case report. Sleep Med 2018;43:1–3.

58. Castelnovo A, Amacker J, Maiolo M, et al. High-density EEG power topography and connectivity during confusional arousal. Cortex 2022;155:62–74.

59. Brás J, Schenck CH, Andrade R, et al. A challenging case of sexsomnia in an adolescent female presenting with depressive-like symptoms. J Clin Sleep Med 2023;19(10):1845–7.

60. Badami V, Avidan A, Schenck C. Hand dominance in sexsomnia: a clue to pathophysiology? Sleep 2023; 46(Supplement_1):A433–4.

61. Irfan M, Schenck CH. Sleep-related orgasms in a 57-year-old woman: a case report. J Clin Sleep Med 2018;14(1):141–4.

62. Kumar V, Grbach VX, Castriotta RJ. Resolution of sexsomnia with paroxetine. J Clin Sleep Med 2020; 16(7):1213–4.

63. Bušková J, Piorecký M, Měrková R. Sexsomnia can be triggered by sleep-related head jerks. Sleep Med 2022;92:12–4.

Somnambulism

Ramona Cordani, MD[a], Regis Lopez, MD, PhD[b], Lucie Barateau, MD, PhD[b],
Sofiene Chenini, MD[b], Lino Nobili, MD, PhD[a], Yves Dauvilliers, MD, PhD[b],*

KEYWORDS

- Somnambulism • NREM parasomnia • Disorders of arousal • Pathophysiology • Dissociated sleep
- Differential diagnosis • Treatment

KEY POINTS

- Somnambulism, a NREM parasomnia, aligns within the spectrum of Disorders of Arousal alongside with confusional arousal and sleep terror.
- NREM parasomnias arise from disrupted boundaries between wakefulness and NREM sleep leading to the coexistence of wake- and sleep-like brain activity during episodes.
- The pathogenesis involves a multifaceted interplay of predisposing, priming, and precipitating factors requiring in-depth investigation (genetic, neurobiology…) to elucidate its origins.
- Diagnostic criteria rely on clinical observations. Identification and integration of objective criteria (SWS fragmentation) into the diagnostic process may enhance diagnostic accuracy.
- Somnambulism can affect various aspects of an individual's well-being. Recognizing and addressing these consequences are paramount in effective management.

SOMNAMBULISM: THE MOST COMPLEX FORM OF DISORDERS OF AROUSAL

Somnambulism, also referred to as sleepwalking (SW), is a condition characterized by a variety of abnormal paroxysmal behaviors during sleep, resulting in walking with an altered state of consciousness and impaired judgment.[1–3] SW is a subtype of non-rapid eye movement (NREM) sleep parasomnias, which encompass disorders occurring mostly during slow-wave sleep (SWS), typically in the first third of the main sleep period.[1] The International Classification of Sleep Disorders, Third Edition Text-Revised (ICSD-3 TR) classifies SW as a disorder of arousal (DOA), distinguishing three primary clinical manifestations, namely confusional arousal (CA), sleep terror (ST), and, precisely, SW.[3] Sexsomnia, also known as sleep-related abnormal sexual behavior or sleep sex, is deemed a subtype of CAs and somnambulism. Moreover, in addition to DOA, NREM parasomnias encompass sleep-related eating disorder, also referred to as sleep eating.[3]

The three forms of DOA exhibit different features, namely in terms of motor activity (eg, CA, unlike SW, occurs with the patient in bed looking around confused), emotions (STs frequently involve intense fear, crying, or screaming), and autonomic reactions (in STs, a heightened autonomic response can result in tachycardia, tachypnea, sweating, skin redness, mydriasis, and increased muscle tone).[3] However, grouping DOA into specific categories may be oversimplified. Rather, a hierarchical continuum seems to connect different behavioral patterns of DOA.[1,4] Even though one of the patterns might predominate, it is not unusual for people with somnambulism to experience ST and CA. Also, studies show that there is a significant connection between a family history of somnambulism and ST, hinting at these conditions being diverse expressions of the same underlying physiologic condition.[1,5]

[a] Department of Neuroscience, Rehabilitation, Ophthalmology, Genetics, Maternal and Child Health, University of Genoa, Genoa, Italy; [b] Department of Neurology, Sleep-Wake Disorders Unit, Gui-de-Chauliac Hospital, CHU Montpellier, INSERM Institute of Neurosciences of Montpellier, University of Montpellier, France
* Corresponding author. Centre national de référence narcolepsie hypersomnies, 80, avenue Augustin Fliche, 34295 Montpellier Cedex 5, France.
E-mail address: y-dauvilliers@chu-montpellier.fr

Sleep Med Clin 19 (2024) 43–54
https://doi.org/10.1016/j.jsmc.2023.10.001

PATHOPHYSIOLOGY

Disruption of boundaries between wakefulness and sleep is assumed to be the fundamental physiologic mechanism responsible for NREM parasomnias. Specifically, compelling data from neuroimaging and electrophysiological evidence suggest the coexistence of wake- and sleep-like activity within cortical and subcortical brain regions during episodes.[1,6–9] In this scenario, the rising complexity of NREM parasomnia events seems to mirror the gradual intricacy and duration of this dissociated state. Moreover, several clinical and experimental findings suggest a dysfunction in SWS regulation.[2,10–13]

Local Dissociation of Sleep and Arousal

Intracerebral stereo-electroencephalography (EEG) investigations conducted in patients with epilepsy during presurgical evaluation have shown that the occurrence of transient dissociated electrophysiological states is an intrinsic feature of NREM sleep.[14] This finding suggested the coexistence of wake and sleep patterns in different cortical areas with the occurrence of local cortical activations (increases in EEG frequency, including alpha and beta rhythms) within the sensorimotor system in synchrony with sleep-like EEG patterns (slow waves) in structures such as the dorsolateral prefrontal cortex, even in the absence of any behavioral manifestations. These phenomena support the hypothesis that NREM parasomnias might result from an imbalance of these two states. During somnambulism, a single study using single-photon emission computed tomography revealed the coexistence of frontoparietal associative cortices deactivation and thalamo-cingulo-cortical pathway activation.[6] These aligns with intra-cerebral EEG recordings of CA, revealing local activations in motor, cingulate (frontal and central cingulate gyrus), insular, temporopolar, and amygdala cortices, along with simultaneous presence of slow waves in frontal and parietal dorsolateral cortices and persistent sleep spindles in the hippocampal cortex.[7,8] Moreover, a noninvasive source imaging EEG study evaluating epochs immediately preceding SW found increased brain activation in the cingulate cortex.[9]

Overall, these findings suggest that the defining traits of NREM parasomnias may be attributed to the activation of the amygdalo-temporo-insular areas (emotional activation) and motor cortex (movements) and the concurrent deactivation of the hippocampal and frontal associative cortices (amnesia and altered consciousness).[1]

Somnambulism and other NREM parasomnia provide a fascinating model illustrating that sleep and wakefulness are not mutually exclusive, sleep is not necessarily a global brain phenomenon, and dissociated electrophysiological behaviors may coexist within the sleeping brain.[15]

The question of whether SW is unique to humans remains unanswered, as there have been no reports of spontaneous episodes in animals, including nonhuman primates.[16] Clarifying this aspect could provide valuable insights into the underlying mechanisms of this phenomenon.

Abnormalities in Regulation of Slow-Wave Sleep

The neurophysiological traits and alterations in sleep continuity in NREM parasomnias are noteworthy. NREM parasomnias typically arise from SWS and are characterized by the persistence of slow waves recorded on surface EEG primarily in the frontal regions along with mixed alpha and fast EEG activities[2] (**Fig. 1**). Hypersynchronous delta wave activity (ie, high-voltage > 150 μV) has often been described in relation to parasomniac episodes that may sometimes precede such episodes but has low specificities for the diagnosis of NREM parasomnia.[1,2] Subjects with somnambulism exhibit NREM sleep instability. Polysomnographic (PSG) studies have demonstrated, in both children and adults, an increased SWS fragmentation characterized by a higher number of awakenings and micro-arousals during SWS, even on episode-free nights.[2,10,11] Moreover, an increase in cyclic alternating pattern rates, another marker of NREM sleep instability, has been found even on nights when parasomnia episodes are absent.[17–19] Quantitative EEG studies highlighted abnormalities in slow-wave activity (SWA), including reduced SWA power, especially during the first NREM period, and altered dynamics of SWA throughout the night.[11,12] These changes are likely due to increased awakenings, affecting the build-up and physiologic decline of SWA during sleep. Furthermore, a high-density EEG study unveiled reduced SWA power in the centro-parietal regions, which likely corresponds to a decrease in SWA within motor, premotor, and cingulate areas.[13]

Another distinctive characteristic on NREM parasomnias pertains to atypical response to sleep deprivation. Unlike healthy subjects who experience a rebound of SWS after sleep deprivation as a consequence of heightened sleep homeostatic pressure, in subject with NREM parasomnias, sleep deprivation tends to result not only in increased rebound of SWS but also increased awakenings from SWS during subsequent recovery sleep and amplifies the likelihood of laboratory-recorded somnambulic events.[20–23] It is worth noting that

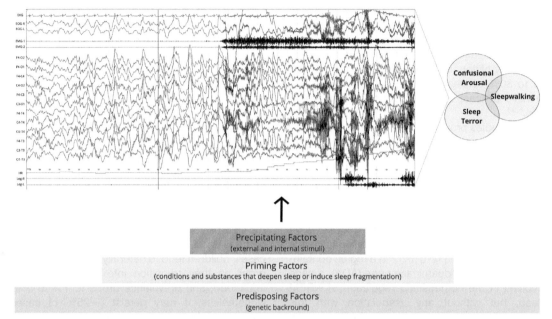

Fig. 1. Pathophysiology of disorders of arousal. According to the "3-P" pathophysiological model, the interplay between predisposing, priming, and precipitating factors promotes somnambulism, sleep terrors, and confusional arousals. In subjects with a predisposing genetic background, conditions and substances known to deepen sleep and/or induce sleep fragmentation may lead to the occurrence of DOA episodes triggered by a wide range of internal and external stimuli. During episodes, the PSG pattern is often characterized by the persistence of slow/mixed EEG activity, associated with motor and autonomic activations. EKG, electrocardiogram; EOG, electrooculogram; EMG, electromyogram; HR, heart rate.

this response to sleep deprivation seems to primarily affect SWS, with reductions in awakenings during N2 and REM sleep.[21] In addition, episodes recorded during recovery sleep are more complex and agitated,[23] suggesting a persistence of abnormal arousal reactions in sleepwalkers after sleep deprivation.

Neurobiology

Altered neurotransmitter activity, specifically gamma-aminobutyric acid (GABA) and serotonin, has been proposed as a potential factor in somnambulism pathophysiology, disrupting the balance between sleep and wakefulness.[1,24–26]

GABA is the primary inhibitory neurotransmitter of the central nervous system with a crucial role in NREM sleep regulation. Findings from transcranial magnetic stimulation in sleepwalkers during wakefulness indicate reduced efficiency of inhibitory circuits in the motor cortex, indicating impaired GABAergic transmission.[24]

Serotonergic dysfunction has also been implicated, supported by evidence of SW induced by selective serotonin reuptake inhibitors (SSRIs) and drugs with affinity for serotonin receptors.[27–29] The association between SW and migraine, which is also associated with impaired serotonin

regulation, further supports this hypothesis.[25,30] In rats, local intracerebral microinjections of serotonin may result in a behavioral awake state with high EEG delta activity resembling SW[26]; however, this has not been replicated and there are no reliable animal models of SW to date.

Despite this evidence, the domain of basic research concerning somnambulism and other types of DOA remains notably limited.

The "3-P" Pathophysiological Model

Somnambulism's pathophysiology involves complex interactions among genetic, neurobiological, and environmental factors. According to the "3-P" pathophysiological model, NREM parasomnias are likely to occur when priming and precipitating factors occur in individuals with a predisposing genetic background[31] (see **Fig. 1**).

Growing evidence supports a genetic predisposition to DOA, with a positive family history recognized in up to 60% of cases in clinical cohorts.[10,32] Familial aggregation studies revealed a higher prevalence of somnambulism among relatives of affected individuals. First-degree relatives have a 10-fold higher likelihood of experiencing SW compared with the general population.[2] To note, the chance increases with the degree of parental history. For children with one parent affected with SW, the likelihood is 47.4%, rising to 61.5% when both parents have an SW history.[5] Interestingly, a strong association of somnambulism with a positive family history of ST has also been shown, as up to 80% of sleepwalkers have been reported to have at least a family history of SW and/or STs.[5,33]

Twin studies provide further insights, with somnambulism being significantly more prevalent in monozygotic than in dizygotic twins.[34–36]

Genome-wide association and candidate gene studies have identified potential genetic variants associated with somnambulism susceptibility, although more research is needed to fully elucidate the genetic underpinnings. A genome-wide survey of an SW family found a significant linkage to chromosome 20q12-q13.12 in a region containing the adenosine deaminase gene (ADA), a gene involved in the homeostatic regulation of NREM sleep, but without any association with this gene.[37] Moreover, the sequence of ADA gene in 251 sleepwalkers did not reveal any association with SW.[38] Another study evaluated the genetic susceptibility regarding the human leukocyte antigen (HLA) region reported that the DQB1*05:01 allele is more common in sleepwalkers than in the general population.[39] A subsequent study confirmed these results demonstrating a high frequency of HLA DQB1*05:01 for different types of NREM parasomnias.[40]

Priming factors include conditions and substances that deepen sleep, hinder the awakening process, and/or induce sleep fragmentation.

Factors that modify sleep encompass sleep deprivation and certain medications including non-benzodiazepine (BDZ) hypnotics (eg, zolpidem, zaleplon, and zopiclone) and lithium.[1,31] In general, drugs that enhance GABA activity at the GABA-A receptor, enhance serotonergic activity, or block the activity of noradrenaline at B-receptors may trigger NREM parasomnias. Furthermore, the association between sodium oxybate and NREM parasomnias has been reported in children and adults treated for narcolepsy,[41,42] as per low-sodium oxybate in adults treated for idiopathic hypersomnia.[43]

On the other hand, factors known to induce or increase sleep fragmentation, such as co-occurring sleep disorders (eg, sleep-disordered breathing and narcolepsy), heightened emotional states pre-sleep, stress, anxiety, fever, and late physical activity, are prone to prime SW episodes.[44,45]

Finally, individuals who experience SW describe a wide range of precipitating factors, including external stimuli like noise or physical contact, as confirmed in studies conducted in sleep laboratory settings. The probability of occurrence of SW when sleeping in unfamiliar locations is difficult to estimate according to patients and studies.[1] Some studies suggest potential internal triggers such as respiratory events or leg movements, although this association remain inconclusive in other research.[1,46]

EPIDEMIOLOGY

Somnambulism is a rather common sleep disorder, especially among children, where prevalence rate ranges from 3% to 14%. In toddlers aged 2.5 to 4 years, the prevalence is approximately 3%, increasing to around 11% at 7 and 8 years. By the age of 10 years, it reaches 13.5%, and then decreases to 12.7% at 12 years.[1,2,5] In most cases, children tend to naturally overcome the disorder as they transition into adolescence and adulthood, and prevalence drops to 1% to 5%.[2] Nonetheless, it may persist (~25% of cases) and, in rare instances, may start in adulthood.[2,5] In addition, self-reported episodes of frequency and severity worsening between adolescence and adulthood have been reported.[47,48] Why somnambulism persists into adulthood in some people but not in others is unclear. Several factors may impact its evolution over time. It is plausible that "primary" forms, which typically manifest during childhood and are characterized by the presence of predisposing factors, may persist into adulthood due to ongoing priming and precipitating factors, thereby reducing the likelihood of remission as the individuals mature. Alongside, children may experience "developmental" SW, marked by infrequent episodes that tend to diminish with age and changes in sleep patterns. Conversely, adult-onset cases are more likely to be secondary to specific treatments or medical conditions. Hence, when assessing de novo adult-onset SW, it is crucial to investigate potential associations with drugs and medical conditions, as previously delineated.

Taken together, literature findings underscore that SW is relatively common throughout life, particularly during childhood. However, accurate prevalence determination is hampered by methodological constraints inherent in detecting and quantifying this behavior. Estimates may not reflect correct prevalence rates even considering that data collection usually relies on informants, and episodes occur during sleep, making them less likely to be witnessed. Consequently, extensive epidemiologic investigations are requisite to comprehensively explore the occurrence and incidence across various life stages and its clinical course.

CLINICAL FEATURES, CURRENT DIAGNOSTIC CRITERIA, AND CLUES FOR DIFFERENTIAL DIAGNOSIS

Somnambulism entails a wide range of activities, from simple to complex behavior with high-level planning and motor control. Sleep talking can also occur. The complex movements encompass seemingly aimless actions, ordinary and habitual behaviors executed at an inappropriate time, or unsuitable and potentially hazardous actions. Episodes of SW in childhood are typically slow and nonviolent, although this is contingent on the specific environmental circumstances. Conversely, in adulthood, episodes often manifest as more complex, restless, vigorous, and prolonged.[2–4,49] They usually stem from CA but can also start abruptly and last from a few seconds to several minutes, typically ending gradually.[4]

It is noteworthy that classification systems, ICSD3-TR and the Diagnostic and Statistical Manual of Mental Disorders, Fifth Edition (DSM-5)[3,49] established the frequent occurrence of amnesia of episodes as a key feature of SW. The available literature, however, presents compelling evidence suggesting that sleepwalkers can recall certain aspects when actively probed. They demonstrate the ability to recall at least parts of episodes by identifying specific behaviors displayed during the episodes, perceptual elements from the environment during events, and reporting experienced emotions (such as fear, anger, frustration, and impotence). These findings collectively challenge the notion of complete amnesia among the adult population. Conversely, children tend to more consistently report experiencing complete amnesia of episodes.[48,50,51]

Another questioned aspect concerns limited or absent dream imagery during episodes. This standpoint lacks robust support when scrutinizing recent scientific literature, which offers evidence of specific mental experiences during such episodes. Of note, in studies focusing on this aspect, more than half of the subjects under investigation reported instances of dreamlike mentation concomitant with nocturnal motor episodes. Some subjects exhibit clear and vivid hallucinatory experiences, featuring "dreamed" objects or characters.[50–55] Based on these findings, some investigators suggest considering partial or complete amnesia and limited or no associated dream imagery (especially in children) as optional supportive but not mandatory criteria.[56]

Finally, the absence of objective diagnostic criteria within the current classification systems is a topic of discussion.[3,49] SW diagnosis relies on clinical criteria gathered through meticulous patient interviews, unlike REM sleep behavior disorder (RBD), which requires also objective assessment (ie, REM sleep without atonia).[3,49] In certain clinical scenarios, video PSG recording may be necessary to rule out differential diagnoses and comorbid sleep disorders.[10] However, SW episodes are observed rarely within a sleep laboratory setting, prompting endeavors to determine the sensitivity and specificity of markers observed in sleep studies and establish quantifiable diagnostic criteria. In this context, SWS fragmentation and slow/mixed arousal indexes have emerged as suitable biomarkers for diagnosing DOA in adults and children.[10,57] Moreover, analysis of behavioral reactions during N3 interruption (ie, opening the eyes at least two times in the same night) has been proposed as sensitive, specific, and reproducible for discriminating patients with DOA from controls.[58]

In the realm of non-PSG examinations, home infrared night video recordings are being explored as a promising method for improving diagnosis of parasomnias in a real-world setting.[59]

Among the intricate array of differential diagnoses, one noteworthy consideration is sleep-related hypermotor epilepsy (SHE) (**Table 1**). This condition is characterized by seizures mainly occurring during NREM sleep, which can manifest as sustained dystonic postures, as well as complex, hyperkinetic, and bizarre motor patterns, sometimes accompanied by affective symptoms or ambulatory behaviors,[60] making differentiation with DOA challenging. Although PSG is the gold standard for diagnosing sleep-related events, it may not be sufficient in making differential diagnosis as DOA or SHE; major episodes may not be recorded during one night recording and interictal and ictal scalp EEG recordings may be uninformative in many SHE patients.[60] A recent study has identified differences in the semeiology of briefest episodes in SHE and DOA, founding that tonic/dystonic and hypermotor patterns, as well as stereotypy, are typical of seizures with paroxysmal arousals in contrast to DOA simple arousal movements.[61] A thorough semiological analysis is crucial but can be complicated by certain clinical features like screaming or walking. Therefore, objective markers are essential for enhancing diagnostic accuracy.

In non-PSG techniques, namely automated and semiautomated movement analysis techniques, a machine learning pipeline based on video analysis has demonstrated an 80% accuracy rate in differentiating DOA and SHE.[62] These preliminary results indicate its potential as a valuable tool to support physicians in a diagnostic process that may require costly resources and specialized

Table 1
Comparison of key features of disorders of arousal and sleep-related hypermotor epilepsy

	DOA	SHE
Gender	M = F	M > F
Age at onset	More common in childhood	Any age, peak in childhood
Family history	Frequent family history of NREM parasomnia	Possible family history of epilepsy
Stereotypic motor pattern	-	+
Mental content	Limited (some evidence)	-
Time of occurrence	Usually, first third of the main sleep period	Anytime
Sleep stage of occurrence	Mainly N3 stage	Primarily N2 stage
PSG findings	Hyper-synchronous slow waves; SWS fragmentation	Interictal and ictal scalp EEG may be uninformative
Frequency	Sporadic	Almost every night
Frequency (per night)	Rare episodes (one major episode, possibly more minor ones)	Several episodes
Evolution over time	Tend to disappear	Stable, increased frequency, rare remission
Consciousness at the end of the episode	Impaired	Variable
Recall	Rare in children, possible in adults	Inconstant

Abbreviations: +, yes; -, no; DOA, disorders of arousal; F, female; M, male; N2, N2 stage of NREM sleep; N3, N3 stage of NREM sleep; PSG, polysomnography; SHE, sleep-related hypermotor epilepsy.

expertise. Further research is warranted to refine and validate this promising approach.[62]

CONSEQUENCES AND COMORBIDITIES

Although often considered a benign condition, somnambulism can present challenges affecting various aspects of individual's life. Recognizing and addressing consequences and related comorbidities are essential components of SW management.

Daytime Adverse Consequences

Excessive daytime sleepiness
The well-documented SWS disruption could result in excessive daytime sleepiness (EDS). Nonetheless, research on the occurrence of EDS yields different findings. For instance, self-report assessment (Epworth Sleepiness Scale [ESS]) found EDS (defined by ESS score > 10) in 40% to 47% of subjects in studies involving patients with SW or SW/ST.[13,32,53,63] However, studies using objective measurements, notably the Multiple Sleep Latency Test (MSLT, recognized as the gold standard for objectively assessing EDS), provided varying results. A study involving a small sample of adult sleepwalkers (10 subjects) revealed EDS, even after episode-free nights, reporting significantly lower mean sleep-onset latencies than controls. Remarkably, 70% had a mean latency of less than 8 minutes (the threshold for objective EDS).[64] Nevertheless, a case-control study involving a larger sample (30 adults with SW/ST) did not corroborate these results. Although confirming that EDS is a frequent complaint based on ESS (~67% scored ESS > 10), it identified only two patients with objective EDS during MSLT. Of note, this research highlighted distinct temporal patterns of sleep latencies during MSLT trials among these patients. Unlike the typical noontime sleepiness observed in controls, patients demonstrated reduced sleep latencies only during the first two trials (at 9:00 and 11:00 AM).[65] Interestingly, EDS was not associated with concomitant sleep disorders, SWS fragmentation or episodes frequency.[63,65] Taken together, these findings suggest that EDS may be an intrinsic feature of DOA.

Cognitive, emotional, and psychiatric symptoms
Sleepwalkers may experience embarrassment, shame, or fear due to their behaviors with consequences on social relationships.[49] Moreover, given the pivotal role of sleep in brain health, cognitive functions, and emotional regulation,[66] it is plausible to suggest that NREM parasomnias elicit adverse effects on cognitive abilities, emotional well-being, and quality of life.

However, compared with other sleep disorders, knowledge of the effect of NREM parasomnia is limited. First, a reduced quality of life in SW has been reported.[32] Regarding cognitive domains, research provides heterogeneous findings. Among DOA, impaired visuospatial working memory and selective visual attention have been described in affected individuals.[67] To delve specifically into somnambulism, a study involving adult patients compared with healthy controls revealed executive function impairment related to inhibitory control following 25 hours of sleep deprivation but not under normal waking conditions.[68] Another study focusing on subjects with SW/ST found no differences in verbal memory consolidation compared with healthy controls, despite more frequent awakenings during SWS and more prolonged wakefulness after sleep onset.[69] Moreover, a study comparing short-term memory and verbal learning among DOA, SHE, and healthy controls revealed no differences between patients and controls, identifying impairment exclusively in SHE subjects. However, it is important to note that this study did not specifically examine SW alone.[70]

Concerning psychological and psychiatric aspects, severe parasomnias may lead to emotional distress, potentially increasing susceptibility to depressive or anxiety disorders.[49] Concurrently, stress, anxiety, and psychiatric disorders could potentially act as priming/precipitating factors, either directly or indirectly, through sleep disruption, sleep deprivation, or medication intake.[31]

The relationship between SW and psychological factors remains insufficiently elucidated, yielding diverse and occasionally conflicting results. In adults, some evidence suggests an increased frequency of depressive and anxious symptoms. For instance, a prospective cohort study, using face-to-face clinical interviews, standardized questionnaires, and PSG, reported such association; however, the study found that the association with depressive symptoms did not remain significant after adjusting for fatigue, somnolence, and insomnia.[32] Labelle and colleagues did not identify any significant link between adult SW and depression or anxiety.[71] Intriguingly, they found that individuals with more psychopathological symptoms were less likely to have a positive SW family history, hinting at reduced genetic influence in such cases. However, the proportion of sleepwalkers reporting childhood versus adult-onset showed no substantial differences within their group. This differs from findings in psychiatric settings, where have been reported an overall SW prevalence of 8.5% and adult-onset in nearly half of sleepwalkers,[72,73] indicating a potential link between somnambulism and psychiatric disorders. Nonetheless, it is important

to consider that these findings rely on clinical evaluations, and further studies are needed to confirm these results and rule out any possible concurrent factors (such as drug intake).

Regarding the pediatric population, association between DOA and anxiety, particularly separation anxiety, has been reported.[74,75] A recent study involving children and adolescents with DOA, including 56% with SW, reported that around one-third of the participants exhibited emotional and behavioral problems, which severity correlated with that of their parasomnia episodes.[76]

Injuries, Safety Risks, and Forensic Implications

SW can pose a serious risk of injury to oneself or others as a result of unintentional actions that may occur during episodes.[2] This condition, along with ST, RBD, and SHE, significantly contributes to sleep-related injuries.[77]

During SW episodes, individuals engage in activities such as climbing through windows, attempting to descend stairs, and leaving the house, with risk of falling, colliding with objects, and being involved in accidents.[78] Data from the literature suggest that a significant proportion of patients do not perceive pain during episodes.[30] This observation might be influenced by recall bias but could help explain why they remain asleep despite injuries. It is crucial to underscore that dangerous actions, including driving a vehicle, suspected self-harm, or even cases of homicide or attempted homicide, have been documented, posing substantial challenges in the realm of forensic investigation.[2,79]

MANAGEMENT

The management of somnambulism primarily aims to reduce episodes frequency and severity, enhancing overall sleep quality and ensuring safety during episodes. Generally, a multifaceted strategy is used, encompassing an educational program, behavioral interventions, environmental adjustments, and pharmacotherapy in more severe cases.

Non-Pharmacological Interventions

Non-pharmacological approaches include various strategies such as providing reassurance to patients and their families, ensuring a safe environment, removing factors that predispose or trigger episodes, using scheduled awakenings, and using psychological interventions.

Reassurance and environmental safety
Initial management involves educating patients, families, and bed partners about the frequent

benign nature of somnambulism, particularly in pediatric cases,[56,78,80] and its often spontaneous favorable clinical course.

Moreover, instructing parents/caregivers on appropriate responses during an episode is pivotal, such as gently guiding the individual back to bed to prevent potential danger.[81] Environmental safety measures are crucial to decrease injury risks. Tailored precautions should be adopted for each patient, such as positioning the bedroom on the ground floor, avoiding bunk bed, using secure locks on windows and doors, and decluttering the bedroom.[80–82]

Scheduled awakenings

For individuals with frequent and predictable episodes, anticipatory awakenings can be considered. They involves waking sleepwalkers slightly before the typical occurrence time (usually 15–20 minutes prior)[2,83] with an efficacy rate of ~ 60%.[83] The goal is to shift the individual into a lighter sleep state, decreasing the likelihood of an episode.

Psychological interventions

Psychological approaches have been suggested with promising results in case series and retrospective studies[82]; however, objective assessments of their efficacy and investigations into their long-term effectiveness are lacking. Cognitive behavioral therapy (CBT), including stimulus control and relaxation techniques, demonstrates efficacy in managing SW, aiding in recognizing and altering maladaptive thoughts and behaviors.[84] A combination of CBT and mindfulness meditation has been reported to be effective in managing somnambulism in individuals with increased stress and anxiety levels.[84] In addition, hypnosis, aiming to induce relaxation, is reported to reduce somnambulism frequency in certain cases.[56]

Management of Priming and Precipitating Factors

Apart from treating the disorder itself, it is crucial to address the underlying priming/precipitating factors. Adhering to the "3-P model" pathogenetic framework, maintaining regular sleep routines to prevent sleep deprivation is imperative.[31,56,84] Moreover, any internal or external stimuli that contribute to trigger episodes should be managed.[81,84] Timely diagnosis and treatment of coexisting sleep disorders are advised. Addressing sleep-disordered breathing, restless legs syndrome, periodic limb movement disorder, and central disorders of hypersomnolence is linked to effective management of NREM parasomnia

(although available investigations do not exclusively focus on SW).[84,85] Finally, reducing or abstaining from caffeine and alcohol consumption close to bedtime, as well as reviewing medications for potential interactions, is recommended.[81,84]

Pharmacologic Interventions

Pharmacologic approaches are considered when frequent episodes persist despite addressing underlying factors, when there is an increased risk of harm and in instances where potential legal consequences arise due to behaviors such as sexual or violent actions.[86] However, knowledge about treatments derives mainly from case reports and retrospective studies, and data mostly lack objective efficacy measures, randomized placebo-controlled studies, and long-term assessments.

Intermediate and long-acting BDZs stand as the prevailing pharmacologic recourse. Their effectiveness may stem from their sedative impacts, SWS decrease, and modulation of cortical arousals.[86] Clonazepam stands out as the primary BDZ of choice, with effectiveness also in managing somnambulism induced by neuroleptics and in cases with harmful behaviors and sleep violence.[77,84] However, evaluating its precise efficacy faces limitations, mainly due to the prominent employment of subjective rather than objective measurements. The first objective evidence of effectiveness in reducing episode frequency was recently provided using home nocturnal infrared video in a small group of adults with NREM parasomnia.[59]

Within BDZs, the effectiveness of diazepam exhibits inconclusive outcomes, whereas reports of improvement with clobazam, alprazolam, temazepam, and flurazepam are limited to anecdotal cases.[80,86]

It is advisable to consider the potential risk of experiencing daytime sleepiness when using BDZs, particularly in situations like driving. Furthermore, given their muscle-relaxing properties, BDZs should be used cautiously when sleep-disordered breathing is present.[86]

When exploring other pharmacologic options, available data are often inconclusive and sometimes contradictory. Antidepressants, both SSRIs and tricyclic antidepressants, have been suggested as potential treatments for SW in some case series but have also been reported as potential triggers for SW.[80,86] Retrospective studies and small case series suggest potential effectiveness of L-5- hydroxytryptophan, melatonin, and melatonin receptor agonists in treating SW.[84,86] However, it is important to consider the limitations of these findings, including their retrospective nature and small sample sizes.

SUMMARY AND FUTURE PERSPECTIVES

The existing body of scientific evidence provides a foundational understanding of somnambulism, but critical areas necessitate further investigation to deepen comprehension of this complex phenomenon.

First, the diagnostic approach relies primarily on clinical criteria, which do not consistently align with current scientific knowledge. Future research should prioritize the establishment of precise and objective criteria that can be integrated into classification systems.

Second, the etiopathological processes, particularly genetic and neurobiological factors, require deeper exploration to shed light on the origins of SW.

In addition, research should focus on elucidating the specific impact of SW on specific cognitive domains and psychological well-being, as current findings are conflicting.

Last, studies using objective measurements are essential to corroborate the effectiveness of treatment options for SW, ensuring optimal management of this disorder.

In conclusion, although our understanding of somnambulism has advanced significantly, these knowledge gaps underscore the importance of ongoing and future research endeavors. Addressing these uncertainties will refine our comprehension, enhance diagnostic precision, and lead to more effective treatments, ultimately improving the well-being of individuals affected by this intriguing sleep disorder.

CLINICS CARE POINTS

- Somnambulism is very common in the general population, from mild and infrequent often in childhood to sometimes seriously damaging episodes in adults.

- The clinical course of somnambulism is often a decrease with age but with large variability.

- Identifiable risk factors for somnambulism episodes (sleep deprivation, drug intake) should be recognized and avoided.

- Differential diagnosis of somnambulism (nocturnal seizures, other parasomnias) must be systematically sought.

- The decision to prescribe pharmacological treatment must be carefully considered in the context of somnambulism.

DISCLOSURE

No disclosure related to this article.

REFERENCES

1. Castelnovo A, Lopez R, Proserpio P, et al. NREM sleep parasomnias as disorders of sleep-state dissociation. Nat Rev Neurol 2018;14(8):470–81.
2. Zadra A, Desautels A, Petit D, et al. Somnambulism: clinical aspects and pathophysiological hypotheses. Lancet Neurol 2013;12(3):285–94.
3. American Academy of Sleep Medicine. International classification of sleep disorders-third edition, text revision (ICSD-3-TR). Darien, IL: American Academy of Sleep Medicine; 2023.
4. Derry CP, Harvey AS, Walker MC, et al. NREM arousal parasomnias and their distinction from nocturnal frontal lobe epilepsy: a video EEG analysis. Sleep 2009;32(12):1637–44.
5. Petit D, Pennestri MH, Paquet J, et al. Childhood sleepwalking and sleep terrors: a longitudinal study of prevalence and familial aggregation. JAMA Pediatr 2015;169(7):653–8.
6. Bassetti C, Vella S, Donati F, et al. SPECT during sleepwalking. Lancet 2000;356(9228):484–5.
7. Terzaghi M, Sartori I, Tassi L, et al. Evidence of dissociated arousal states during NREM parasomnia from an intracerebral neurophysiological study. Sleep 2009;32(3):409–12.
8. Terzaghi M, Sartori I, Tassi L, et al. Dissociated local arousal states underlying essential clinical features of non-rapid eye movement arousal parasomnia: an intracerebral stereo-electroencephalographic study. J Sleep Res 2012;21(5):502–6.
9. Januszko P, Niemcewicz S, Gajda T, et al. Sleepwalking episodes are preceded by arousal-related activation in the cingulate motor area: EEG current density imaging. Clin Neurophysiol 2016;127(1):530–6.
10. Lopez R, Shen Y, Chenini S, et al. Diagnostic criteria for disorders of arousal: a video-polysomnographic assessment. Ann Neurol 2018;83(2):341–51.
11. Espa F, Ondze B, Deglise P, et al. Sleep architecture, slow wave activity, and sleep spindles in adult patients with sleepwalking and sleep terrors. Clin Neurophysiol 2000;111(5):929–39.
12. Gaudreau H, Joncas S, Zadra A, et al. Dynamics of slow-wave activity during the NREM sleep of sleepwalkers and control subjects. Sleep 2000;23(6):755–60.
13. Castelnovo A, Riedner BA, Smith RF, et al. Scalp and source power topography in sleepwalking and sleep terrors: a high-density EEG study. Sleep 2016;39(10):1815–25.
14. Nobili L, Ferrara M, Moroni F, et al. Dissociated wake-like and sleep-like electro-cortical activity during sleep. Neuroimage 2011;58(2):612–9.

15. Siclari F, Tononi G. Local aspects of sleep and wakefulness. Curr Opin Neurobiol 2017;44:222–7.

16. Kantha SS. Is somnambulism a distinct disorder of humans and not seen in non-human primates? Med Hypotheses 2003;61(5–6):517–8.

17. Parrino L, Ferri R, Bruni O, et al. Cyclic alternating pattern (CAP): the marker of sleep instability. Sleep Med Rev 2012;16(1):27–45.

18. Zucconi M, Oldani A, Ferini-Strambi L, et al. Arousal fluctuations in non-rapid eye movement parasomnias: the role of cyclic alternating pattern as a measure of sleep instability. J Clin Neurophysiol 1995; 12(2):147–54.

19. Guilleminault C, Kirisoglu C, da Rosa AC, et al. Sleepwalking, a disorder of NREM sleep instability. Sleep Med 2006;7(2):163–70.

20. Borbély AA, Baumann F, Brandeis D, et al. Sleep deprivation: effect on sleep stages and EEG power density in man. Electroencephalogr Clin Neurophysiol 1981;51(5):483–95.

21. Zadra A, Pilon M, Montplaisir J. Polysomnographic diagnosis of sleepwalking: effects of sleep deprivation. Ann Neurol 2008;63(4):513–9.

22. Pilon M, Montplaisir J, Zadra A. Precipitating factors of somnambulism: impact of sleep deprivation and forced arousals. Neurology 2008;70(24):2284–90.

23. Joncas S, Zadra A, Paquet J, et al. The value of sleep deprivation as a diagnostic tool in adult sleepwalkers. Neurology 2002;58(6):936–40.

24. Oliviero A, Della Marca G, Tonali PA, et al. Functional involvement of cerebral cortex in adult sleepwalking. J Neurol 2007;254(8):1066–72.

25. Juszczak GR, Swiergiel AH. Serotonergic hypothesis of sleepwalking. Med Hypotheses 2005;64(1): 28–32.

26. Cape EG, Jones BE. Differential modulation of high-frequency γ-electroencephalogram activity and sleep–wake state by noradrenaline and serotonin microinjections into the region of cholinergic basalis neurons. J Neurosci 1998;18(7):2653–66.

27. Stallman HM, Kohler M, White J. Medication induced sleepwalking: a systematic review. Sleep Med Rev 2018;37:105–13.

28. de Filippis R, Guinart D, Rania M, et al. Olanzapine-related somnambulism: a systematic review of literature and a case report of anorexia nervosa. J Clin Psychopharmacol 2021;41(6):658–66.

29. Gouverneur A, Ferreira A, Morival C, et al. A safety signal of somnambulism with the use of antipsychotics and lithium: a pharmacovigilance disproportionality analysis. Br J Clin Pharmacol 2021;87(10):3971–7.

30. Lopez R, Jaussent I, Dauvilliers Y. Pain in sleepwalking: a clinical enigma. Sleep 2015;38(11):1693–8.

31. Pressman MR. Factors that predispose, prime and precipitate NREM parasomnias in adults: clinical and forensic implications. Sleep Med Rev 2007; 11(1):5–30. discussion 31-33.

32. Lopez R, Jaussent I, Scholz S, et al. Functional impairment in adult sleepwalkers: a case-control study. Sleep 2013;36(3):345–51.

33. Kales A, Soldatos CR, Bixler EO, et al. Hereditary factors in sleepwalking and night terrors. Br J Psychiatry 1980;137:111–8.

34. Hublin C, Kaprio J. Genetic aspects and genetic epidemiology of parasomnias. Sleep Med Rev 2003; 7(5):413–21.

35. Bakwin H. Sleep-walking in twins. Lancet 1970; 2(7670):446–7.

36. Hublin C, Kaprio J, Partinen M, et al. Prevalence and genetics of sleepwalking: a population-based twin study. Neurology 1997;48(1):177–81.

37. Licis AK, Desruisseau DM, Yamada KA, et al. Novel genetic findings in an extended family pedigree with sleepwalking. Neurology 2011;76(1):49–52.

38. Fournier S, Dauvilliers Y, Warby SC, et al. Does the adenosine deaminase (ADA) gene confer risk of sleepwalking? Journal of Sleep Research 2022; 31(4). https://doi.org/10.1111/jsr.13537.

39. Lecendreux M, Bassetti C, Dauvilliers Y, et al. HLA and genetic susceptibility to sleepwalking. Mol Psychiatry 2003;8(1):114–7.

40. Heidbreder A, Frauscher B, Mitterling T, et al. Not only sleepwalking but NREM parasomnia irrespective of the type is associated with HLA DQB1*05: 01. J Clin Sleep Med 2016;12(04):565–70.

41. Lecendreux M, Poli F, Oudiette D, et al. Tolerance and efficacy of sodium oxybate in childhood narcolepsy with cataplexy: a retrospective study. Sleep 2012;35(5):709–11.

42. Wang YG, Swick TJ, Carter LP, et al. Safety overview of postmarketing and clinical experience of sodium oxybate (Xyrem): abuse, misuse, dependence, and diversion. J Clin Sleep Med 2009; 5(4):365–71.

43. Morse AM, Dauvilliers Y, Arnulf I, et al. Long-term efficacy and safety of low-sodium oxybate in an open-label extension period of a placebo-controlled, double-blind, randomized withdrawal study in adults with idiopathic hypersomnia. J Clin Sleep Med 2023; jcsm:10698.

44. Howell MJ. Parasomnias: an updated review. Neurotherapeutics 2012;9(4):753–75.

45. Leu-Semenescu S, Maranci JB, Lopez R, et al. Comorbid parasomnias in narcolepsy and idiopathic hypersomnia: more REM than NREM parasomnias. J Clin Sleep Med 2022;18(5):1355–64.

46. Lopez R, Dauvilliers Y. Is restless legs syndrome involved in ambulation related to sleepwalking? Sleep 2016;39(4):955–6.

47. Kalantari N, McDuff P, Pilon M, et al. Self-reported developmental changes in the frequency and characteristics of somnambulistic and sleep terror episodes in chronic sleepwalkers. Sleep Med 2022; 89:147–55.

48. Idir Y, Oudiette D, Arnulf I. Sleepwalking, sleep terrors, sexsomnia and other disorders of arousal: the old and the new. J Sleep Res 2022;31(4):e13596.
49. American Psychiatric Association. Diagnostic and statistical manual of mental disorders. 5th Edition. American Psychiatric Association; 2013. https://doi.org/10.1176/appi.books.9780890425596.
50. Castelnovo A, Loddo G, Provini F, et al. Mental activity during episodes of sleepwalking, night terrors or confusional arousals: differences between children and adults. NSS 2021;13:829–40.
51. Baldini T, Loddo G, Sessagesimi E, et al. Clinical features and pathophysiology of disorders of arousal in adults: a window into the sleeping brain. Front Neurol 2019;10:526.
52. Castelnovo A, Loddo G, Provini F, et al. Frequent, complex and vivid dream-like/hallucinatory experiences during NREM sleep parasomnia episodes. Sleep Med 2021;82:61–4.
53. Oudiette D, Leu S, Pottier M, et al. Dreamlike mentations during sleepwalking and sleep terrors in adults. Sleep 2009;32(12):1621–7.
54. Uguccioni G, Golmard JL, de Fontréaux AN, et al. Fight or flight? Dream content during sleepwalking/sleep terrors vs. rapid eye movement sleep behavior disorder. Sleep Med 2013;14(5):391–8.
55. Longe O, Omodan A, Leschziner G, et al. Non-REM parasomnias: a scoping review of dreams and dream-like mentation. Croat Med J 2022;63(6):525–35.
56. Mainieri G, Loddo G, Provini F, et al. Diagnosis and management of NREM sleep parasomnias in children and adults. Diagnostics 2023;13(7):1261.
57. Lopez R, Laganière C, Chenini S, et al. Video-polysomnographic assessment for the diagnosis of disorders of arousal in children. Neurology 2021;96(1):e121–30.
58. Barros A, Uguccioni G, Salkin-Goux V, et al. Simple behavioral criteria for the diagnosis of disorders of arousal. J Clin Sleep Med 2020;16(1):121–8.
59. Lopez R, Barateau L, Chenini S, et al. Home nocturnal infrared video to record non-rapid eye movement sleep parasomnias. Journal of Sleep Research 2023;32(2). https://doi.org/10.1111/jsr.13732.
60. Proserpio P, Loddo G, Zubler F, et al. Polysomnographic features differentiating disorder of arousals from sleep-related hypermotor epilepsy. Sleep 2019;42(12):zsz166.
61. Loddo G, Baldassarri L, Zenesini C, et al. Seizures with paroxysmal arousals in sleep-related hypermotor epilepsy (SHE): dissecting epilepsy from NREM parasomnias. Epilepsia 2020;61(10):2194–202.
62. Moro M, Pastore VP, Marchesi G, et al. Automatic video analysis and classification of sleep-related hypermotor seizures and disorders of arousal. Epilepsia 2023;64(6):1653–62.
63. Desautels A, Zadra A, Labelle MA, et al. Daytime somnolence in adult sleepwalkers. Sleep Med 2013;14(11):1187–91.
64. Montplaisir J, Petit D, Pilon M, et al. Does sleepwalking impair daytime vigilance? J Clin Sleep Med 2011;7(2):219.
65. Lopez R, Jaussent I, Dauvilliers Y. Objective daytime sleepiness in patients with somnambulism or sleep terrors. Neurology 2014;83(22):2070–6.
66. Krause AJ, Simon EB, Mander BA, et al. The sleep-deprived human brain. Nat Rev Neurosci 2017;18(7):404–18.
67. Ferini-Strambi L, Galbiati A, Marelli S, et al. Disorders of arousal: evaluation of neurocognitive function in 69 consecutive patients. Sleep 2017;40(suppl_1):A274.
68. Labelle MA, Dang-Vu TT, Petit D, et al. Sleep deprivation impairs inhibitory control during wakefulness in adult sleepwalkers. J Sleep Res 2015;24(6):658–65.
69. Uguccioni G, Pallanca O, Golmard JL, et al. Is sleep-related verbal memory consolidation impaired in sleepwalkers? J Sleep Res 2015;24(2):197–205.
70. Puligheddu M, Congiu P, Figorilli M, et al. Neuropsychological and behavioral profile in sleep-related hypermotor epilepsy (SHE) and disorders of arousal (DOA): a multimodal analysis. JCM 2023;12(1):374.
71. Labelle MA, Desautels A, Montplaisir J, et al. Psychopathologic correlates of adult sleepwalking. Sleep Med 2013;14(12):1348–55.
72. Lam SP, Fong SYY, Yu MWM, et al. Sleepwalking in psychiatric patients: comparison of childhood and adult onset. Aust N Z J Psychiatry 2009;43(5):426–30.
73. Waters F, Moretto U, Dang-Vu TT. Psychiatric illness and parasomnias: a systematic review. Curr Psychiatr Rep 2017;19(7):37.
74. Petit D, Touchette E, Tremblay RE, et al. Dyssomnias and parasomnias in early childhood. Pediatrics 2007;119(5):e1016–25.
75. Laberge L, Tremblay RE, Vitaro F, et al. Development of parasomnias from childhood to early adolescence. Pediatrics 2000;106(1):67–74.
76. Castelnovo A, Turner K, Rossi A, et al. Behavioural and emotional profiles of children and adolescents with disorders of arousal. J Sleep Res 2021;30(1):e13188.
77. Schenck CH, Milner DM, Hurwitz TD, et al. A polysomnographic and clinical report on sleep-related injury in 100 adult patients. Am J Psychiatr 1989;146(9):1166–73.
78. Mason TBA, Pack AI. Pediatric parasomnias. Sleep 2007;30(2):141–51.
79. Siclari F, Khatami R, Urbaniok F, et al. Violence in sleep. Brain 2010;133(12):3494–509.
80. Attarian H. Treatment options for parasomnias. Neurol Clin 2010;28(4):1089–106.
81. Tinuper P, Bisulli F, Provini F. The parasomnias: mechanisms and treatment. Epilepsia 2012;53(Suppl 7):12–9.

82. Ntafouli M, Galbiati A, Gazea M, et al. Update on nonpharmacological interventions in parasomnias. PGM (Postgrad Med) 2020;132(1):72–9.

83. Kotagal S. Treatment of dyssomnias and parasomnias in childhood. Curr Treat Options Neurol 2012; 14(6):630–49.

84. Drakatos P, Marples L, Muza R, et al. NREM parasomnias: a treatment approach based upon a retrospective case series of 512 patients. Sleep Med 2019;53:181–8.

85. Gurbani N, Dye TJ, Dougherty K, et al. Improvement of parasomnias after treatment of restless leg syndrome/periodic limb movement disorder in children. J Clin Sleep Med 2019;15(05):743–8.

86. Proserpio P, Terzaghi M, Manni R, et al. Drugs used in parasomnia. Sleep Med Clin 2018;13(2):191–202.

Sleep-Related Eating Disorder

Melissa C. Lipford, MD*, R. Robert Auger, MD

KEYWORDS

- Parasomnia • Sleep-related eating disorder • SRED • Nocturnal eating • Night-eating syndrome

KEY POINTS

- Sleep-related eating disorder (SRED) is an NREM parasomnia characterized by recurrent amnestic episodes of eating/drinking.
- SRED is most commonly seen in association with a separate untreated sleep disorder but can be idiopathic.
- Identification/treatment of accompanying sleep disorders is the mainstay of treatment.
- Data are limited with respect to management of idiopathic or refractory cases of SRED, but research of topiramate has yielded promising results.

INTRODUCTION

Sleep-related eating disorder (SRED) is a non-rapid eye movement (NREM) sleep parasomnia, which can be considered a subtype of sleepwalking. SRED is characterized by recurrent episodes of eating and drinking following partial arousals from sleep. Afflicted individuals are typically amnestic of the behavior the following day or have only partial recall. This disorder is associated with adverse physical and mental health as well as social embarrassment and negative impact on quality of life. It can arise spontaneously or be provoked by certain medications.

SRED should be distinguished from night eating syndrome (NES), a condition in which excessive nocturnal eating occurs in fully awake individuals. SRED was first described by Schenck and colleagues in 1991 via a case series of 19 predominantly female adult patients.[1] Since the original description, understanding of the clinical and polysomnographic features has advanced, but the disorder remains underrecognized and is frequently challenging to manage. This review will describe the clinical characteristics of SRED as well as diagnostic and management modalities. The features of SRED versus NES will also be differentiated.

CLINICAL CHARACTERISTICS AND DIAGNOSTIC CRITERIA

The cardinal feature of SRED includes arousals from sleep during which food (and/or drink) is rapidly ingested. The arousal typically occurs a few hours after sleep onset (generally in the first half of the night), and the majority of patients report nightly episodes. Some endorse multiple eating episodes nightly. Each episode may last from a few to more than 10 minutes.[1] The formal *International Classification of Sleep Disorders* (third edition) diagnostic criteria are summarized in **Table 1**. Noteworthy features include the lack of conscious knowledge while eating and/or drinking and partial to complete morning amnesia of the events. Additionally, in over 65% of these patients, there is a history of consumption of strange foods or non-food substances during episodes.[2] For example, consumption of raw bacon, coffee grounds, and cigarettes has been reported. There may be a preference toward higher calorie or carbohydrate-laden foods, eventually contributing to weight gain. Interestingly, alcohol is almost never consumed during SRED episodes, and a history of alcohol use during episodes may suggest an alternative etiology. The eating may appear out of control or compulsive, and the foods consumed often do not represent the individual's

Center for Sleep Medicine, Mayo Clinic, 200 First Street Southwest, Rochester, MN 55905, USA
* Corresponding author.
E-mail address: Lipford.Melissa@mayo.edu

Sleep Med Clin 19 (2024) 55–61
https://doi.org/10.1016/j.jsmc.2023.10.013
1556-407X/24/© 2023 Elsevier Inc. All rights reserved.

sleep.theclinics.com

Table 1
Diagnostic criteria for sleep-related eating disorder

1.	Recurrent episodes of involuntary/unconscious nocturnal eating that occur after an arousal
2.	At least 1 of the following are associated with the eating episodes:
a.	Consumption of strange foods or non-food substances
b.	Sleep-related injuries or potential injuries while in the act of preparing food or searching for food
c.	Adverse health consequences from the nocturnal eating episodes
3.	Partial or complete amnesia regarding the eating episodes, and lack of awareness during episodes
4.	The episodes are not better explained by another comorbid sleep disorder, medical disorder, psychiatric disorder, or medication/substance use.

Data from the International Classification of Sleep Disorders. 3rd edition, text revision. Darien, IL: American Academy of Sleep Medicine 2023.

food preferences. In fact, consumption of foods to which one is allergic can occur.[3]

Persons may engage in nocturnal food preparation behaviors including chopping, cooking, or baking. These can potentially result in personal injury or property damage. Food may be spilled in the home or brought back into bed. Upon awakening, individuals typically have varying degrees of amnesia of episodes. The evidence of a messy kitchen, food stains, or wrappers and crumbs in the bed may be the means by which amnestic individuals become aware of their SRED episodes. Individuals frequently report satiety upon waking and secondary morning anorexia.

If woken amid an episode, individuals may appear agitated or confused. A preceding sensation of hunger is typically not reported by patients who have been woken during these behaviors. Compensatory next day behaviors such as food restriction or increased exercise may be employed. Additionally, some patients try to curb behaviors by locking the refrigerator or cabinets. Self-induced vomiting, which can be associated with daytime eating disorders, is typically absent in SRED patients.[4]

Health Ramifications

Patients with SRED may suffer from unrefreshing sleep and daytime fatigue. In 44% of patients,

weight gain and obesity result from the consumption of excessive calories during sleep. Associated metabolic sequelae such as diabetes or hyperlipidemia may eventually arise.[4,5] Patients with SRED may also engage in potentially unhealthy means of weight loss including severe daytime caloric restriction.[3]

Accidents during food preparation can lead to serious injuries in SRED patients. Approximately one-third of patients have reported hurting themselves during events. Reports describe patients burning themselves during cooking or spilling hot foods/liquids onto themselves. Patients have lacerated their hands while chopping foods. Poisoning or gastrointestinal injury can occur from the consumption of toxic or non-food substances.[3,5–7] Dental pathology can also arise in these patients from eating excessively high-sugar foods at night, biting into hard foods, or returning to bed with food still in the mouth.[6]

Mood-related ramifications are another serious concern stemming from SRED. Understandably, the condition can cause stress to the patient and their family. Montgomery and Haynes and colleagues reported frequent feelings of shame and helplessness in SRED patients.[8] Difficulties in losing weight due to factors outside of one's control are a driver of psychological distress. In addition, episodes may be associated with social stigma and intimate partner-related embarrassment. SRED patients commonly report a comorbid history of anxiety or depression,[7,9] with 1 case-series documenting 70% of SRED respondents with a history of depression.[10]

DEMOGRAPHICS AND GENETIC FACTORS

As is typical for most NREM parasomnia behaviors, the onset of SRED is more common among young individuals. It typically presents between 22 and 39 years of age and there is a female predominance, with women making up 60% to 83% of cases.[3,7] The disease tends to have a chronic course with delay to diagnosis as evidenced by a case series describing a duration of symptoms between 4 and 15 years prior to SRED identification.[3,5,11]

The exact prevalence of SRED is unknown. Survey studies of college students and those referred to a sleep clinic have reported 0.5% to 5% to meet criteria for SRED. These numbers may potentially represent an underestimation, given the low overall awareness of SRED.[6]

It is unclear whether there is a genetic component to SRED. There are data demonstrating familial relationships; in 4 case series, between 19% and 27% of SRED subjects had family members with similar symptoms.[4,5,10,12] A case report also documents a female with SRED whose fraternal twin sister and father also had the disorder.[13] This is not surprising, given the genetic predilections in other parasomnia behaviors including somnambulism. Familial relationships are also frequent in daytime eating disorders.[14]

Pathophysiology

Physiologic studies have not been performed in patients with SRED. In those with concomitant sleep disorders, it has been suggested that arousals may provoke varying levels of consciousness, prompting somnambulism and sleep-related eating in predisposed individuals.[4] A videopolysomnographic study described recurrent swallowing and chewing movements during NREM sleep in 29 of 35 patients (83%).[15] Some investigators have proposed that dopaminergic mechanisms may be involved in the pathophysiology of the condition.[12]

RISK FACTORS AND POTENTIAL TRIGGERS

While SRED can be idiopathic, it is most linked with other sleep, medical, or mood disorders, or triggered by medications. Case series of SRED show associations with comorbid sleep disorders as well as with sedative-hypnotic medication use. A childhood history of sleepwalking (somnambulism) is particularly frequent; in fact, SRED can be considered a form of sleepwalking.[16] In a survey-based study, over 30% of responders with restless legs syndrome also had symptoms of SRED.[17] SRED has also been associated with obstructive sleep apnea, narcolepsy, and circadian rhythm sleep-wake disorders. SRED may overlap with other parasomnia disorders, including REM sleep behavior disorder.[3]

A higher prevalence of SRED is also noted among those with daytime eating disorders such as anorexia or bulimia. Nine to 17% of individuals enrolled in an eating disorders treatment program reported SRED, and a separate study cited up to 40% of eating disorder patients meeting criteria.[1,3–5] Secondary daytime restriction of caloric intake often occurs in these patients who eat large volumes of food at night. Unfortunately, daytime food restriction can exacerbate SRED symptoms.[3]

Psychiatric disease is also commonly present in patients with SRED. A case series by Winkelman and colleagues, reported 70% of SRED patients with a history of depression.[10] Generalized anxiety disorder (18%) may also be present. Up to 16% of patients associate the onset of SRED symptoms with a stressful life event, and stress is also a trigger for more frequent events. Additionally, 24% of patients with SRED have a comorbid or prior history of substance abuse.[2,4,5]

Medication Triggers

Many medications have been associated with SRED, and the high prevalence of comorbid psychiatric disease may be in part related. SRED induced by zolpidem has been described in multiple case series, which is not surprising given associations between sedative-hypnotics and other NREM parasomnias. In these reports, some patients developed SRED de novo with exposure to zolpidem and others with a prior history of SRED developed worsening and/or frequency of symptoms (including degree of amnesia) subsequent to exposure. Zolpidem use among patients with restless legs may further increase the incidence of SRED.[18] Other medications have also been linked to SRED including benzodiazepines, antipsychotics, and anticholinergics.[5,19,20] In a review from Komada and colleagues involving 30 patients with SRED, events were associated with sedative hypnotics among one-third.[21] In a series from Winkelman and colleagues, the majority (70%) of the 37 patients reported use of psychotropic drugs.[4] Discontinuation of presumed offending agents and treatment of comorbid sleep disorders can lead to resolution of SRED.[22–24]

SRED has also been reported to occur following cessation of cigarettes, alcohol, or illicit substances. The condition has also been observed among those with encephalitis or autoimmune hepatitis.[3]

DIFFERENTIAL DIAGNOSIS AND DISTINCTION BETWEEN SLEEP-RELATED EATING DISORDER AND NIGHT EATING SYNDROME

Night eating syndrome (NES), originally described in 1955, shares many clinical features with SRED, thus a careful clinical history is needed to distinguish between the 2 entities.[25] See **Table 2** for a summarization of the distinctions between SRED and NES. NES is a primary eating disorder in which nocturnal eating occurs with full consciousness and recall. These patients typically either eat prior to going to bed or awaken with an intense desire to eat. They may consume a third to a half of their daily calories at night after the evening meal. Patients frequently endorse initiation or maintenance insomnia and are unable to fall asleep until food ingestion occurs. NES patients may have cravings for specific foods at night (often high-caloric carbohydrate-laden foods), and consumption of non-food substances does not occur. Morning anorexia is also common.[26] While SRED is relatively uncommon, NES may impact 1% to 4% of

Table 2
Distinctions between sleep-related eating disorder and night eating syndrome

	SRED	NES
Prevalence	Uncommon	Relatively common
Degree of Recall of Events	Amnestic	Full recall
Awareness During Events	Unconscious/unaware of behaviors	Awake and conscious of eating
Timing of Episodes	After falling asleep; usually first half of the night	Can occur prior to bed or at any time during the night
Consumption of Strange or Non-Food Substances	Yes	No
Morning Anorexia	Yes	Yes
Comorbid Sleep Disorders	Common	Uncommon
Comorbid Eating Disorders	Common	Common
Comorbid Mood Disorders	Yes	Yes
Adverse Health Ramifications	Yes	Yes

the overall population and manifest in 6% to 16% of obese persons. Similar to daytime eating disorders, NES is more common in females (66% and83% of cases).[27,28] As with SRED, episodes of NES are more frequent in the setting of stressful life events. Both conditions are highly associated with other psychiatric pathology, such as anxiety and depression. In both conditions, problematic weight gain as well as extensive and at times harmful methods to lose weight are employed (purging behaviors, excessive exercise, severe daytime caloric restriction). There does not appear to be a relationship between NES and other sleep disorders as is seen with SRED.[7]

NES and SRED can be difficult to tease apart in some cases. SRED patients may have partial awareness of nocturnal eating and NES patients have reported reduced awareness of nocturnal eating in the setting of concurrent sedative-hypnotic use.[6,21] Options for treatment of NES remain limited. Small studies have shown benefit with sertraline and topiramate and behavioral treatments are also utilized.[29,30]

Other conditions that may mimic symptoms of SRED include bulimia nervosa with nocturnal eating and binge eating disorder. Kleine–Levin syndrome, a recurrent hypersomnia, can present with inappropriate nighttime eating (during wakefulness), but its symptom complex of bizarre behaviors, hypersexuality, and typical occurrence among young males create a straightforward distinction from SRED. Patients with peptic ulcer disease or hypoglycemic states may also eat at night to curb symptoms, but the ancillary features of these conditions should also make it relatively easy to separate from SRED.[6]

CLINICAL EVALUATION AND POLYSOMNOGRAPHY FINDINGS

Ascertaining the diagnosis of SRED relies most heavily on taking a thorough sleep, medical, and psychiatric history. It is essential to seek corroborative history from a witness, such as a spouse, partner, or roommate if possible. It is important to query for a thorough description of events. This should include time of night, degree of associated awareness during the event, morning recall, and descriptors of the patient during the event (ie, were they disoriented, making slowed or strange movements, or responding incoherently to questioning?). A review of all medications is required, particularly inquiries targeting use of sedative hypnotics or psychiatric medications. Querying for a prior history of parasomnia behaviors dating back to childhood as well as a history of comorbid eating disorders is also essential. Triggers should be assessed such as sleep deprivation, recent stressors, alcohol use, and smoking cessation; inquiries should target symptoms suggestive of comorbid sleep disorders such as obstructive sleep apnea or restless legs syndrome. It is important to assess each patient's relationship with food and body weight to determine whether a separate eating disorder is present, in which case they should be referred for appropriate management. Asking about any unsafe or potentially unsafe activities or consumption of non-food or toxic substances is extremely important toward developing a plan that enhances patient safety.

Polysomnography Findings

Polysomnography is not required to make a diagnosis of SRED, as it is a clinical diagnosis. However, polysomnography can be very helpful to exclude other comorbid sleep disorders and to ascertain for other parameters that may disrupt sleep and lend to parasomnia behaviors. These include sleep-disordered breathing at any level of severity or periodic limb movements with associated arousals. SRED may or may not be captured during polysomnography. To increase the likelihood of capturing an event, placing food at the bedside is recommended. A full 16-lead electroencephalography montage may be considered in patients who have comorbid seizure disorders, seizure risk factors, or stereotypic nocturnal events. In prior studies capturing SRED events, polysomnography has demonstrated mixed sleep/wake features with overall electroencephalography background slowing. Events often arise from slow-wave sleep but have been documented from all NREM stages. Video recordings have demonstrated patients ambulating with eyes open, making slowed movements, and appearing confused. A study from Vetrugno and colleagues demonstrated sleeping SRED patients making masticatory movements during NREM sleep.[15]

MANAGEMENT OPTIONS FOR SLEEP-RELATED EATING DISORDER

Management strategies for SRED are based primarily on anecdotal evidence as well as a few small clinical trials. A recent study from Winkelman and colleagues demonstrated efficacy of topiramate in treating this disorder. The investigation consisted of 34 patients with SRED symptoms dating back at least 6 months and who had at least 3 episodes weekly. Subjects were randomized to either placebo or topiramate (with max dosing of 300 mg) and followed over 13 weeks. In the topiramate group, SRED symptom frequency reduced significantly (from 75% to 33% of nights). Weight loss was also demonstrated in the topiramate group.[31] Adverse effects associated with topiramate include paresthesias, somnolence, impaired cognition, mood disturbances, and renal stones.[32] Antidepressant therapies such as sertraline, paroxetine, or fluvoxamine have also been reported in the literature with some success.[33]

Treatments for resulting obesity may be necessary in SRED patients, particularly in those who develop morbid obesity. Weight loss medications may be considered. Caution should be undertaken in employment of medications that have stimulant properties, as these may increase nocturnal arousals and potentially compound the issue. In these patients, detailed discussion of the condition should be undertaken prior to considering bariatric surgery, as SRED events could potentially lead to additional complications in the postoperative setting.

Identification and treatment of comorbid sleep disorders and addressing psychological stressors and/or psychiatric disease are paramount. Tapering potentially offending medications may also be necessary. **Table 3** summarizes management strategies for SRED.

DISCUSSION AND SUMMARY

Sleep-related eating disorder (SRED) is a non-rapid-eye movement (NREM) parasomnia characterized by recurrent episodes of eating/drinking following partial arousals from sleep, with associated partial or complete amnesia. It is important to distinguish SRED from nocturnal eating syndrome,

Table 3
Management of sleep-related eating disorder

Pharmacologic interventions	Topiramate appears effective, based on small clinical trials. Dosing up to a max of 300 mg nightly has been shown to be beneficial Antidepressant agents have been anecdotally shown to reduce frequency of events
Avoiding precipitating factors	• Sedative hypnotics • Antipsychotics • Anticholinergics • Stimulants • Alcohol use • Sleep deprivation
Treatment of comorbid sleep disorders	• Restless legs syndrome • Obstructive sleep apnea • Irregular sleep-wake schedule
Treatment of comorbid psychiatric disorders	• Anxiety • Depression • Daytime eating disorders (anorexia, bulimia)

an eating disorder of wakefulness that requires unique expertise for evaluation and management.

Adverse health consequences and impairments in quality of life from SRED are common. A significant number of those afflicted incur weight gain and associated metabolic sequelae.[4,5] More directly, accidents during food preparation amidst confusional arousals can lead to serious injuries, in addition to poisoning or gastrointestinal injury related to consumption of toxic or non-food substances.[3,5–7] Mood-related ramifications are also common, ranging from embarrassment and shame to discreet psychiatric diagnoses.

While the condition can be idiopathic, it is most seen in association with an unrecognized/untreated arousal-producing comorbid sleep disorder and/or in association with psychoactive medications. Related, management consists predominantly of addressing comorbidities and removing potentially offending medications. While a thorough clinical history is often sufficient, additional sleep testing may be necessary to identify coexisting sleep disorders and/or other phenomena that may contribute to arousals.

Limited data suggest benefit from topiramate and other medications in idiopathic or otherwise refractory cases. Further research is required to better understand the factors that incite or exacerbate SRED, which will in turn propel more sophisticated treatment trials.

DISCLOSURE

The authors report no commercial or financial conflicts of interest.

REFERENCES

1. Schenck CH, Hurwitz TD, Bundlie SR, et al. Sleep-related eating disorders: polysomnographic correlates of a heterogeneous syndrome distinct from daytime eating disorders. Sleep 1991;14:419–31.
2. Auger RR. Sleep-related eating disorders. Psychiatry (Edgmont) 2006;3:64–70, 2945843.
3. American Academy of Sleep Medicine. International classification of sleep disorders. 3rd edition. Darien, IL: American Academy of Sleep Medicine; 2023. text revision.
4. Winkelman JW. Clinical and polysomnographic features of sleep-related eating disorder. J Clin Psychiatry 1998;59:14–9.
5. Schenck CH, Hurwitz TD, O'Connor KA, et al. Additional categories of sleep-related eating disorders and the current status of treatment. Sleep 1993;16:457–66.
6. Kryger MH. Chapter 117: sleep-related cardiac risk. In: Kryger MH, Roth T, Goldstein CA, editors. Principles and practice of sleep medicine. 7th edition. London, UK: Elsevier; 2022.
7. Winkelman JW, Johnson EA, Richards LM. Sleep-related eating disorder. Handb Clin Neurol 2011;98:577–85.
8. Montgomery L, Haynes LC. What every nurse needs to know about nocturnal sleep-related eating disorder. J Psychosoc Nurs Ment Health Serv 2001;39:14–20.
9. Winkelman JW, Herzog DB, Fava M. The prevalence of sleep-related eating disorder in psychiatric and non-psychiatric populations. Psychol Med 1999;29:1461–6.
10. Winkelman JW. Sleep-related eating disorder: the dateline dataset (abstract). Sleep Res 1997;31.
11. Winkelman JW. Nocturnal binge eating is a familial disorder (abstract). Sleep Res 1993;68.
12. Provini F, Albani F, Vetrugno R, et al. A pilot double-blind placebo-controlled trial of low-dose pramipexole in sleep-related eating disorder. Eur J Neurol 2005;12:432–6.
13. De Ocampo J, Foldvary N, Dinner DS, et al. Sleep-related eating disorder in fraternal twins. Sleep Med 2002;3:525–6.
14. Hudson JI, Lalonde JK, Berry JM, et al. Binge-eating disorder as a distinct familial phenotype in obese individuals. Arch Gen Psychiatry 2006;63:313–9.
15. Vetrugno R, Manconi M, Ferini-Strambi L, et al. Nocturnal eating: sleep-related eating disorder or night eating syndrome? A videopolysomnographic study. Sleep 2006;29:949–54.
16. Brion A, Flamand M, Oudiette D, et al. Sleep-related eating disorder versus sleepwalking: a controlled study. Sleep Med 2012;13:1094–101.
17. Howell MJ, Schenck CH. Restless nocturnal eating: a common feature of Willis-Ekbom Syndrome (RLS). J Clin Sleep Med 2012;8:413–9.
18. Irfan M, Schenck CH, Howell MJ. NonREM disorders of arousal and related parasomnias: an updated review. Neurotherapeutics 2021;18:124–39.
19. Lu ML, Shen WW. Sleep-related eating disorder induced by risperidone. J Clin Psychiatry 2004;65:273–4.
20. Paquet V, Strul J, Servais L, et al. Sleep-related eating disorder induced by olanzapine. J Clin Psychiatry 2002;63:597.
21. Komada Y, Takaesu Y, Matsui K, et al. Comparison of clinical features between primary and drug-induced sleep-related eating disorder. Neuropsychiatr Dis Treat 2016;12:1275–80.
22. Morgenthaler TI, Silber MH. Amnestic sleep-related eating disorder associated with zolpidem. Sleep Med 2002;3:323–7.
23. Najjar M. Zolpidem and amnestic sleep related eating disorder. J Clin Sleep Med 2007;3:637–8.
24. Schenck CH. Clinical and research implications of a validated polysomnographic scoring method for REM sleep behavior disorder. Sleep 2005;28:917–9.

25. Stunkard AJ, Grace WJ, Wolff HG. The night-eating syndrome; a pattern of food intake among certain obese patients. Am J Med 1955;19:78–86.

26. Allison KC, Lundgren JD, O'Reardon JP, et al. Proposed diagnostic criteria for night eating syndrome. Int J Eat Disord 2010;43:241–7.

27. Kucukgoncu S, Midura M, Tek C. Optimal management of night eating syndrome: challenges and solutions. Neuropsychiatr Dis Treat 2015;11:751–60. PMC4371896.

28. Rand CS, Macgregor AM, Stunkard AJ. The night eating syndrome in the general population and among postoperative obesity surgery patients. Int J Eat Disord 1997;22:65–9.

29. O'Reardon JP, Allison KC, Martino NS, et al. A randomized, placebo-controlled trial of sertraline in the treatment of night eating syndrome. Am J Psychiatr 2006;163:893–8.

30. Winkelman JW. Treatment of nocturnal eating syndrome and sleep-related eating disorder with topiramate. Sleep Med 2003;4:243–6.

31. Winkelman JW, Wipper B, Purks J, et al. Topiramate reduces nocturnal eating in sleep-related eating disorder. Sleep 2020;43. https://doi.org/10.1093/sleep/zsaa060.

32. Merative MIcromedex®. Micromedex assistant. Ann Arbor, MI: Merative US L.P; 2023. Available at: https://www.micromedexsolutions.com/home/dispatch. Accessed: October 14, 2023.

33. Miyaoka T, Yasukawa R, Tsubouchi K, et al. Successful treatment of nocturnal eating/drinking syndrome with selective serotonin reuptake inhibitors. Int Clin Psychopharmacol 2003;18:175–7.

Sleep Terrors

Muna Irfan, MBBS

KEYWORDS

- Sleep terrors • Non-REM parasomnia • Pavor nocturnus • Night terrors • Disorder of arousal

KEY POINTS

- STs are NREM parasomnias under umbrella of disorders of arousal and hence share similar pathophysiological mechanism.
- They arise mostly out of N3 and are associated with abnormal SWA but can also occur in N2.
- They are most prevalent in pediatric age group and dissipate with age, are generally benign but rarely can be disruptive or lead to daytime fatigue.
- The parasomnia is clinically manifested by abrupt partial awakening with little or no recollection from NREM sleep, with behaviors representing intense fear such as crying and screaming associated with autonomic hyperactivity.
- Sleep state dissociation underlies the pathophysiology where sleep slow wave activity is noted in frontoparietal regions and awake like fast activity in motor and cingulate areas of brain thus explaining the physical manifestation of lack of awareness and motor activity with manifestation of fear.
- Interplay of predisposing factors in conjunction with priming factors may increase homeostatic drive and precipitating factors cause fragmentation of slow wave sleep resulting in partial arousals.
- Careful historical account, timing, and description of the nocturnal events with associated features can help with diagnosis. Polysomnogram is required only if other co-morbid sleep disorders such as OSA or PLMD are suspected.
- Management includes alleviation of precipitating factors, treatment of comorbid sleep disorders and ensuring regular sleep schedule with sufficient sleep. Parental and family reassurance, safety measures and scheduled awakenings are mainstay of treatment.
- If episodes are disruptive, pharmacologic agents such as clonazepam, other benzodiazepine, antidepressants TCA (imipramine, clomipramine), SSRIs (paroxetine, fluoxetine), mirtazapine, melatonin, ramelteon and in pediatric age group L hydroxytryptophan can be trialed.

 Video content accompanies this article at http://www.sleep.theclinics.com.

INTRODUCTION

Sleep terrors (STs) are parasomnias arising out of non-Rem stage of sleep, characterized by precipitous incomplete arousal from N3 sleep with intense fear manifested by inconsolable crying and screaming. They are usually associated with agitation and autonomic hyperactivity. They are classified under disorders of arousal (DOA) and hence share similar diagnostic general criteria and pathophysiological mechanism.[1] Typically, there is partial or complete amnesia for the episode. Associated symptoms of autonomic activation are noted in the form of mydriasis, diaphoresis, tachycardia, tachypnea, and flushing of skin. There may be partial fragmented dream imagery of frightening nature,[2] but vivid recall is not noted.

DIAGNOSTIC CRITERIA

The general diagnostic criteria for DOA are listed in **Box 1** and criteria for ST in **Box 2**.

Department of Neurology, University of Minnesota, Minneapolis Veterans Affairs Healthcare System, 1816 Ellie Court, Eagan, MN 55122, USA
E-mail address: irfan007@umn.edu

Sleep Med Clin 19 (2024) 63–70
https://doi.org/10.1016/j.jsmc.2023.12.004
1556-407X/24/Published by Elsevier Inc.

The nocturnal behaviors usually occur in the initial part of night generally out of N3 but can also arise out of N2; duration may last from few minutes to longer and can be associated with other DOA such as sleep walking (SW). The behaviors, though usually benign, on rare occasions may result in aggressive behavior if family members/caregivers try to intervene. Upon awakening, the individual is usually disoriented and confused. Sleep related choking is also a rare manifestation of ST where individual perceives abrupt distressing choking sensation without any airway blockage arising from partial arousal from N3 sleep.[1]

DEMOGRAPHICS

STs are much more prevalent in pediatric population than adolescent and adults. Variable prevalence has been reported, ranging in children 1 to 12 years of age at 1% to 6.5%[1] but higher rates of 14% or more up to 25% have also been reported.[3] In adults prevalence of 2.2% has been reported with range of 2.3% to 2.6% in 15 to 64 year old and declines to 1% in older than 65 year old.[1] In pediatric population, it is more common in

males but no gender predilection is noted in adult group.[2,4]

PATHOPHYSIOLOGY

Exact etiopathological mechanism has not been proven but several developmental neuromaturational, environmental, and familial factors have been implicated.[5] Higher percentage of slow wave sleep (SWS) in children and resolution with age points to developmental factors. Immature GABA ergic activity and cholingeric inhibitory circuits may lead to abnormal activity associated with ST. Self-limiting nature of ST in many cases with the changes in sleep architecture suggest neurodevelopmental maturation factors. Persistence into adulthood is generally due to interplay of factors increasing SWS and some affecting Non-REM instability. The pathway can be summarized well as cascading interplay of predisposing, priming, and perpetuating factors in which genetic predisposition, immature brain circuitry provide backdrop, and priming and precipitating factors, such as sleep deprivation and central nervous system (CNS) suppressants, deepen homeostatic sleep drive, and superimposed external or internal factors (environmental stimulation, obstructive sleep apnea [OSA]) and so on can induce cortical arousals.[6] CNS acting medications which can increase SWS and enhance sedation, such as neuroleptics, sedatives/hypnotics, stimulants, clonidine, cocaine, and opiates can also induce ST.[4]

Sleep state dissociation also explains the pathophysiological basis of ST. During these behaviors, slow wave activity (SWA) is noted in frontoparietal association cortex and hippocampus (governing awareness and recollection), and faster activity is noted in the motor cortex, limbic cortex, and amygdala (movement and emotions), thus indicating dissociation from full sleep into state where certain brain regions are in sleep while others are active.[6]

A recent study explored the phenomenon of NREM arousal related slow wave synchronization and discovered that slow wave synchronization process occurs abnormally during periods of high SWA in these parasomnias and is associated with higher SWA after movement. These findings suggest that abnormal timing of arousal related slow wave synchronization may underlie the occurrence of DOA.[7]

Serotonergic dysfunction has also been suggested due to its role in SWS generation, arousal, and motoric activity. This theory lends itself to the notion that L-5-hydroxytryptophan could help reduce frequency of STs.

Genetic predilection is also suggested. A prospective study of twins showed ST being explained by 2 component model at 18 months (43.7% additive genetic effects and 56.3% non-shared environmental effect) and at 30 months (41.5% additive genetic effects and 58.5% non-shared environmental effect) which suggests heritability.[8] Also high prevalence of human leukocyte antigen (HLA) DQB1*04 and HLA DQB1*05:01 has been linked to ST.[9,10]

CLINICAL PRESENTATION

The clinical presentation of ST in pediatric age group is generally very unsettling for the parents. The child would acutely arise from sleep in the earlier third of night with inconsolable crying and screaming in a frightened state. It may result in motoric activity or ambulatory behavior of running or bolting in a state of dread. It is associated with autonomic activity such as pupillary dilatation, tachycardia, tachypnea, and cutaneous vasodilatation. The individual may appear disoriented and confused during the episode, and efforts to redirect and intervene may aggravate agitation further leading to physical resistance. Episode may last from seconds to several minutes with individual eventually returning to bed. There is no recollection of the event by the individual, and usually the behaviors are brought to attention by family members. While active vivid dream mentation is not present, instances of vague frightening imagery have been reported. Similarly, individuals are disoriented without any clear recollection of the event, though vague ambiguous information may be retained.[5] The linked Video 1 clip demonstrates ST in an adult induced by loud noise.

CLINICAL EVALUATION

Accurate account of semiology of the nocturnal behavior obtained from patient, parents and family members in case of children and bedpartner of adult patients, is key to clinical diagnosis. Sleep diary detailing various factors/habits affecting the timing of sleep wake can also be revealing. History to assess symptoms for comorbid sleep disorders such as OSA and physical examination to assess physical signs and presentation suggestive of sleep conditions can help with detection and management of contributing factors. Detailed account of triggers such as external factors disrupting sleep, such as noise, and priming and predisposing factors such as sleep deprivation, comorbid disorders such as insomnia and restless legs syndrome (RLS) may facilitate identification and alleviation of these conditions. Meticulous medication reconciliation can also help recognize incriminating agents.

Questionnaires

There are few screening tools available in the form of questionnaires, which can aid in assessment.

Munich Parasomnia Screening (MUPS) is a self-administered 21 question screening questionnaire assessing different behaviors, DOAs and includes 1 question on STs. MUPS has sensitivity of 83% to 100% and specificity of 89% to 100% for DOA.[11]

Paris Arousal Disorder Scale is another self-administered tool comprising of 17 questions with score of greater than 13/50 delineating STs and SW from controls. It has sensitivity of 83.6% and specificity of 89.5%.[12]

A recently proposed Arousal Disorder Questionnaire, which is a 2 part form based on International classification of Sleep-3 criteria, demonstrated sensitivity of 73% (95% CI: 60–82) and specificity of 96% (95% CI:89–98).[13]

Polysomnographic Evaluation

Even though polysomnography (PSG) is not mandatory for diagnosis of ST, comprehensive video PSG recording can help evaluate other coexistent disorders such as OSA and other differential diagnosis. The video recording of the nocturnal behaviors can clarify the emergence of these behaviors from N3 or less frequently from N2 stage of sleep. Auditory stimulation can increase the yield of the event occurring during the PSG but lack of capture of events does not exclude the diagnosis. A study investigating adrenergic activity in patients with SW/ST, demonstrated that the N3 arousals were associated with a 33% increase in heart rate, a 57% decrease in pulse wave amplitude (indicating a major vasoconstriction), a 24% increase in respiratory rate and a doubling of respiratory amplitude. Notably, tachycardia and vasoconstriction started 4 seconds before motor arousal. Arousals arising from parasomnia were associated with greater tachycardia, vasoconstriction, and polypnea than quiet arousals, with pre-arousal gradual increases in heart rate and vasoconstriction and autonomic arousal occurring 4 s before motor arousal from N3 sleep in patients which suggests higher adrenergic reaction than in controls.[6] A PSG clip is shown in **Fig. 1** demonstrating increase in heart rate denoted by open blue arrow and abnormal slowing of electroencephalogram (EEG) activity denoted by solid blue arrow right before ST related arousal.

Sleep macro architectural changes

Findings in literature regarding sleep macroarchitectural changes in ST and DOA are mixed. Decrease in N1 and N2, longer SWS, shorter latency

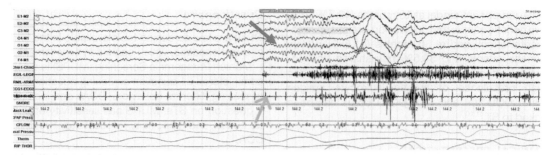

Fig. 1. Hypersynchronization of slow wave activity before arousal associated with Sleep Terror: The attached figure illustrates a 60-s epoch of polysomnographic recording. The closed blue arrow points to the synchronization of electrocerebral waves in EEG leads C3-M2, C4-M1, O1-M2, M2-O1, F4-M1, right before arousal associated with sleep terror. The open green arrow points to an increase in heart rate captured by ECG1-ECG2.

to SWA, and increase REM have been reported. Increased fragmentation of sleep has also been noted with a study proposing microarousal scoring method through SWS fragmentation index at threshold of 6.8/h being 80% sensitive and specific for DOA.[14] Another recent study suggested EEG abnormalities in K complex of Stage II sleep noted more in pediatrics as compared to adults.[13]

Sleep microarchitectural changes

Studies have also shown an increase in cyclic alternating pattern (CAP), increase in number of CAP cycles and arousal occurring with EEG synchronization. CAP is periodic transient cyclically occurring electrocerebral oscillations in NREM sleep, distinct from background EEG, which mark sleep state instability.[15] This depth of architectural assessment is generally labor intensive and hence is performed in research domain.

Electroencephalographic recording of arousals

Hypersynchronous Delta (HSD), which is, continuous high voltage slow wave delta activity greater than 150mv, has also been observed to occur right before the NREM parasomnias and ST.[16]

Intracranial EEG recording in research studies has shown SWA from frontoparietal associative cortices and fast frequency low voltage activity in motor and limbic region.[6]

One study proposed classification of SWS fragmentation as fast, slow, or mixed pattern per hour of SWS with higher slow/mixed arousal index7/hr in DOA but these scoring methods are not pragmatic for clinical application.[14]

Home Video Recording

Due to technological advances, patients' family members can have access to recording on digital devices, which can provide valuable information for clinical evaluation and may suffice in context of appropriate clinical information.

DIFFERENTIAL DIAGNOSIS

Various other conditions can mimic ST but accurate description, nature of behaviors, clinical findings, and associated features can help distinguish these.[17] They are enlisted in **Box 3**, and differentiating clinical characteristics are summarized in **Table 1**.

REM sleep behavior disorder is a REM parasomnia characterized by dream enactment behavior of vocalization, yelling, screaming, and rapid jerky movement enacting vivid dreams of hostile connotation. The differentiating features include occurrence in later part of the night and vivid dream recall. PSG findings of REM sleep without atonia is hallmark finding and thus can help in diagnosis.[18]

Trauma associated sleep disorders were described by Mysliwiec characterized by disruptive nocturnal behaviors in NonREM and REM in conjunction with nightmares emanating from prior trauma. The temporal association of onset with prior trauma as instigating factor is characteristic feature, which can help separate from ST. Similarly, post-traumatic stress disorder related nightmares are also themed at causal traumatic event

---

Box 3
Conditions mimicking ST

REM sleep disorder

Trauma associated sleep disorders/PTSD related sleep disturbance

Sleep related epilepsy [nocturnal frontal lobe epilepsy]

Nightmare disorder

Confusional arousal

Nocturnal panic attacks

Sleep related dissociative disorder

Table 1
Clinical characteristics, behavioral manifestation and associated findings of some common conditions imitating ST

Condition	Behavior	Amnesia	Autonomic Symptoms	Timing	Duration	Sleep Stage
ST	Fearful, inconsolable crying, agitated	+	+	First half	Several minutes	NREM(3)3,N2
RBD	Dream enactment behaviors(elaborate movements/ vocalizations)	-	-	Latter	Seconds-minutes	REM
TASD	Nightmares and disruptive nocturnal behaviors, limb jerks, twitches	−/+	+	Any	Variable	Any
SHE	Stereotypic rhythmic, rocking, thrusting movement,	+	+	Any	Several minutes	N1,N2>N3
CA	Confused awakening in the bed	+	-	First	few minutes	NREM(N3,N2)

Abbreviations: CA, Confusional arousal; RBD, REM sleep behavior disorder; SHE, Sleep related hypermotor epilepsy; ST, Sleep terror; TASD, Trauma associated sleep disorders.

and hence can be differentiated from ST based on nature of dreams.[19]

Sleep related hypermotor epilepsy formerly called nocturnal frontal lobe epilepsy can be identified based on semiology and recurrent nocturnal epileptic activity. Ictal activity in this condition is characterized by recurrent repetitive stereotypical behaviors of bicycling or running movements, rocking, thrusting, dystonic posturing, and other bizarre behaviors lasting for seconds to minutes with little or no post-ictal confusion. The ictal spells occur mostly in N1 and N2 as opposed to ST which tend to happen in N3. Extended EEG montage with PSG can record ictal activity but on occasion when seizure foci may be very deep and localized; the electrocerebral activity may not be picked up by scalp electrodes. Such cases should be evaluated further in epilepsy monitoring unit.[20]

Other DOA of arousal such as confusional arousal (CA) can be differentiated by lack of autonomic symptoms such as mydriasis, tachycardia, tachypnea, diaphoresis usually associated with ST. In CA, the individual partially awakens from sleep but appears confused and disoriented while remaining in bed.

Nocturnal panic attacks can occur in patients with significant anxiety and distress, but the individual will recollect the occurrence and the anxious distress of feeling fear and doom while patients with ST will not themselves be perturbed by the event.

Sleep related dissociative disorders are result of some psychological conflict or physical or emotional abuse where elaborate nocturnal behaviors result from maladaptive defense mechanism of suppressing conscious recollection of the past trauma/conflict.[21] Detailed history, and behavioral and psychological evaluation can help delineate these from ST.

MANAGEMENT

Management of ST is based on identifying the priming and precipitating factors. Addressing the causes of sleep deprivation and any precipitating factors such as stress, caffeine use, changes in sleep schedule, any incriminating medications and comorbid sleep disorders is very important.[22,23] Various behavioral and pharmacologic approaches are discussed as following.

Behavioral Management

Behavioral strategies should be employed in all cases of ST regardless of age and in most instances conservative approach is sufficient.

Family counseling

Parents and family members in case of children and bedpartner in case of adults should be counseled and reassured about the benign nature of the condition and provided education to ensure good sleep structure and adequate sleep environment with less interruptions.

Precipitating factors

Any precipitating factors such as caffeine use and influences disrupting sleep should be avoided. Co-morbid sleep disorders such as OSA, RLS, and others should be addressed to consolidate sleep and decrease homeostatic drive.

Safety measures

Environmental safety should be prioritized. Ensuring patients' sleeping environment free of injurious objects, fastened windows and secure front door is necessary. By-stander education of family members, especially ones sharing the bedroom, is very important. They should be advised not to physically restrain or intervene as efforts to redirect the individual may result in paradoxic physical aggression.

Scheduled awakenings

If ST are frequent or distressful to the family occurring at predictable timing, scheduled awakenings 15 to 30 mins before the timing of event can be performed consistently for 1 to 4 weeks. Detailed protocol for scheduled awakening is elaborated in **Box 3**. Based on same principle vibrating devices under bedsheets activated by parents smart phone at timed interval can also achieve same results.[24]

Scheduled Aawakening Pprotocol for DOA	
1	*Keep track of individual's sleep patterns for 2 weeks* Record bedtime, awake time, and timing of parasomnia activity
2	*Once consistent sleep pattern is established, calculate the interval from sleep time to parasomnia activity.* Scheduled awakening should occur 15--30 minutes before the timing of event.
3	*At the designated time, awaken the individual* with light touch or gentle verbal prompt.
4	*Once the individual awakens fully (is able to respond) allow to return to sleep.*

- Practice consistently for 2--4 weeks.
- Use this approach only in cases where consistent sleep pattern is noted.
- If parasomnia event occurs earlier than planned awakening, move the arousal 15 minutes earlier than occurrence

Other behavioral interventions

Hypnosis has also been attempted to help relieve ST with some evidence.[25] Other behavioral interventions include coping strategies, relaxation therapy and psychotherapy especially in cases where individuals may be dealing with significant distress.[26]

Table 2 Treatment modalities for ST[23,25,28–30]	
Behavioral Management	Family Counseling Alleviation of precipitating factors Safety measures Scheduled awakening Hypnosis, relaxation therapy, psychotherapy
Pharmacologic management	Clonazepam, other benzodiazepines (diazepam, lorazepam, midazolam) 5-Hydroxytryptophan or L tryptophan Antidepressants (paroxetine, imipramine, clomipramine), paroxetine, melatonin, ramelteon

Pharmacologic Intervention

While in most cases behavioral management is adequate, in clinical scenario of disruptive ST resulting in significant distress, injury or daytime sleepiness, pharmacologic agents may be tried.

Clonazepam

Clonazepam is the most studied agent for treatment of DOA including ST. The mechanism of action is by virtue of suppression of N3 fragmentation and transition into lighter stages. It should be initiated in dose of 0.125 mg and gradually escalating to 0.5 or 1 mg titrating to effect if not limited by side effects. It should be taken 60 to 90 minutes before bedtime and 4 to 6 weeks after resolution of STs, gradual taper can be considered.[27]

Schenck and colleagues demonstrated sustained resolution in 86% of patients of SW and ST with clonazepam and other benzodiazepines when followed longitudinally for 3.5 years.[28]

5 hydroxytryptophan

L-tryptotyphan has shown improvement in 84% of patients in doses of 500 to 4500 mg (mean dose of 2400 mg) according to pediatric studies. The proposed mechanism of action is by modulation of arousal mechanism.[29] These studies support the use of 5-hydroxytryptophan and its precursor tryptophan in pediatric population.

Antidepressants

Other medications used for ST include tricyclic antidepressants (imipramine and clomipramine), selective serotonin inhibitors (Paroxetine, fluoxetine), trazodone, mirtazapine, melatonin, and ramelteon.[2,23,30]

Various intervention strategies have been summarized in **Table 2**.

CLINICS CARE POINTS

- ST are more common in children with prevalence ranging from 1% to 6.5% in 1 to 12 years of age group but higher rates up to 25% have also been reported.

- In adults, prevalence is lower at 2.2% with a range of 2.3% to 2.6% in 15 to 64-year-old, declining to 1% in older than 65-year-old.

- In pediatric age group it occurs more in males but in adults no gender preponderance is noted.

- According to ICSD-3 RT, the ST should meet the general criteria of DOA and are characterized by episodes of abrupt terror, typically beginning with an alarming vocalization such as frightening scream with intense fear and signs of autonomic arousal, including mydriasis, tachycardia, tachypnea, and diaphoresis.

- CNS acting medications such as neuroleptics, sedatives/hypnotics, stimulants, clonidine, cocaine and opiates can induce ST by increasing SWS and enhancing sedation.

- Interaction of predisposing genetics and immature neurodevelopmental circuitry, priming factors such as sleep deprivation and CNS suppressants deepening sleep drive with superimposed factors (noise, OSA etc.) can induce partial cortical arousals as substrate of ST.

- Human Leukocyte Antigen (HLA) DQB1*04 and HLA DQB1*05:01 have been linked to ST.

- There is partial or complete amnesia of the event by the individual and usually the behaviors are observed by family members. There is no vivid dream mentation, but instances of vague frightening imagery can be experienced.

- ST generally occur in first third of night arising from N3 or N2, last for few minutes and can be more disruptive to family members than the individual.

- Management is focused on alleviating precipitating factors, treating comorbid conditions, counseling and safety.

- Scheduled awakenings can help decrease frequency in pediatric cases.

- In disruptive cases, clonazepam can be used in doses of 0.125 mg to 1 mg.

- 5-hydroxytryptophan and its precursor tryptophan has been shown positive trend in pediatric studies in doses of 500 to 4500 mg.

DISCLOSURE

No conflict of Interest to disclose.

SUPPLEMENTARY DATA

Supplementary data related to this article can be found online at https://doi.org/10.1016/j.jsmc.2023.12.004.

REFERENCES

1. American Academy of Sleep Medicine. International classification of sleep disorders. 3rd edition. Revis Darien; 2023. text.
2. Leung AKC. Sleep terrors: an updated review. Curr Pediatr Rev 2022. https://doi.org/10.2174/18756336mtaxpndi61.
3. Petit D, Pennestri MH, Paquet J, et al. Childhood sleepwalking and sleep terrors: a longitudinal study of prevalence and familial aggregation. JAMA Pediatr 2015;169(7):653–8.
4. Irfan M, Schenck CH, Howell MJ. NonREM disorders of arousal and related parasomnias: an updated review. Neurotherapeutics 2021. https://doi.org/10.1007/s13311-021-01011-y.
5. Idir Y, Oudiette D, Arnulf I. Sleepwalking, sleep terrors, sexsomnia and other disorders of arousal: the old and the new. J Sleep Res 2022. https://doi.org/10.1111/jsr.13596.
6. Terzaghi M, Sartori I, Tassi L, et al. Evidence of dissociated arousal states during NREM parasomnia from an intracerebral neurophysiological study. Sleep 2009;32(3):409–12. https://doi.org/10.1093/sleep/32.3.409.
7. Cataldi J, Stephan AM, Marchi NA, et al. Abnormal timing of slow wave synchronization processes in non-rapid eye movement sleep parasomnias. Sleep 2022;45(7).
8. Nguyen BH, Pérusse D, Paquet J, et al. Sleep terrors in children: a prospective study of twins. Pediatrics 2008. https://doi.org/10.1542/peds.2008-1303.
9. Heidbreder A, Frauscher B, Mitterling T, et al. Not only sleepwalking but NREM parasomnia irrespective of the type is associated with HLA DQB1*05:01. J Clin Sleep Med 2016;12(4):565–70.
10. Irfan M, Schenck CH, Howell MJ. Non-rapid eye movement sleep and overlap parasomnias. Continuum 2017;23(4):1035–50. https://doi.org/10.1212/CON.0000000000000503. Sleep Neurology.
11. Fulda S, Hornyak M, Müller K, et al. Development and validation of the Munich parasomnia screening (MUPS). Somnologie - Schlafforsch und Schlafmedizin 2008. https://doi.org/10.1007/s11818-008-0336-x.
12. Arnulf I, Zhang B, Uguccioni G, et al. A scale for assessing the severity of arousal disorders. Sleep 2014;37(1). https://doi.org/10.5665/sleep.3322.

13. Loddo G, La Fauci G, Vignatelli L, et al. The Arousal Disorders Questionnaire: a new and effective screening tool for confusional arousals, Sleepwalking and Sleep Terrors in epilepsy and sleep disorders units. Sleep Med 2021;80:279–85.

14. Lopez R, Shen Y, Chenini S, et al. Diagnostic criteria for disorders of arousal: a video-polysomnographic assessment. Ann Neurol 2018. https://doi.org/10.1002/ana.25153.

15. Zucconi M, Ferini-Strambi L. NREM parasomnias: arousal disorders and differentiation from nocturnal frontal lobe epilepsy. Clin Neurophysiol 2000;111.

16. Camaioni M, Scarpelli S, Gorgoni M, et al. EEG patterns prior to motor activations of parasomnias: a systematic review. Nat Sci Sleep 2021;713–28.

17. Provini F, Tinuper P, Bisulli F, et al. Arousal disorders. Sleep Med 2011;12(Suppl 2):S22–6.

18. Irfan M, Howell MJ. Rapid eye movement sleep behavior disorder: overview and current perspective. Curr Sleep Med Reports 2016;2(2):64–73.

19. Brock MS, Matsangas P, Creamer JL, et al. Clinical and polysomnographic features of trauma associated sleep disorder. J Clin Sleep Med 2022;18(12):2775–84.

20. Tinuper P, Bisulli F, Cross JH, et al. Definition and diagnostic criteria of sleep-related hypermotor epilepsy. Neurology 2016;86(19):1834–42.

21. American Academy of Sleep Medicine. Darien, IL, . International classification of sleep disorders. 3rd edition. Am Acad Sleep Med.; 2014.

22. Varghese R, Irfan M. Delirium versus dementia: a diagnostic conundrum in clinical practice. Psychiatr Ann 2017;47(5). https://doi.org/10.3928/00485713-20170411-02.

23. Mainieri G, Loddo G, Provini F, et al. Diagnosis and management of NREM sleep parasomnias in children and adults. Diagnostics 2023;13(7):1261.

24. Gigliotti F, Esposito D, Basile C, et al. Sleep terrors-A parental nightmare. Pediatr Pulmonol 2022;57(8):1869–78.

25. Hauri PJ, Silber MH, Boeve BF. The treatment of parasomnias with hypnosis: a 5-year follow-up study. J Clin Sleep Med 2007. https://doi.org/10.5664/jcsm.26858.

26. Laganière C, Gaudreau H, Pokhvisneva I, et al. Sleep terrors in early childhood and associated emotional–behavioral problems. J Clin Sleep Med 2022. https://doi.org/10.5664/jcsm.10080.

27. Kotagal S. Parasomnias of childhood. Curr Opin Pediatr 2008;20(6):659–65.

28. Schenck CH, Mahowald MW. Long-term, nightly benzodiazepine treatment of injurious parasomnias and other disorders of disrupted nocturnal sleep in 170 adults. Am J Med 1996;100(3):333–7.

29. Van Zyl LT, Chung SA, Shahid A, et al. L-tryptophan as treatment for pediatric non-rapid eye movement parasomnia. J Child Adolesc Psychopharmacol 2018. https://doi.org/10.1089/cap.2017.0164.

30. Irfan, Muna, Liendo A. Sleep Terrors. Encyclopedia of Sleep and Circadian Rhythms. 2nd Edition. Encyclopedia of Sleep and Circadian Rhythms; 2022. Encyclopedia of Sleep and Circadian Rhythms.

Rapid Eye Movement Sleep Behavior Disorder
Clinical Presentation and Diagnostic Criteria

Brandon M. Jones, MD, MS[a], Stuart J. McCarter, MD[b],*

KEYWORDS

- Rapid eye movement sleep behavior • Parasomnia • Parkinsonism • Dementia
- Rapid eye movement sleep without atonia

KEY POINTS

- Rapid eye movement (REM) sleep behavior disorder (RBD) classically presents with repetitive complex motor behavior during sleep with associated dream mentation.
- RBD is largely a disorder of older individuals, although dream enactment behaviors may manifest at any age, with many individuals reporting symptom onset in their 20s or 30s.
- REM sleep without atonia is best evaluated in the chin or flexor digitorum superficialis muscles.

INTRODUCTION

Rapid eye movement (REM) sleep is characterized by vivid dream mentation accompanied by skeletal muscle paralysis to prevent abnormal motor activity associated with dream content. In 1965, Michel Jouvet demonstrated the loss of typical REM sleep–associated skeletal muscle paralysis with associated abnormal behaviors despite persistent electroencephalographic REM sleep in cats following lesioning of the dorsal pons.[1] In the early 1980s, Carlos Schenck and Mark Mahowald encountered their first patient with a history of violent behaviors during sleep at the University of Minnesota with polysomnography (PSG) demonstrating the loss of normal REM sleep muscle paralysis and concurrent abnormal motor activity. In 1986, they published a series of 4 patients with similar findings, coining the term "REM sleep behavior disorder (RBD)."[2] In this article, we will focus on the clinical presentation, etiologic considerations, and diagnosis of RBD. A separate article on the management of RBD in this issue will present the treatment options based on a recent practice guideline.

CLINICAL PRESENTATION OF RAPID EYE MOVEMENT SLEEP BEHAVIOR DISORDER

The classic patient with RBD presents to sleep clinics with recurrent, violent motor activity and vocalization mirroring dream content. Dreams are often quite vivid and typically contain a confrontational theme such as fighting, being attacked, or being chased, although more than half of RBD patients are completely unaware of their behaviors.[3,4] Thus, collateral history from a bedpartner is a vital component in the evaluation of patients with sleep disorders, especially RBD. While attack-themed or chase-themed dream mentation is commonly reported in the literature, dream enactment behaviors mirroring dream content of playing sports, musical instruments, performing household chores, or activities from the workplace are also frequent.[5] Since these are less disruptive, they may be less likely to be considered abnormal and underreported. Additionally, patients or bedpartners may not volunteer this information, either because they believe dream enactment to be a normal phenomenon or out of embarrassment.

[a] Department of Neurology, Mayo Clinic, 200 1st Street SW, Rochester, MN 55905, USA; [b] Department of Neurology; Center for Sleep Medicine, Mayo Clinic, 200 1st Street SW, Rochester, MN 55905, USA
* Corresponding author.
E-mail address: mccarter.stuart@mayo.edu

Sleep Med Clin 19 (2024) 71–81
https://doi.org/10.1016/j.jsmc.2023.10.004

Typical dream enactment behaviors include running, kicking, punching, swearing, and some patients may leave the bed. Because of this, injuries to both patients and bedpartners are common, with some studies reporting between 50% and 96% of individuals with some degree of injury to themselves or bedpartners from dream enactment behaviors.[2,4,6–8] While most injuries are mild, approximately 12% are severe (subdural hematomas, fractures, lacerations) and require medical attention (**Fig. 1**).[7] The frequency of dream enactment behaviors is variable and unpredictable, with some individuals experiencing episodes multiple times per night while others may act out their dreams less than once per year. Use or withdrawal from substances, such as withdrawal from alcohol, or exposure to specific medications as well as times of heightened stress may influence the frequency of RBD. While significant dream enactment episodes are variable, many patients may demonstrate minor "REM behavioral events" which are visible episodes with minor purposeful motor behaviors during REM sleep or excess of elementary motor events such as recurrent muscle twitches are common and may be evident with close observation of an individual's sleep.[9]

Given the increased proportion of REM sleep during the second half of the night, RBD episodes are more likely to occur in the early morning hours, although the time of night behaviors occur is not specific for RBD. Unlike non-REM parasomnia behaviors, RBD episodes are typically brief, lasting seconds to less than 1 minute, although periods of normal REM muscle paralysis may interrupt dream enactment behaviors resulting in a prolonged-appearing episode of waxing and waning severity. Unfortunately, predicting potentially injurious behaviors is difficult as the frequency of dream enactment behaviors does not predict future injuries.[7] It is not uncommon for RBD symptom severity to escalate over time and then spontaneously improve, particularly as parkinsonism or cognitive impairment develops.

EPIDEMIOLOGY OF RAPID EYE MOVEMENT SLEEP BEHAVIOR DISORDER

RBD is largely a disorder of older individuals, although dream enactment behaviors may manifest at any age, with many individuals reporting symptom onset in their 20s or 30s. Pediatric RBD can be seen, primarily in narcolepsy type 1 where it may represent dissociation of REM sleep, but is rare and not well understood.[10] Most large cohort studies on RBD, including the largest multicenter study of 1280 RBD patients, have reported a significant older male predominance of approximately 80% with an average age at diagnosis of 66 years old.[11] Epidemiologic studies of PSG-confirmed RBD have reported a 1% to 2% prevalence in the general population, although population-based studies suggest the presence of dream enactment behaviors in between 5% and 13% of adults over the age of 60, showing increasing prevalence with increasing age.[12–15] Despite the reported male predominance in most cohort studies of RBD, studies on PSG-proven RBD have demonstrated an equal male/female ratio, particularly if RBD is diagnosed before the age of 50 years as women with RBD tend to be younger than men at RBD diagnosis (Alexandres and colleagues, unpublished observations, 2023).[12]

Postulated reasons for the male/female discrepancy in RBD have included less violent dream enactment behaviors in women compared with men as well as the fact the women have a longer life expectancy, and thus are less likely to have a bedpartner to report abnormal behaviors at night.[12] However, when comparing 372 men and women who were diagnosed with isolated RBD within the same month, there were no differences in injury frequency or RBD as the reason for sleep referral (Alexandres and colleagues, unpublished observations, 2023). It may be that the sex discrepancy in Lewy body spectrum disease, the underlying etiology of RBD in the majority of cases, explains the reported sex differences in RBD cohorts, but further work is needed to understand differences between men and women with RBD.[16]

ETIOLOGY OF RAPID EYE MOVEMENT SLEEP BEHAVIOR DISORDER

Initially considered to be only a unique and interesting parasomnia, Schenck and Mahowald keenly recognized that many patients they initially identified later developed parkinsonism or dementia, with 38% of patients "phenoconverting" 10 years after their initial report in 1986. This number grew to 81% 26 years after diagnosis, with all patients developing alpha-synucleinopathy neurodegenerative diseases, the majority of whom developed Parkinson's disease (PD) or dementia with Lewy bodies (DLB).[17,18] Several studies, including a large multicenter study, have confirmed the strong association between RBD and alpha-synucleinopathy neurodegenerative diseases with a phenoconversion rate of 6.6% per year, or 73% 12 years after initial RBD diagnosis in the "typical" older male RBD population.[11,19] How this number applies to younger RBD patients remains poorly understood. Recent data published in abstract form suggest the

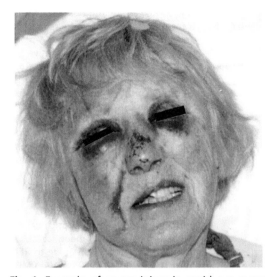

Fig. 1. Example of severe injury in rapid eye movement (REM) sleep behavior disorder. Photograph of a 74-year-old patient with REM sleep behavior disorder (RBD) who suffered significant orofacial trauma after diving out of bed during a dream enactment episode. This highlights the severity of injuries that can occur in individuals with RBD. (Used with permission from: Sleep and Its Disorders. Avidan, Alon Y., Bradley and Daroff's Neurology in Clinical Practice, 101, 1664-1744.e9. Copyright © 2022, Elsevier Inc. All rights reserved.)

annualized phenoconversion rate in those aged less than 60 years old at RBD diagnosis appears significantly lower than the previously reported 6% to 7% risk per year, highlighting a strong driver of age in phenoconversion.[20]

When RBD is diagnosed in individuals without parkinsonism, cognitive impairment, or severe autonomic dysfunction, it is considered "isolated RBD (iRBD)" whereas individuals who developed dream enactment behaviors at the same time or after the development of other cognitive, motor, or autonomic symptoms are considered "secondary/symptomatic" RBD. Underlying alpha-synucleinopathies are the most common cause of RBD but may present distinctly in different clinical syndromes. For instance, RBD occurs in 90% of patients with multiple system atrophy (MSA) and may develop prior to motor or autonomic symptoms in this case, but it is rare to identify iRBD patients who go on to develop MSA.[11,21] On the other hand, 40% to 50% of PD patients and 80% of DLB patients have RBD.[22,23] The majority of iRBD patients will develop PD or DLB, with a slight predilection for DLB which may be related to the heterogenous etiologies of PD. RBD may occur in other conditions including narcolepsy type 1 and some autoimmune encephalopathies such

as Iglon5-related disease, anti-ma2, LGi1, CASPR2, and dipeptidyl-peptidase-like protein 6 encephalitis.[24,25] Lesions to the pons or medulla from stroke, hemorrhage, demyelination, or tumors may also cause acute onset RBD, although other neurologic deficits are usually apparent in these cases.[26] (**Fig. 2**) RBD has been reported in other neurodegenerative diseases such as Alzheimer's disease and progressive supranuclear palsy, although Lewy body copathology likely explains RBD in these groups.[27] RBD has also been reported in spinocerebellar atrophy type 3 and myotonic dystrophy type 2.[28,29]

Serotonergic medications are commonly implicated in the development of RBD.[30] Specifically asking about an association with the initiation of or dose increase of serotonergic medications, specifically antidepressants, is necessary in RBD patients as dose reduction or changing medications may improve or resolve RBD symptoms.[31] Serotonergic medications directly increase REM sleep muscle activity even in the absence of dream enactment behaviors and likely unveil RBD in patients who are predisposed to develop it later in life[17,30] (**Fig. 3**).

DIAGNOSIS OF RAPID EYE MOVEMENT SLEEP BEHAVIOR DISORDER

RBD is diagnosed based on criteria established by the International Classification of Sleep Disorders (ICSD-3)[32] which include (1) repeated episodes of sleep-related vocalization and/or complex motor behaviors; (2) these behaviors are documented by PSG to occur during REM sleep or, based on clinical history of dream enactment, are presumed to occur during REM sleep; (3) polysomnographic recording demonstrates REM sleep without atonia (RSWA); and (4) the disturbance is not better explained by another sleep disorder, mental disorder, medication, or substance abuse. PSG demonstrating the presence of RSWA is core to confirming a diagnosis, as individuals who meet criteria 1 and 2 but either PSG is not available or does not demonstrate RSWA can be considered "probable" RBD.[32] Given the prognostic implications of a diagnosis of RBD, PSG should be performed whenever possible for optimal confidence in RBD diagnosis.[33]

When reviewing the PSG in a patient with suspected RBD, 2 separate aspects require consideration. The first is the identification of RSWA. Identification of RSWA requires at least some portion of normal REM atonia so that a baseline can be established (**Fig. 4**). Some patients with RBD may never demonstrate normal REM muscle atonia. In these cases REM sleep can be identified

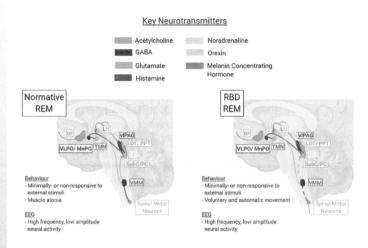

Fig. 2. Key brain regions and neurotransmitters involved in the regulation and maintenance of the REM sleep stage under healthy normative or pathologic RBD conditions. In RBD, dysfunction within the SubC → VMM → spinal motor neuron pathway results in a lack of REM atonia (depicted with *dotted line*). BF, basal forebrain; LC, locus coeruleus; LDT/PPT, laterodorsal tegmentum/pedunculopontine tegmentum; LH, lateral hypothalamus; Subc/PC, subcoeruleus/pre-locus coeruleus; TMN, tuberomammillary nucleus; vlPAG, ventrolateral periaqueductal gray; VLPO/MnPO, ventrolateral preoptic nucleus/median preoptic nucleus; VMM, ventromedial medulla. (Used with permission from Roguski A, Rayment D, Whone AL, Jones MW, Rolinski M. A Neurologist's Guide to REM Sleep Behavior Disorder. Front Neurol. 2020 Jul 8;11:610. https://doi.org/10.3389/fneur.2020.00610. PMID: 32733361; PMCID: PMC7360679.)

through review of the electroencephalogram (EEG) and electrooculogram leads to identify the typical EEG features of REM sleep and REMs.[34–36] In these rare cases, the level of muscle activity during stage N3 sleep can also be used as a baseline for "normal" atonia.[34–36] As arousals related to sleep-disordered breathing during REM sleep cause increased muscle activity during REM sleep, evaluation for the presence of RSWA should only be done if sleep-disordered breathing is absent or if it has been adequately treated.[9] The second vitally important aspect in the evaluation of the PSG in RBD patients is review of time-synchronized audio and video for motor activity and vocalizations associated with RSWA. The camera should have the ability to zoom and be placed so the entire bed can be viewed with the patient in any position.[9] While complex violent dream enactment behaviors are not subtle, these are infrequently captured during PSG. Minor limb jerks and elementary semipurposeful limb movements such as repetitive finger and wrist flexion, known as "hand babbling," are common in patients with RBD and occur at a much higher frequency with consistent night-to-night activity when compared with complex motor activity.[37] While the presence of minor excessive motor jerks or simple elementary movements are not sufficient for a diagnosis of RBD by the American Academy of Sleep Medicine (AASM) ICSD-3 criteria in the absence of a dream enactment history, their presence along with RSWA is strongly suggestive of underlying

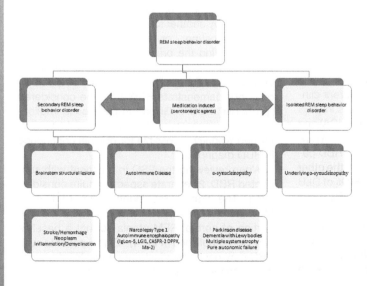

Fig. 3. Etiologic breakdown of rapid eye movement sleep behavior disorder. The majority of isolated REM sleep behavior disorder (RBD) is caused by presumed underlying alpha-synucleinopathy neurodegenerative diseases. However, the use of serotonergic medications (primarily antidepressants) often causes RBD in the absence of other neurologic signs or symptoms and in the majority of cases likely "unmasks" a latent underlying alpha-synucleinopathy in patients with isolated RBD. However, in some cases serotonergic medications can trigger RBD that resolves with discontinuation of the medication. Thus medication-induced RBD exists on a spectrum between isolated and secondary RBD.

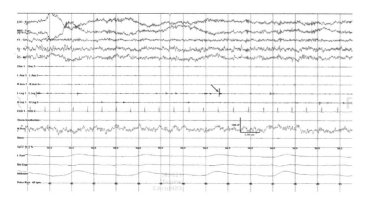

Fig. 4. 30-s epoch of REM sleep demonstrating normal rapid eye movement (REM) muscle atonia. Note the brief burst of muscle activity lasting less than 150 milliseconds (*red arrow*) which is consistent with fragmentary myoclonus but meets criteria for a phasic muscle burst by REM sleep without atonia. These brief bursts are a normal phenomenon in the leg electromyography leads, but contributes to inaccuracy of the leg muscles when scoring REM sleep without atonia.

RBD, even in the absence of clinical history. Additional guidance on evaluation on the review of video-PSG in patients with suspected RBD for research purposes can be found in recent International REM Sleep Behavior Disorder Study Group publications.[9,38]

QUANTIFICATION OF RAPID EYE MOVEMENT SLEEP WITHOUT ATONIA

Determination of the presence or absence of RSWA is an evolving field. In clinical sleep labs, the submentalis or mentalis muscle along with the tibialis anterior has classically been used for the evaluation of RSWA. However, recent data suggest the flexor digitorum superficialis (FDS) is the most sensitive and specific muscle for a diagnosis RBD and the least prone to artifactual RSWA. Historically and in most clinical practices, the determination of RSWA has been based on qualitative review of PSG. However, the last 20 years have seen an explosion of manual and automated quantitative RSWA analysis methodologies, which are based on the original quantitative methodology proposed by Lapierre and Montplaisir in 1992 with various nuanced differences.[39]

Manual quantification of RSWA allows for accurate scoring of RSWA and exclusion of muscle activity associated with arousal or sleep-disordered breathing. However, it is very time consuming and laborious, making it difficult to implement in clinical practice. Due to the prognostic implications associated with a diagnosis of RBD, quantitative cutoffs for a diagnosis of RBD rather than a qualitative yes/no assessment of RSWA are vitally important. Manual quantification methods of scoring RSWA share largely the same tenants and the AASM scoring criteria for RSWA have also adopted these methodologies.[9] Proposed cutoffs for a diagnosis of RBD using various methodologies have been previously reported.[9,35,36,40]

In brief, RSWA is somewhat arbitrarily defined as 2 separate activity types: short bursts lasting 0.1 to 15 seconds (**Fig. 5**), depending on the criteria used, known as "phasic/transient" muscle activity, and longer, low-amplitude bursts of activity lasting greater than 15 seconds, known as "tonic" muscle activity (**Fig. 6**).[9,35,36,40] It should be pointed out there is no clear physiologic evidence supporting different mechanisms generating phasic and tonic muscle activity. Finally, most manual quantitative RSWA analysis methodologies have added a third category, "any" muscle activity, which is the presence of either phasic or tonic muscle activities, in other words, the sum total of all RSWA in a specific muscle.[35,36]

RSWA is scored in each muscle individually and then activity from each muscle can be combined with other muscles. For practical purposes, RSWA can be scored based on the presence of a 3-s "mini-epoch" or 30-s epoch time base. Mini-epochs or epochs are scored as "RSWA positive" or "RSWA negative." An overall RSWA percentage is calculated as the number of mini-epochs or epochs with RSWA divided by those without RSWA.[35,36,40] Interestingly, despite slightly different definitions of each muscle activity type used in each methodology, cutoffs for an RBD diagnosis are largely similar. Broadly speaking, phasic chin muscle activity of 10% to 15% is greater than 80% sensitive and greater than 90% specific for RBD, while chin "any" muscle activity of 18% to 21% is greater than 85% and 95% sensitive and specific for RBD.[9] Interestingly, the 95th percentile of chin muscle activity in normal individuals throughout the lifespan is 9.1%, suggesting that at RSWA level of greater than 10% in the chin is likely pathologic.[41] Tonic muscle activity typically is measured only in the chin as it is less likely to happen in the limbs. Tonic cutoff levels are somewhat variable, with different groups reporting chin tonic cutoff rates of between 1%

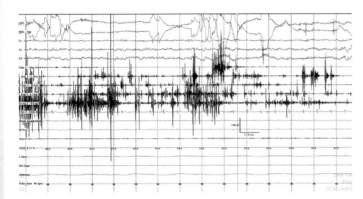

Fig. 5. 30-s epoch of rapid eye movement (REM) sleep demonstrating diffuse phasic bursts of REM sleep without atonia in all 4 limbs, and, to a much lesser extent the chin.

and 8% with greater than 95% sensitivity and specificity.[9] However, in the authors' experience, the presence of any tonic muscle activity is abnormal and strongly suggestive of RBD. Additional direct measurement of duration of individual muscle bursts can be helpful in cases of diagnostic uncertainty, as RBD patients often have longer duration of muscle bursts than non-RBD patients.[35,36]

The anterior tibialis is generally considered to be much less specific for RBD, likely due to other processes which could influence RSWA, such as L5 radiculopathies, fragmentary myoclonus (see **Fig. 4**), or periodic limb movements of sleep (PLMS) with intrusion into REM. It should be pointed out that PLMS with intrusion into REM sleep is not uncommon in RBD patients and likely reflects dysregulated muscle control in RBD patients.[9] Additionally, serotonergic agents seem to preferentially affect the anterior tibialis muscles through unclear mechanisms.[30] Thus when encountering an RBD patient with significant anterior tibialis RSWA, review of their medication list for these medications is recommended, and considering transitioning to an alternative medication in difficult-to-control RBD could be considered.

There is growing evidence that FDS is the most sensitive and specific muscle for an RBD diagnosis as well as the muscle least prone to artifacts with good inter-rater reliability.[38] The Sleep Innsbruck Barcelona group has proposed a combined metric utilizing the submentalis and FDS muscle activity of 27.2% as the optimal cutoff for RBD diagnosis with a sensitivity of 90.4% to 100% and specificity of 88% to 100%, which has also been adopted by the AASM ICSD-3 criteria, although this is based on 30-s epochs.[32,40] When considering this cutoff, a positive 30-s epoch is defined as containing at least 5 positive 3-s mini-epochs. Optimal cutoffs for FDS RSWA are still being established; however, a cutoff of between 11% and 17% bilateral FDS any RSWA has been reported to be at least 90% sensitive and up to 100% specific for RBD.[40,42]

There are a number of different automated methodologies for the scoring of RSWA, all with differing algorithms.[9] In general, these are fairly accurate, particularly in more straightforward cases of RBD without sleep-disordered breathing. Pros of the automated analyses include significantly less manpower and time involved in scoring RSWA; however, it is difficult to exclude RSWA

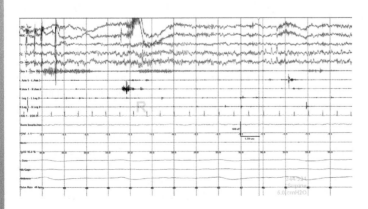

Fig. 6. 30-s epoch of rapid eye movementsleep demonstrated sustained tonic muscle activity in the chin.

from arousals or sleep-disordered breathing, thus RSWA may be scored inaccurately and lead to a false diagnosis if not reviewed manually. Further, these automated analyses software are not integrated with clinical sleep software, so offline processing is required. Ideally, a combined method of automated RSWA analysis with manual review for confirmation will be clinically available in the near future to allow for more efficient and accurate diagnosis of RBD.

Due to the resource-intensive nature of PSG, alternative methods to identify RBD have been studied, although none of these are yet acceptable for RBD diagnosis. Wrist actigraphy has recently been shown to correlate closely with PSG-confirmed RBD in PD patients, although more study is needed before this can be considered for routine clinical use.[43]

CLINICAL EVALUATION OF PATIENTS WITH SUSPECTED RAPID EYE MOVEMENT SLEEP BEHAVIOR DISORDER

Due to the strong association between RBD and alpha synucleinopathies, all patients should be evaluated for autonomic, motor, and cognitive dysfunction.[44,45] Patients with iRBD commonly complain of hyposmia or anosmia, constipation, orthostatic intolerance or syncope, erectile dysfunction, and urinary urgency.[46] Symptoms range from mild to severe, including frank orthostatic hypotension and urinary retention, particularly in those with evolving multiple system atrophy. Assessment of orthostatic blood pressure should be done in patients with complaints of orthostatic intolerance. Motor complaints in IRBD are often mild if present, with some complaining of subtle balance or motor slowing that may not be perceptible on neurologic examination. Subtle abnormalities may be found on quantitative motor testing such as Purdue pegboard testing or Timed Up and Go testing.[47] Cognitive complaints are variable. In the authors experience, these occur mostly when trying to pay attention and multitasking, which sometimes precludes maintaining gainful employment despite normal bedside testing.[48] It is not uncommon for formal neuropsychometric testing to be normal due to a preserved ability to maintain focus on single tasks which falls apart in the real world due to multiple distractions. The best test for assessment of subtle cognitive deficits in iRBD is trails making B, which has shown good predictive ability for the development of future cognitive impairment.[48]

In general, neuroimaging is not required in most patients with iRBD. However, due to the potential

for lesional RBD, sudden onset RBD symptoms in conjunction with other neurologic symptoms such as cranial nerve abnormalities, weakness, or sensory loss requires brain imaging to rule out alternative pathologies as the cause of RBD in these rare cases.[26]

DIFFERENTIAL DIAGNOSIS OF RAPID EYE MOVEMENT SLEEP BEHAVIOR DISORDER

Multiple conditions can mimic RBD which require exclusion (**Table 1**).

Obstructive sleep apnea (OSA; pseudo-RBD): Patients present with similar complaints of abnormal motor activity during sleep with varying frequency and severity, with or without dream recall. Symptoms of sleep-disordered breathing are typically present. PSG will demonstrate sleep apnea with normal preserved REM atonia, although this can only be confidently assessed once sleep-disordered breathing is treated. Symptoms typically fully resolve with the resolution of OSA. However, comorbid OSA and RBD is not uncommon and the treatment of OSA can improve RBD symptoms but will generally not fully resolve them.[49]

Non-REM parasomnias (confusional arousals, sleepwalking): Non-REM parasomnias including confusional arousals and sleepwalking may mimic RBD. PSG is required to differentiate non-REM parasomnias from RBD. Clinically, sleep walking is typically less violent, less associated with dream recall, and events are longer in duration than RBD. It is rare for RBD patients to leave the bed and continue acting out their dreams since most RBD patients awaken after falling out of bed. Sleepwalking and confusional arousals may be more likely to arise earlier in the night as well due to increased slow-wave sleep during the first half of the night.[49]

Nocturnal Epilepsy: Typically presents with stereotyped behaviors, classically with significant lower extremity involvement (ie, bicycling movements) in classic nocturnal frontal lobe epilepsy. Unlike patients with RBD who are immediately aware of their surroundings upon awakening, patients with nocturnal epilepsy are more likely to present with postictal confusion and wandering, along with other symptoms such as urinary incontinence and tongue biting, which are usually absent in RBD. The Frontal Lobe Epilepsy and Parasomnias Scale may be useful in differentiating nocturnal epilepsy from confusional arousals and RBD with a reported sensitivity of 70% and specificity of 100%.[50] Confirmation of seizures or epileptiform activity on sleep EEG or PSG is required for diagnosis.

Table 1
Differential diagnosis of rapid eye movement sleep behavior disorder

	RBD	OSA	Non-REM Parasomnias (Sleepwalking, Confusional Arousals)	Nocturnal Epilepsy	PTSD/TASD	PLMD	Nightmare Disorder
Age of onset	Middle-age, elderly	Adulthood	Childhood and young adults, rarely older adults	Childhood and young adults, rarely older adults	Adulthood	Adulthood	Children, young adults
Sleep stage	REM	NREM/REM	NREM	NREM	REM > NREM	NREM/REM	NREM/REM
Timing of behaviors	Second half of sleep period	Any time	First half of sleep period	Any time, possible predilection for 1st half of sleep period	Any Time	Any time	Any time
Semiology	Complex, brief, apparent goal-directed behaviors	Less purposeful or goal-directed than RBD	Variable, can be goal-directed but usually less jerky and brief compared with RBD (sleep walking), or flailing and less purposeful (confusional arousal)	Stereotyped, often excessive leg movements (bicycling)	Complex, brief, apparent goal-directed behaviors (TASD), less purposeful/ nonspecific or nongoal directed (PTSD)	Repetitive, relatively stereotyped movements occurring periodically usually isolated to the legs, rarely involving upper extremities or torso	No motor activity
RSWA	++	-	+/-	-	+	-	-
Sleep-related injury	++	-	+/-	+/-	+	-	-
Dream recall	++	+	+/-	-	+	+/-	-
Duration of symptoms	0–60 s	0–60 s	5–10 min, can be longer	3–5 min	0–60 s	Varies	Varies

Abbreviations: NREM, non-rapid eye movement; OSA, obstructive sleep apnea; PLMD, periodic limb movement disorder; PTSD, post-traumatic stress disorder; RBD, rapid eye movement sleep behavior disorder; REM, rapid eye movement; RSWA, rapid eye movement sleep without atonia; TASD, trauma-associated sleep disorder.

Post-traumatic stress disorder/trauma-associated sleep disorder: Requires a history of traumatic experience. Typically dream content mirrors the prior trauma but not always.[51] Quantitative analysis of REM muscle tone has shown RSWA, although typically this is not present to the same degree as that seen in RBD.[52] Please see the most UpToDate review of this topic in this issue of Sleep Medicine Clinics by Daniel Barone.

Periodic limb movement disorder (PLMD): PLMS are stereotyped, repetitive triple flexion movements of the lower extremities occurring during non-REM sleep which can be mistaken for dream enactment behaviors by bedpartners. Vivid dream recall is less common and the upper extremities are usually not involved, although in severe cases, there may be full body movement and upper extremity involvement. PSG in PLMD typically demonstrates periodic limb movements that resolve during REM sleep although these may extend into REM sleep in some cases. The majority of abnormal complex behaviors occur due to the limb movement–induced arousal.[53] RSWA is absent in the chin EMG.

Nightmare disorder: Will present with vivid dreams usually without associated motor behaviors although hypermotor activity may occur with arousal. RSWA is absent on PSG.

SUMMARY

RBD remains a fascinating parasomnia with varied presentations of dramatic, complex behaviors with loud vocalizations and vivid terrifying dreams to more minor jerks or semipurposeful movements with more pleasant dreams or no dream recall at all. Dream enactment behaviors are often not voluntarily discussed by patients or spouses so specifically questioning patients and bedparters for the presence of dream enactment is vital during clinical interview of patients. Timely and accurate diagnosis of RBD is vital, not only because of the importance of initiation of treatment to reduce risk of injury, but also given the prognostic implications of a diagnosis of iRBD. All patients with RBD should have a careful neurologic examination to detect subtle evidence of parkinsonism or cognitive impairment as well as to look for other abnormalities that could suggest a structural cause for their symptoms. Review of the PSG to confirm RSWA is central to an accurate diagnosis of RBD while also ruling out mimics. Patients often demonstrate REM behavioral events during PSG which are smaller amplitude jerks or semipurposeful movements during REM sleep, and careful video review is often required to detect these.

Manual quantification of RSWA remains a gold standard for diagnosis in research settings and only be done when there is no concurrent sleep-disordered breathing that may cause falsely elevated RSWA. A general rule of thumb for review of PSG for suspected RBD patients is that a chin RSWA levels of greater than 10% should be considered abnormal and is strongly suggestive of RBD and tonic RSWA is almost always abnormal. The FDS is evolving as the diagnostic muscle of choice for RBD diagnosis due to high sensitivity and specificity as well as limited risk of artifacts, although this muscle is not widely available in sleep clinics. The anterior tibialis muscle is highly prone to artifacts and should not be used as the only muscle for diagnosis of RBD when evaluating for RSWA.

CLINICS CARE POINTS

- The majority of RBD patients are unaware of their behaviors; collateral history from bedpartner or observer should always be obtained.
- Polysomnographic demonstration of RSWA is required for the diagnosis of RBD and determination of RSWA should only be done once sleep-disordered breathing is adequately treated to prevent false diagnosis.
- Most patients demonstrate minor REM behavioral events of elementary jerking or semipurposeful movements like repetitive finger and wrist flexion, known as "hand babbling," during overnight PSG which supports a diagnosis of RBD
- The chin (mentalis/submentalis) muscle and FDS muscles are the most sensitive and specific for RBD when evaluating RSWA, while the anterior tibialis is not specific and artifact prone.
- More than 10% to15% of any RSWA in the chin muscle is abnormal and the presence of tonic RSWA is almost always considered abnormal
- All patients with RBD require a detailed neurologic examination and close observation for the development of parkinsonism or cognitive impairment as well as other neurologic abnormalities that would suggest a structural cause for their RBD. Neuroimaging (specifically brain MRI) is recommended in patients with focal neurologic signs on examination (excluding parkinsonism); however, the majority of patients with RBD do not require neuroimaging.

DISCLOSURE

Dr Jones and Dr McCarter report no disclosures.

REFERENCES

1. Jouvet M, Delorme F. Locus coeruleus et sommeil paradoxal. C R Soc Biol 1965;159:895–9.
2. Schenck CH, Bundlie SR, Ettinger MG, et al. Chronic behavioral disorders of human REM sleep: a new category of parasomnia. Sleep 1986;9(2):293–308.
3. Fernandez-Arcos A, Iranzo A, Serradell M, et al. The clinical phenotype of idiopathic rapid eye movement sleep behavior disorder at presentation: a study in 203 consecutive patients. Sleep 2016;39(1):121–32.
4. Frauscher B, Gschliesser V, Brandauer E, et al. REM sleep behavior disorder in 703 sleep-disorder patients: the importance of eliciting a comprehensive sleep history. Sleep Med 2010;11(2):167–71.
5. Oudiette D, DeCock VC, Lavault S, et al. Nonviolent elaborate behaviors may also occur in REM sleep behavior disorder. Neurology 2009;72(6):551–7.
6. McCarter SJ, Boswell CL, St Louis EK, et al. Treatment outcomes in REM sleep behavior disorder. Sleep Med 2013;14(3):237–42.
7. McCarter SJ, St Louis EK, Boswell CL, et al. Factors associated with injury in REM sleep behavior disorder. Sleep Med 2014;15(11):1332–8.
8. Olson EJ, Boeve BF, Silber MH. Rapid eye movement sleep behaviour disorder: demographic, clinical and laboratory findings in 93 cases. Brain 2000;123(Pt 2):331–9.
9. Cesari M, Heidbreder A, St Louis EK, et al. Video-polysomnography procedures for diagnosis of rapid eye movement sleep behavior disorder (RBD) and the identification of its prodromal stages: guidelines from the International RBD Study Group. Sleep 2022;45(3). https://doi.org/10.1093/sleep/zsab257.
10. Lloyd R, Tippmann-Peikert M, Slocumb N, et al. Characteristics of REM sleep behavior disorder in childhood. J Clin Sleep Med 2012;8(2):127–31.
11. Postuma RB, Iranzo A, Hu M, et al. Risk and predictors of dementia and parkinsonism in idiopathic REM sleep behaviour disorder: a multicentre study. Brain 2019;142(3):744–59.
12. Haba-Rubio J, Frauscher B, Marques-Vidal P, et al. Prevalence and determinants of rapid eye movement sleep behavior disorder in the general population. Sleep 2018;41(2). https://doi.org/10.1093/sleep/zsx197.
13. Kang SH, Yoon IY, Lee SD, et al. REM sleep behavior disorder in the Korean elderly population: prevalence and clinical characteristics. Sleep 2013;36(8):1147–52.
14. Boeve BF, Molano JR, Ferman TJ, et al. Validation of the Mayo Sleep Questionnaire to screen for REM sleep behavior disorder in a community-based sample. J Clin Sleep Med 2013;9(5):475–80.
15. Boot BP, Boeve BF, Roberts RO, et al. Probable rapid eye movement sleep behavior disorder increases risk for mild cognitive impairment and Parkinson disease: a population-based study. Ann Neurol 2012;71(1):49–56.
16. Chiu SY, Wyman-Chick KA, Ferman TJ, et al. Sex differences in dementia with Lewy bodies: focused review of available evidence and future directions. Parkinsonism Relat Disord 2023;107:105285.
17. Schenck CH, Boeve BF, Mahowald MW. Delayed emergence of a parkinsonian disorder or dementia in 81% of older men initially diagnosed with idiopathic rapid eye movement sleep behavior disorder: a 16-year update on a previously reported series. Sleep Med 2013;14(8):744–8.
18. Schenck CH, Bundlie SR, Mahowald MW. Delayed emergence of a parkinsonian disorder in 38% of 29 older men initially diagnosed with idiopathic rapid eye movement sleep behaviour disorder. Neurology 1996;46(2):388–93.
19. Iranzo A, Fernandez-Arcos A, Tolosa E, et al. Neurodegenerative disorder risk in idiopathic REM sleep behavior disorder: study in 174 patients. PLoS One 2014;9(2):e89741.
20. Alexandres C, McCarter S, Tabatabai G, et al. Clinical features and phenoconversion risk in women with isolated REM sleep behavior disorder [abstract]. Mov Disord 2023;38(suppl 1).
21. Palma JA, Fernandez-Cordon C, Coon EA, et al. Prevalence of REM sleep behavior disorder in multiple system atrophy: a multicenter study and meta-analysis. Clin Auton Res 2015;25(1):69–75.
22. Ferman TJ, Boeve BF, Smith GE, et al. Inclusion of RBD improves the diagnostic classification of dementia with Lewy bodies. Neurology 2011;77(9):875–82.
23. Poryazova R, Oberholzer M, Baumann CR, et al. REM sleep behavior disorder in Parkinson's disease: a questionnaire-based survey. J Clin Sleep Med 2013;9(1):55–9.
24. Iranzo A. Sleep and neurological autoimmune diseases. Neuropsychopharmacology 2020;45(1):129–40.
25. Gadoth A, Devine MF, Pittock SJ, et al. Sleep disturbances associated with DPPX autoantibodies: a case series. J Neurol 2023;270(7):3543–52.
26. McCarter SJ, Tippmann-Peikert M, Sandness DJ, et al. Neuroimaging-evident lesional pathology associated with REM sleep behavior disorder. Sleep Med 2015;16(12):1502–10.
27. Boeve BF, Silber MH, Ferman TJ, et al. Clinicopathologic correlations in 172 cases of rapid eye movement sleep behavior disorder with or without a coexisting neurologic disorder. Sleep Med 2013;14(8):754–62.

28. Friedman JH. Presumed rapid eye movement behavior disorder in Machado-Joseph disease (spinocerebellar ataxia type 3). Mov Disord 2002;17(6):1350–3.

29. Shepard P, Lam EM, St Louis EK, et al. Sleep disturbances in myotonic dystrophy type 2. Eur Neurol 2012;68(6):377–80.

30. McCarter SJ, St Louis EK, Sandness DJ, et al. Antidepressants increase REM sleep muscle tone in patients with and without REM sleep behavior disorder. Sleep 2015;38(6):907–17.

31. Howell M, Avidan AY, Foldvary-Schaefer N, et al. Management of REM sleep behavior disorder: an American Academy of Sleep Medicine systematic review, meta-analysis, and GRADE assessment. J Clin Sleep Med 2023;19(4):769–810.

32. AAoS Medicine. International classification of sleep disorders. 3rd edition. Darien, IL: American Academy of Sleep Medicine; 2014.

33. Cesari M, Heidbreder A, St Louis EK, et al. Polysomnographic diagnosis of REM sleep behavior disorder: a change is needed. Sleep 2023;46(1). https://doi.org/10.1093/sleep/zsac276.

34. Frauscher B, Iranzo A, Hogl B, et al. Quantification of electromyographic activity during REM sleep in multiple muscles in REM sleep behavior disorder. Sleep 2008;31(5):724–31.

35. McCarter SJ, St Louis EK, Duwell EJ, et al. Diagnostic thresholds for quantitative REM sleep phasic burst duration, phasic and tonic muscle activity, and REM atonia index in REM sleep behavior disorder with and without comorbid obstructive sleep apnea. Sleep 2014;37(10):1649–62.

36. McCarter SJ, St Louis EK, Sandness DJ, et al. Diagnostic REM sleep muscle activity thresholds in patients with idiopathic REM sleep behavior disorder with and without obstructive sleep apnea. Sleep Med 2017;33:23–9.

37. Sixel-Doring F, Schweitzer M, Mollenhauer B, et al. Intraindividual variability of REM sleep behavior disorder in Parkinson's disease: a comparative assessment using a new REM sleep behavior disorder severity scale (RBDSS) for clinical routine. J Clin Sleep Med 2011;7(1):75–80.

38. Cesari M, Heidbreder A, Bergmann M, et al. Flexor digitorum superficialis muscular activity is more reliable than mentalis muscular activity for rapid eye movement sleep without atonia quantification: a study of interrater reliability for artifact correction in the context of semiautomated scoring of rapid eye movement sleep without atonia. Sleep 2021;44(9). https://doi.org/10.1093/sleep/zsab094.

39. Lapierre O, Montplaisir J. Polysomnographic features of REM sleep behavior disorder: development of a scoring method. Neurology 1992;42(7):1371–4.

40. Frauscher B, Iranzo A, Gaig C, et al. Normative EMG values during REM sleep for the diagnosis of REM sleep behavior disorder. Sleep 2012;35(6):835–47.

41. Feemster JC, Jung Y, Timm PC, et al. Normative and isolated rapid eye movement sleep without atonia in adults without REM sleep behavior disorder. Sleep 2019;42(10). https://doi.org/10.1093/sleep/zsz124.

42. Leclair-Visonneau L, Feemster JC, Bibi N, et al. Contemporary diagnostic visual and automated polysomnographic REM sleep without atonia thresholds in isolated REM sleep behavior disorder. J Clin Sleep Med 2023. https://doi.org/10.5664/jcsm.10862.

43. Raschella F, Scafa S, Puiatti A, et al. Actigraphy enables home screening of rapid eye movement behavior disorder in Parkinson's disease. Ann Neurol 2023;93(2):317–29.

44. Roguski A, Rayment D, Whone AL, et al. A Neurologist's Guide to REM sleep behavior disorder. Front Neurol 2020;11:610.

45. St Louis EK, Boeve BF. REM sleep behavior disorder: diagnosis, clinical implications, and future directions. Mayo Clin Proc 2017;92(11):1723–36.

46. Hogl B, Stefani A, Videnovic A. Idiopathic REM sleep behaviour disorder and neurodegeneration - an update. Nat Rev Neurol 2018;14(1):40–55.

47. Postuma RB, Gagnon JF, Bertrand JA, et al. Parkinson risk in idiopathic REM sleep behavior disorder: preparing for neuroprotective trials. Neurology 2015;84(11):1104–13.

48. Genier Marchand D, Montplaisir J, Postuma RB, et al. Detecting the cognitive prodrome of dementia with lewy bodies: a prospective study of rem sleep behavior disorder. Sleep 2017;40(1). https://doi.org/10.1093/sleep/zsw014.

49. Antelmi E, Lippolis M, Biscarini F, et al. REM sleep behavior disorder: mimics and variants. Sleep Med Rev 2021;60:101515.

50. Manni R, Terzaghi M, Repetto A. The FLEP scale in diagnosing nocturnal frontal lobe epilepsy, NREM and REM parasomnias: data from a tertiary sleep and epilepsy unit. Epilepsia 2008;49(9):1581–5.

51. Brock MS, Powell TA, Creamer JL, et al. Trauma associated sleep disorder: clinical developments 5 Years after discovery. Curr Psychiatr Rep 2019;21(9):80.

52. Feemster JC, Steele TA, Palermo KP, et al. Abnormal rapid eye movement sleep atonia control in chronic post-traumatic stress disorder. Sleep 2022;45(3). https://doi.org/10.1093/sleep/zsab259.

53. Gaig C, Iranzo A, Pujol M, et al. Periodic limb movements during sleep mimicking REM sleep behavior disorder: a new form of periodic limb movement disorder. Sleep 2017;40(3). https://doi.org/10.1093/sleep/zsw063.

Rapid Eye Movement Sleep Behavior Disorder
Management and Prognostic Counseling

Roneil Malkani, MD, MS[a,b,*]

KEYWORDS

- Rapid eye movement sleep behavior disorder • Neurodegeneration • Treatment
- Prognostic counseling • Parkinson disease • Dementia • Clonazepam • Melatonin

KEY POINTS

- Management of rapid eye movement sleep behavior disorder (RBD) entails pharmacologic and nonpharmacologic means to reduce the risk of sleep-related injuries to oneself and bedpartner, vivid or disruptive dreams, and bedpartner sleep disruption.
- Safety precautions to protect the sleep environment, such as padding nearby furniture or the floor, lowering the mattress, or installing a bedrail, are necessary to reduce risk of sleep-related injury and should be reviewed with patients at diagnosis and regularly thereafter.
- Pharmacologic management includes low-dose clonazepam, melatonin, transdermal rivastigmine, and pramipexole.
- The choice of pharmacologic agent may depend on the frequency and severity of dream-enactment episodes and be weighed against the risk of treatment-emergent adverse events such as cognitive dysfunction, sedation, and gait instability.
- Isolated RBD confers a high lifetime risk of neurodegenerative diseases. A patient-centered approach to risk disclosure preserving the patient's autonomy to know or not know is recommended.

INTRODUCTION

Rapid eye movement (REM) sleep behavior disorder (RBD) involves malfunction of the brainstem mechanisms of REM sleep, resulting in vivid or disruptive dreams, physical manifestations of dream mentation, or dream-enactment behaviors, which can lead to injuries to oneself or bedpartner. In addition, one with RBD may experience vivid and even frightening dreams. Video polysomnography (vPSG) is required for diagnosis to confirm the presence of REM sleep without atonia (RSWA) and exclude mimics such as obstructive sleep apnea (sleep apnea pseudo-RBD) and periodic limb movements in sleep (periodic limb movement pseudo-RBD).[1] If the diagnosis is consistent with RBD but vPSG is not available, then a diagnosis of probable RBD can be made. In some patients, RSWA is seen without historical or videographic evidence of dream-enactment behaviors or other clear cause. This has been termed isolated RSWA or "subclinical" RBD which may be a prodrome of RBD. Since there are no clinical symptoms, symptomatic treatment is not warranted, but such patients should be monitored for development of dream enactment. Once the diagnosis has been preliminarily made or confirmed, the next step is to initiate management to improve symptoms and reduce the risk of injury and sleep disruption.

a Department of Neurology, Northwestern University Feinberg School of Medicine, Chicago, IL, USA;
b Neurology Service, Jesse Brown Veterans Affairs Medical Center, 820 South Damen Avenue, Damen Building, 9th Floor, Chicago, IL 60612, USA
* Neurology Service, Jesse Brown Veterans Affairs Medical Center, 820 South Damen Avenue, Damen Building, 9th Floor, Chicago, IL 60612.
E-mail address: r-malkani@northwestern.edu

Sleep Med Clin 19 (2024) 83–92
https://doi.org/10.1016/j.jsmc.2023.12.001
1556-407X/24/Published by Elsevier Inc.

sleep.theclinics.com

Recent data support the presence of unique phenotypes of RBD. Isolated RBD (iRBD), previously referred to as idiopathic RBD, occurs in isolation without any other clear cause. This type is strongly associated with the future development and "phenoconversion" to neurodegenerative disorders over several years. Secondary (or symptomatic) RBD refers to RBD in the setting of other neurologic diseases such as Parkinson disease (PD) or narcolepsy. Drug-induced RBD may also occur, typically with antidepressants, such as the serotonin selective reuptake inhibitors (SSRIs) and serotonin norepinephrine reuptake inhibitors (SNRIs).

This review will discuss management strategies, including safety precautions and medications, for RBD and the importance and potential approaches in prognostic counseling of neurodegeneration risk for patients with iRBD.

DISCUSSION
Management Overview

Management of RBD encompasses counseling on the diagnosis, education on safety precautions, and consideration of nonpharmacologic and pharmacologic strategies. In addition to informing the patient of the presence of the diagnosis, including the course and risk of injury, there should be some discussion on the dreams. Many patients report having aggressive or violent dream imagery such as arguing with someone or defending oneself from an attacker or animal. These dreams can be disturbing, and patients may wonder if the content is a window into their inner psyche or subconscious, leading to further distress which they may not volunteer. However, such themes run across many with RBD and do not reflect the patient's personality, and indicating such is relieving to patients. Depending on the severity, treatment may start prior to polysomnographic confirmation to limit the risk of injury prior to the study. Because many treatments have been studied across isolated and secondary RBD, both will be included in the discussion on use across specific RBD types for certain treatments as applicable.

There are several important outcomes to evaluate and follow in patients undergoing treatment for RBD. The most critical outcomes to monitor are the frequency and intensity of dream-enactment behaviors and treatment-related adverse events.[2] In addition, these events worsen the patient's sleep quality and increase bedpartner sleep disruption. Vivid dreams further disrupt sleep quality and cause insomnia. While bedpartners will often sleep in separate rooms due to the disruption or potential injury, many will continue to sleep in the same bed or wish to return to sharing the bed, in which case the bedpartner's sleep disruption and potential injury should also be monitored. Not all patients will have the same degree or frequency of various symptoms. For example, dream enactment may be reported once every several months to several times nightly. The longitudinal change of RSWA has also been studied but is not routinely conducted in clinical practice. It is unclear if improvements in RSWA are associated with other important outcomes. The clinician should also monitor for adverse events from treatment, in particular development or worsening of daytime sleepiness and sedation, gait instability, and cognitive dysfunction, which may be seen with many of the treatments.

Of utmost importance for patients with iRBD is a disease modification treatment to slow or halt the progression of neurodegeneration. Unfortunately, to date there are no proven treatments available that modify disease course. In the meantime, regular exercise has the potential for disease modification and should be recommended.[3]

Safety Precautions

Once the diagnosis of RBD (or even probable RBD) is established, the most immediate goal is to reduce the risk of injury. Therefore, even prior to polysomnographic diagnosis, safety precautions to improve safety of the sleep environment must be reviewed with the patient or caregiver at each visit.[2] Such recommendations may include padding or moving away bedside furniture, padding the headboard or walls by the bed, cushioning the floor with a rug or mat, removing nearby glass/metal fixtures and sharp objects that could be injurious, including firearms, lowering the mattress, and adding a bedrail. Bedpartners who wish to continue sleeping in the same bed may need to add a pillow barrier between the patient and themselves to reduce their own risk of injury.

Some patients who have vigorous dream-enactment behaviors may not tolerate or respond to medications. In such instances, it is prudent to consider additional safety measures, such as a pressurized bed and Posey alarm. One small study showed that such an alarm customized with a familiar calming voice that activated during particularly active RBD episodes significantly reduced sleep-related injuries.[4] No adverse events were noted with the bed alarm.

Medication Management

There are many medication options for RBD symptoms that should be considered for most patients given that a single severe event could lead to serious injury.[5] Pharmacologic treatments are summarized in **Table 1**. While there is little evidence on combination therapy, it is common practice to combine treatments if the response to monotherapy is inadequate.

Melatonin is a neurohormone secreted by the pineal gland with a key role in modulating circadian rhythms, attenuating the wake-promoting signal generated by the suprachiasmatic nucleus. While its mechanism in improving RBD remains elusive, one possibility is through its effects on the circadian rhythm. Many observational studies support its use in reducing dream-enactment behaviors in RBD.[5] The only randomized controlled crossover trial on melatonin immediate release (IR) was in 8 RBD patients and found overall improvement.[6] Some studies also suggest it may reduce the severity of RSWA. Based on these data, melatonin IR has conditional approval for its use by the American Academy of Sleep Medicine RBD Management Practice Guidelines of 2023.[2] Melatonin is typically started at 3 mg nightly and titrated as needed to 15 mg nightly. Most patients noted improvement with 6 to 9 mg nightly. Potential side effects of melatonin include daytime sleepiness, nightmares or vivid dreams, and headaches. In many countries, melatonin is regulated, dosing is standardized, and it requires a prescription. However, in the United States, melatonin is not government regulated and is regarded as a nutraceutical and is available over the counter. As a result, the amount of melatonin may vary from what is noted on the bottle and even from lot to lot. Clinicians should therefore reconsider the formulation of melatonin if RBD symptoms suddenly worsen in temporal association with the new melatonin formulation or if symptoms do not improve.

Melatonin also comes in an extended-release or prolonged-release (PR) formulation. Two clinical trials assessed melatonin PR at various doses from 2 to 6 mg nightly in RBD, mainly iRBD. Neither trial noted improvement in RBD clinical outcomes, and one did not find improvement in RSWA.[7,8] However, another approach could be using melatonin PR in a "chronobiotic protocol." A retrospective review reported on melatonin PR 2 mg given at a fixed time 30 minutes before bedtime. Melatonin improved the RBD symptoms within the first month. Those who took it for at least 6 months showed persistent improvement even after stopping it, while those who took it for 1 to 3 months had a gradual return of symptoms after stopping it.[9] The persistent effect suggests a possible chronobiotic effect.

Clonazepam was the first medication noted to improve disruptive dream-enactment behaviors in RBD.[10] It is a long-acting benzodiazepine that may improve RBD symptoms through gamma-aminobutyric acid (GABA)-ergic inhibition of spinal motor neurons,[11] though it does not appear to restore muscle atonia or improve RSWA.[12] One randomized controlled trial and several observational studies have been published including those with iRBD and secondary RBD and have shown significant improvements in dream-enactment behavior frequency and intensity.[5,13] Clonazepam is dosed 0.25 to 1 mg nightly, though some may require higher doses to reduce RBD symptoms. Interestingly, patients can be given low-dose clonazepam for many years without concern for developing tolerance.[14] Given its mechanism, side effects include sedation, daytime sleepiness, gait imbalance, and cognitive impairment. As a result, caution should be used when considering clonazepam in patients with balance or cognitive dysfunction. Many patients with iRBD will develop PD or dementia with Lewy bodies (DLB), and those on clonazepam may need to transition to another treatment for RBD.[2]

Rivastigmine is a cholinesterase inhibitor used primarily in Alzheimer's disease and DLB. Its oral form causes gastrointestinal symptoms including vomiting and diarrhea, but the transdermal (TD) patch formulation bypasses these side effects. Two randomized crossover trials, including a total of 37 participants, found that TD rivastigmine 4.6 mg reduced dream-enactment behavior frequency over 7 to 9 weeks in patients with PD[15] or mild cognitive impairment,[16] who did not previously respond to treatment with melatonin or clonazepam. While the 4.6 mg dose was tested, TD rivastigmine can be dosed up to 13.3 mg daily for dementia. Side effects include skin irritation, daytime sleepiness, mild nausea, and orthostatic hypotension. Since bradycardia can result from the cholinergic effects of rivastigmine, an electrocardiogram should be performed prior to initiating therapy. This medication may be particularly helpful in patients who cannot use or tolerate clonazepam due to cognitive dysfunction.

Pramipexole is a dopamine receptor agonist used to improve motor symptoms of PD and restless legs syndrome. Its mechanism in RBD treatment is unclear since dopamine deficiency is not a feature underlying RBD. Several observational studies and one open-label trial in iRBD showed a significant reduction in RBD episodes with a low dose (mean 0.21 mg/day, range 0.125–0.375 mg/day).[17] For this purpose, pramipexole can be initiated at 0.125 mg at bedtime and titrated for symptoms. The limited available data on pramipexole for secondary RBD have shown mixed results. Side effects of pramipexole include daytime sleepiness, orthostatic hypotension, nausea, impulse control behaviors, and confusion.

Table 1
Summary of medication management options for rapid eye movement sleep behavior disorder

	Daily Dose	Frequency	RBD Types Represented in Clinical Trials	Adverse Events	AASM Recommendation[2]
Melatonin IR	3–15 mg	Nightly	iRBD, PD, narcolepsy	Sleepiness, headache, nausea	Conditional for iRBD and secondary RBD
Melatonin PR	2 mg	30 min before bedtime	iRBD, PD	Sleepiness, headache, nausea	Conditional for iRBD and secondary RBD
Clonazepam	0.25–1.0 mg[a]	Nightly	iRBD, PD, DLB, MSA, narcolepsy	Sleepiness, cognitive impairment	Conditional for iRBD and secondary RBD
Transdermal rivastigmine	4.6–13.3 mg	Every 24 h	Treatment resistant: PD or MCI	Skin irritation, nausea, diarrhea, vomiting, headache, bradycardia	Conditional for iRBD and secondary RBD
Pramipexole	0.125–2.0 mg	Nightly	iRBD	Nausea, orthostatic hypotension, sleepiness, confusion	Conditional for iRBD
Safinamide	50 mg	Daily	PD	Nausea, anxiety, headache, sleepiness, dyskinesias	
Sodium oxybate	4.5–9.0 g	Divided twice nightly	Treatment resistant: iRBD and PD	Anxiety, dizziness, anorexia, increased sweating, difficulty, cognitive impairment	
Memantine	5–20 mg	Daily, titrated to 10 mg twice daily	Dementia due to PD or DLB	Headache, dizziness, daytime sleepiness	
Drug discontinuation	N/A	N/A	Drug-induced RBD	Worsening of mood disorder	Conditional for drug-induced RBD

Abbreviations: AASM, American Academy of Sleep Medicine; DLB, dementia with lewy bodies; IR, immediate release; iRBD, isolated rapid eye movement sleep behavior disorder; MCI, mild cognitive impairment; MSA, multiple system atrophy; PD, Parkinson disease; PR, prolonged release.
[a] Higher doses may be needed.

Memantine is an N-methyl-D-aspartate receptor antagonist used in Alzheimer's disease. One randomized clinical trial of memantine up to 20 mg/day in patients with PD dementia and DLB who had probable RBD found decreased physical activity in the memantine group. However, the clinical outcome measure used is not a typical one used to assess RBD behaviors, and RBD diagnosis was not confirmed by vPSG in these patients, limiting interpretation of this study's findings.[18] Memantine is initiated at 5 mg in the morning and gradually titrated to 10 mg twice daily. Although not observed in the trial, common side effects of memantine include daytime sleepiness, dizziness, and headache.

Sodium oxybate is a sodium salt of gamma-hydroxybutyrate, an endogenous metabolite of the neurotransmitter $GABA_B$ receptor complex which is currently used to manage excessive daytime sleepiness, cataplexy, and disturbed nocturnal sleep in the setting of narcolepsy. It consolidates sleep and promotes slow-wave sleep. The use of sodium oxybate has previously been explored in previous case reports documenting the management of patients with RBD in the setting of narcolepsy or PD noted improvement in RBD symptoms.[5] A recent randomized clinical trial examined the application of sodium oxybate 4.5-9 g nightly in 2 divided doses versus placebo for RBD symptoms in 12 patients with iRBD and 12 patients with RBD due to PD. While no statistical differences between groups were observed, both the sodium oxybate and placebo groups improved in symptom frequency, highlighting the potential placebo responsiveness of RBD.[19]

Safinamide is a monoamine oxidase-B inhibitor with dopaminergic and nondopaminergic effects and is used in the treatment of PD. A randomized controlled crossover study of safinamide 50 mg in patients with symptomatic RBD in the setting of PD showed improvement in RBD episodes and the severity of RSWA after 3 months of use.[20] Side effects include nausea, anxiety, headache, daytime sleepiness, and increased dyskinesias.

Several other medications have been reported in either case series or small uncontrolled studies. These include anticonvulsants such as carbamazepine and gabapentin, antipsychotics, antidepressants such as paroxetine, and the melatonin receptor agonist, ramelteon.[5] Further data are needed to determine the potential of these medications for RBD.

RBD can be induced or worsened by various medications, particularly antidepressants such as (SSRI and SNRI medications. When drug-induced RBD is suspected, discontinuation of the offending agent should be considered in the appropriate case.[2] The benefits regarding RBD of stopping the medication need to be weighed against the potential risks of worsening mood and should be done in partnership with the patient's treating provider, for example their psychiatrist. Furthermore, it can take several weeks to months to see the resolution of dream-enactment behaviors. For those who require antidepressant therapy, bupropion has not been associated with RBD symptoms. In patients who successfully discontinue serotonergic antidepressants and have a resolution of RBD symptoms, a follow-up vPSG may be entertained to reevaluate the presence of RSWA, but longitudinal follow-up is still warranted to follow neurologic status.

PROGNOSTIC COUNSELING
Neurodegeneration Risk with Isolated Rapid Eye Movement Sleep Behavior Disorder

Several years after the discovery of RBD came the finding that those with the isolated form (iRBD) have a higher long-term risk of neurodegenerative diseases.[21] Since then, multiple cohorts have found very high lifetime risk of neurodegenerative diseases, particularly the α-synucleinopathies, a group of neurodegenerative diseases that include idiopathic PD, DLB, and multiple systems atrophy. The latency from diagnosis to phenoconversion (diagnosis of neurodegenerative disease) can be quite long, spanning even decades, although RBD symptoms can emerge even at or after the time of neurodegenerative diagnosis. About half of iRBD patients will be diagnosed with a neurodegenerative disease by about 8 years[22,23] and up to 91% by 14 years.[22] The annual conversion rate is 6.3%, though this is not linear.[23] The long latency reflects that these diseases develop insidiously over many years, with significant neurodegeneration having occurred prior to symptom onset. More recent data demonstrate that the only independent predictor of phenoconversion risk was the age at RBD at the time of diagnosis with the following observations: age less than 50 years may represent the lowest phenoconversion rates at about 1% per year, 2% per year risk of phenoconversion for 50 to 60 year age bracket, 4% per year for those 60 to 70 years of age, and 6% per year for those older than 70 (Alexandres, McCarter, Boeve, Silber, and St. Louis, 2023, unpublished data).

Diagnosis of these diseases is clinical, dependent on symptoms and signs of the disease, and sometimes with confirmation on pathologic testing. Further research has identified various risk markers to predict neurodegeneration course and timing of diagnosis. The most prominent risk factors include quantitative motor testing, abnormal dopamine transporter imaging, cognitive dysfunction, loss of olfaction, and erectile dysfunction.

Controversy in Prognostic Counseling

Despite the known and high lifetime risk of neurodegeneration, there is no consensus on risk disclosure, and this topic remains controversial for several reasons. First, the latency to neurodegenerative disease diagnosis can be several years, creating uncertainty of the future and risk prediction. Though the lifetime risk of neurodegeneration is high, a patient with iRBD may succumb to another illness prior to developing a neurodegenerative disease. Second, there are no disease-modifying therapies that are proven to reduce this risk. This contrasts with other diseases in which a known risk factor lends to risk-reduction treatments, such as mastectomy for women with the BRCA gene. It is uncomfortable for providers to disclose risk of terminal diseases without a way to cure them or lower their risk. Third, RBD may not be the presenting complaint for a patient, but it was uncovered during the interview. Other sleep-related complaints including sleep apnea or insomnia may be the patient's primary concern. One study of RBD patients found that 11% presented for another issue. This may happen because some patients may not be aware of the behaviors or recognize them as abnormal, and if the patient is not concerned then providers may be less enthusiastic about disclosing neurodegeneration risk.

Only a few studies have examined provider perspectives and clinical practice behaviors on risk disclosure in iRBD. In a Turkish study of neurologists, 15.3% favored disclosure for all patients, 6.8% favored no disclosure for all, while 77.9% favored disclosure under certain circumstances, particularly the patient's wish to know or if affected the management plan. However, the percentage of providers against disclosure decreased when reminded about recommendations of diet and exercise to possibly reduce neurodegeneration risk.[24] Another study consulted with 17 experts across 10 countries aimed to develop some guidance on risk disclosure. 41% recommended disclosure in all cases, while 41% would disclose if the patient expressed desire to know about the risks. Furthermore, while 41% would provide details of the risk, most recommended to use more vague terms depending on how much the patient wants to know, such as "significantly increased risk" or "higher risk."[25] Despite the fact that some patients may not want to know about their risk,

few providers appear to give patients the option. One study surveying sleep specialists on their disclosure practices found that only 31.8% asked the patient their preference on risk disclosure.[26] Many providers may not disclose at all. In one study examining clinical documentation, only 55% of iRBD patient records had documentation of prognostic counseling on neurodegeneration.[27]

There is a growing body of literature on patient perspectives on risk disclosure. One study examined patients with PD on their view on early diagnosis of PD, including about knowing the risks of PD prior to diagnosis. Almost half of patients would have wanted to know the risk, though that proportion increased to 85% if disclosure included instructions on lifestyle changes that may affect neurodegeneration risk.[28] Two recent studies examined iRBD patient experiences with risk disclosure. In one study of 31 patients with iRBD enrolled in a cohort study in the United Kingdom, about one-third were not told by their providers, though 90% would have liked to receive prognostic information. About 60% said it should be at the time of RBD diagnosis, and most wanted it to come from the provider making the RBD diagnosis. The other study examined 81 participants enrolled in a cohort study in the United States showed similar results, with 82% wanting to know about the neurodegeneration risk, and 75% reporting that they would lose trust in their provider if risk was not discussed. Interestingly, only 10% preferred to be asked about their preferences prior to risk disclosure.[29] It should be noted that these patients were part of a cohort study and were already aware of the risks.[30]

Approach to Prognostic Counseling

There are several ethical principles to consider in risk disclosure: beneficence, nonmaleficence, and autonomy. Beneficence requires that physicians act in the best interest of the patient. Risk disclosure gives patients the opportunity to plan for the future, consider risk-reduction strategies, and participate in clinical trials. Nonmaleficence requires that clinicians should do no harm, and risk disclosure may induce anxiety or hopelessness in the absence of disease-modifying therapies. Beneficence and nonmaleficence are often aligned, such as in the case of BRCA gene and preventative mastectomy or of colon cancer genetic risk and more frequent colonoscopy screenings. However, in the case of iRBD, these principles can be at odds with each other. Autonomy refers to the patient's right to self-determination and decision-making, and informed consent is an important component to maintain autonomy. Specifically, patients need to

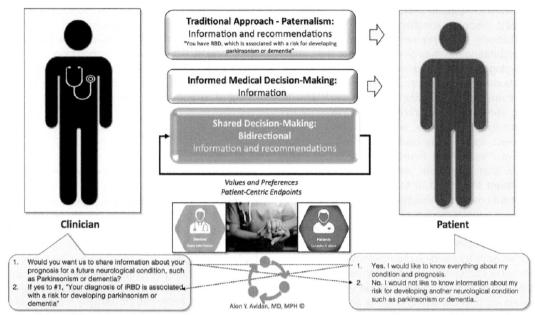

Fig. 1. Shared decision-making model in patients with isolated rapid eye movement (REM) sleep behavior disorder compared to traditional communication methods. Shared decision-making uses a patient-centered approach in which clinicians and patients work together to tailor the sharing of information and management strategies, incorporating the patient's preferences and values, and pursue the best plan for individual clinical situations. (Image courtesy of Alon Avidan, MD, MPH.)

be informed about risks of neurodegenerative diseases to make decisions for the future. However, autonomy also requires that patients have the right to know (or not know) about risks. While some patients want to know to take advantage of potential benefits of knowing, others may wish to not be concerned about risks they cannot mitigate.

There are 2 general methods to approach this situation: "disclosure" and "watchful waiting."[31] With risk disclosure, the patient is provided with information on the link between RBD and neurodegeneration. The advantage of this method is that it respects the patients' right to know about their health and allows patients to life-plan (eg, save finances for future care, fulfill life goals, advance care planning), participate in clinical trials of potential disease-modifying therapies, and be monitored for early neurologic diagnosis. The disadvantages include inducing more anxiety, despair, or stigma associated with impending disease, particularly when there is uncertainty as to when it may occur and in the absence of disease-modifying treatments. With watchful waiting, the clinician withholds risk information unless the patient requests it. While this may address the disadvantage of disclosure, if patients learn of the links between RBD and neurodegeneration through other means such as the Internet, the patient-clinician relationship may be damaged.

A preferable method is a shared decision-making approach (**Fig. 1**), in which patients are presented with the option of knowing or not knowing about risks.[25,31] With this, patients may be asked what they know about RBD and where they learned it. If they are not aware, they can be informed that RBD may be associated with future health risk in their lifetime and then they may be asked if they want to know more. The amount and detail of the information provided should be tailored to the needs of the patient. The clinician can also evaluate the risk based on the presence of other risk markers and monitor for signs and symptoms of neurodegenerative diseases. In patients who do not wish to know, a watchful waiting approach can be followed. The discussion can be approached again at a future visit, and if still not desired, the clinician can offer to discuss it later if the patient wishes.

FUTURE DIRECTIONS

Much research should be done for symptomatic treatment of RBD. First, the evidence for the medications discussed above is based on observations studies with only a few randomized controlled trials. Some studies, such as with sodium oxybate, show a strong placebo response. Therefore, there is great need for vigorous randomized controlled trials in RBD (isolated and secondary) to establish efficacy. Second, mechanisms for most of the medications, including melatonin are unclear, and understanding this may give insight into the pathophysiology of RBD. Third, while the preponderance of data on melatonin support the use of IR formulation, there is still little evidence to support PR melatonin. The chronobiotic protocol with low-dose PR melatonin[9] should be replicated and further explored, as this may clarify melatonin's mechanism of effect in RBD. Fourth, while there are treatments that can work well in RBD, there are significant limitations in tolerability, especially in those with neurodegenerative diseases, due to balance or cognitive dysfunction. New treatments that do not worsen these issues or cause significant daytime sleepiness are needed. Fifth, since most studies have focused on dream-enactment behaviors but not other clinical outcomes associated with RBD, future studies should include additional outcomes such as disturbing dreams and bedpartner sleep disruption.[5]

Beyond symptomatic treatment for RBD, the "holy grail" is to find neuroprotective or disease-modifying therapies to slow or halt the progression of neurodegeneration in iRBD patients. This population is at high risk but does not yet have sufficient pathology to have symptoms. Many clinical trials of potential disease-modifying agents in patients with PD have failed, though at that stage it may have been too late for those agents to slow disease progression. Clinical trials in RBD are needed to see if the neurodegenerative process can be altered in the prodromal stage, but given the long latency to neurodegenerative disease diagnosis, reliable biomarkers sensitive to disease progression will be vital to such efforts. Furthermore, given the number patients needed for such a trial, it will take a multicenter approach.[23]

Finally, guidelines on risk disclosure for neurodegeneration are needed. Much information is available on the Internet, so many patients are learning about this risk even if clinicians do not inform their patients. While some have attempted to do so,[25] a more formal consensus panel that includes sleep specialists, neurologists, ethicists, and patients would be helpful to develop more widely accepted or official guidelines.

SUMMARY

Once the diagnosis of RBD is suspected or established, management includes first and foremost discussion of sleep environment modification to reduce risk of sleep-related injuries. Various medications are recommended, particularly low-dose clonazepam, melatonin, rivastigmine, and pramipexole. The choice of medication may vary based on the associated disease and cognitive or balance dysfunction and may change from iRBD to secondary RBD. Given the strong long-term risks associated with iRBD, disease-modifying treatments are desperately needed to slow or halt the onset of neurodegenerative diseases.

CLINICS CARE POINTS

- Management of RBD symptoms focuses on preventing sleep-related injury to oneself and bedpartner and reducing disturbing dreams.
- At diagnosis and each visit, clinicians should review strategies to improve bedroom safety, such as moving away or padding bedside furniture, removing potentially injurious objects, lowering the mattress, installing a bedrail, and padding the floor.
- Medications are often used to reduce RBD symptoms and include low-dose clonazepam, melatonin, TD rivastigmine, and pramipexole. Drug discontinuation for drug-induced RBD should be considered if the benefit to risk ratio is favorable.
- Melatonin is the first-line treatment for those with cognitive dysfunction or postural instability.
- Patients with iRBD on clonazepam who eventually develop neurodegenerative diseases may need to change to another medication if they develop cognitive dysfunction or postural instability.
- RBD is associated with a high lifetime risk of neurodegenerative diseases, with 50% developing such a condition within 8 years. Patients should be monitored for neurodegenerative diseases for early diagnosis.
- Prognostic counseling for neurodegenerative diseases should be patient-entered and use a shared decision-making approach to protect the patient's autonomy while also balancing the principles of beneficence and nonmaleficence.

ACKNOWLEDGMENTS

This material is the result of work supported with resources and the use of facilities at the Jesse Brown VA Medical Center, Chicago, Illinois. The views expressed in this article are those of the authors and do not necessarily reflect the position or policy of the Department of Veterans Affairs or the US government.

DISCLOSURE

Dr R. Malkani has nothing to disclose.

REFERENCES

1. American Academy of Sleep Medicine. International classification of sleep disorders. 3rd edition. Darien, IL: American Academy of Sleep Medicine; 2014.
2. Howell M, Avidan AY, Foldvary-Schaefer N, et al. Management of REM sleep behavior disorder: an American Academy of Sleep Medicine clinical practice guideline. J Clin Sleep Med 2023;19(4):759–68.
3. McCarter SJ, Boeve BF, Graff-Radford NR, et al. Neuroprotection in idiopathic REM sleep behavior disorder: a role for exercise? Sleep 2019;42(6):zsz064.
4. Howell MJ, Arneson PA, Schenck CH. A novel therapy for REM sleep behavior disorder (RBD). J Clin Sleep Med 2011;7(6):639–644a.
5. Howell M, Avidan AY, Foldvary-Schaefer N, et al. Management of REM sleep behavior disorder: an American Academy of Sleep Medicine systematic review, meta-analysis, and GRADE assessment. J Clin Sleep Med 2023;19(4):769–810.
6. Kunz D, Mahlberg R. A two-part, double-blind, placebo-controlled trial of exogenous melatonin in REM sleep behaviour disorder. J Sleep Res 2010; 19(4):591–6.
7. Gilat M, Coeytaux Jackson A, Marshall NS, et al. Melatonin for rapid eye movement sleep behavior disorder in Parkinson's disease: a randomised controlled trial. Mov Disord 2020;35(2):344–9.
8. Jun JS, Kim R, Ryun JI, et al. Prolonged-release melatonin in patients with idiopathic REM sleep behavior disorder. Ann Clin Transl Neurol 2019; 6(4):716–22.
9. Kunz D, Stotz S, Bes F. Treatment of isolated REM sleep behavior disorder using melatonin as a chronobiotic. J Pineal Res 2021;71(2):e12759.
10. Schenck CH, Bundlie SR, Ettinger MG, et al. Chronic behavioral disorders of human REM sleep: a new category of parasomnia. Sleep 1986;9(2):293–308.
11. Brooks PL, Peever JH. Impaired GABA and glycine transmission triggers cardinal features of rapid eye movement sleep behavior disorder in mice. J Neurosci 2011;31(19):7111–21.
12. Ferri R, Zucconi M, Marelli S, et al. Effects of long-term use of clonazepam on nonrapid eye movement sleep patterns in rapid eye movement sleep behavior disorder. Sleep Med 2013;14(5):399–406.
13. Shin C, Park H, Lee WW, et al. Clonazepam for probable REM sleep behavior disorder in Parkinson's disease: a randomized placebo-controlled trial. J Neurol Sci 2019;401:81–6.
14. Schenck CH, Mahowald MW. Long-term, nightly benzodiazepine treatment of injurious parasomnias and other disorders of disrupted nocturnal sleep in 170 adults. Am J Med 1996;100(3):333–7.
15. Di Giacopo R, Fasano A, Quaranta D, et al. Rivastigmine as alternative treatment for refractory REM behavior disorder in Parkinson's disease. Mov Disord 2012;27(4):559–61.
16. Brunetti V, Losurdo A, Testani E, et al. Rivastigmine for refractory REM behavior disorder in mild cognitive impairment. Curr Alzheimer Res 2014;11(3):267–73.
17. Sasai T, Matsuura M, Inoue Y. Factors associated with the effect of pramipexole on symptoms of idiopathic REM sleep behavior disorder. Parkinsonism Relat Disord 2013;19(2):153–7.
18. Larsson V, Aarsland D, Ballard C, et al. The effect of memantine on sleep behaviour in dementia with Lewy bodies and Parkinson's disease dementia. Int J Geriatr Psychiatry 2010;25(10):1030–8.
19. During EH, Hernandez B, Miglis MG, et al. Sodium oxybate in treatment-resistant rapid-eye-movement sleep behavior disorder. Sleep 2023;46(8):zsad103.
20. Plastino M, Gorgone G, Fava A, et al. Effects of safinamide on REM sleep behavior disorder in Parkinson disease: a randomized, longitudinal, cross-over pilot study. J Clin Neurosci 2021;91:306–12.
21. Schenck CH, Bundlie SR, Mahowald MW. Delayed emergence of a parkinsonian disorder in 38% of 29 older men initially diagnosed with idiopathic rapid eye movement sleep behaviour disorder. Neurology 1996;46(2):388–93.
22. Iranzo A, Fernandez-Arcos A, Tolosa E, et al. Neurodegenerative disorder risk in idiopathic REM sleep behavior disorder: study in 174 patients. PLoS One 2014;9(2):e89741.
23. Postuma RB, Iranzo A, Hu M, et al. Risk and predictors of dementia and parkinsonism in idiopathic REM sleep behaviour disorder: a multicentre study. Brain 2019;142(3):744–59.
24. Kayis G, Yilmaz R, Arda B, et al. Risk disclosure in prodromal Parkinson's disease - a survey of neurologists. Parkinsonism Relat Disord 2023;106:105240.
25. Schaeffer E, Toedt I, Köhler S, et al. Risk disclosure in prodromal Parkinson's disease. Mov Disord 2021; 36(12):2833–9.
26. Teigen LN, Sharp RR, Hirsch JR, et al. Specialist approaches to prognostic counseling in isolated REM sleep behavior disorder. Sleep Med 2021;79:107–12.
27. Feinstein MA, Sharp RR, Sandness DJ, et al. Physician and patient determinants of prognostic counseling in idiopathic REM sleep-behavior disorder. Sleep Med 2019;62:80–5.
28. Schaeffer E, Rogge A, Nieding K, et al. Patients' views on the ethical challenges of early Parkinson disease detection. Neurology 2020;94(19):e2037–44.

29. Gossard TR, Teigen LN, Yoo S, et al. Patient values and preferences regarding prognostic counseling in isolated REM sleep behavior disorder. Sleep 2023;46(1):zsac244.

30. Pérez-Carbonell L, Simonet C, Chohan H, et al. The views of patients with isolated rapid eye movement sleep behavior disorder on risk disclosure. Mov Disord 2023;38(6):1089–93.

31. Malkani RG, Wenger NS. REM sleep behavior disorder as a pathway to dementia: if, when, how, what, and why should physicians disclose the diagnosis and risk for dementia. Curr Sleep Med Rep 2021;7(3):57–64.

Trauma-Associated Sleep Disorder

Daniel A. Barone, MD

KEYWORDS

- Parasomnia • Trauma • Rapid eye movement behavior disorder • Post-traumatic stress disorder
- Nightmares • Sleep disorder

KEY POINTS

- Trauma-associated sleep disorder (TASD) is a proposed parasomnia that develops following a traumatic event, consisting of clinical features of trauma-related nightmares, disruptive nocturnal behaviors, and autonomic disturbances.
- TASD shares similarities with post-traumatic stress disorder, and diagnostic criteria with rapid eye movement sleep behavior disorder.
- The underlying pathophysiology of TASD and how it relates to other parasomnias are not well understood.
- Proposed treatment includes prazosin and management of comorbid sleep disorders.

INTRODUCTION

Nightmares and disruptive nocturnal behaviors that develop after traumatic experiences are known to overlap with other parasomnias. Trauma-associated sleep disorder (TASD) is a proposed parasomnia[1] that develops following a traumatic event, consisting of clinical features of trauma-related nightmares, disruptive nocturnal behaviors, and autonomic disturbances,[2] sharing similarities with post-traumatic stress disorder (PTSD) and diagnostic criteria with rapid eye movement (REM) behavior disorder (RBD). The purpose of this article is to characterize and highlight the clinical features of this condition and note the proposed treatments and areas of further research need.

BACKGROUND

Those who have survived a traumatic experience, both with or without PTSD, often report various sleep disturbances; these consist of trauma-related nightmares, autonomic hyperarousal, and excessive movements.[1] The sleep disturbances that follow a traumatic experience are predictors for physical and psychiatric symptoms, with a bidirectional relationship between sleep, mood, and anxiety.[3] TASD is distinct from PTSD and RBD, although it shares features with both.[1,4,5]

The most notable distinction among the symptoms of TASD (compared with nightmares, for example) is the presence of dream enactment behavior (DEB), occurring with excessive movements and complex vocal and motor behaviors during sleep (both in non-REM (NREM) and REM),[5] and loss or dysregulation of normal REM sleep atonia (appearing similarly to that seen in RBD).[6] See **Box 1** for conditions that should be included in a differential diagnosis of sleep enactment behaviors.

The differences of these disorders can usually be identified with detailed history taking, but a video-monitored polysomnographic study is often warranted.

Additionally, in TASD, the DEB and other symptoms occur in close temporal proximity to trauma; this, plus other features that would be unusual in RBD, are present, such as a nightmare theme and presentation at a much younger age.[5,6] Furthermore, symptoms of hyperarousal are a key feature of TASD, and serve as a main differentiator from the potential neurodegenerative changes in idiopathic RBD.[5]

Symptoms consistent with TASD are not uncommon in military personnel or veterans with combat exposure.[8] The first reports of TASD

Weill Cornell Center for Sleep Medicine, Weill Cornell Medicine, New York-Presbyterian, 425 East 61st Street, 5th Floor, New York, NY 10065, USA
E-mail address: dab9129@med.cornell.edu

Sleep Med Clin 19 (2024) 93–99
https://doi.org/10.1016/j.jsmc.2023.10.005
1556-407X/24/© 2023 Elsevier Inc. All rights reserved.

included young, active duty military personnel[1] who presented with trauma-related nightmares, disruptive nocturnal behaviors such as DEB, and autonomic hyperactivity following combat-related trauma.[2] However, there now exist reports in older veterans with likely TASD,[6,8,9] which bolster the notion that this condition is not a transient phenomenon, but rather a chronic sleep disorder.[2]

A recent study describing the prevalence, demographics, and clinical characteristics of probable TASD in post-9/11 veterans, found that more than 1 out of 10 post-9/11 veterans (12.1%, 95% confidence interval [CI]: 11.1% to 13.2%) report symptoms consistent with TASD.[10] There did not appear to be a difference between among male and female veterans with regards to prevalence, but a small difference regarding race was observed, with a slightly higher proportion of Black or African American individuals among those with probable TASD. Additionally, veterans with probable TASD were more likely to list Army as their current or most recent branch, which is consistent with other data[11] demonstrating that sleep disorders are more frequently diagnosed in those who have served in the Army, possibly related to higher rate of deployments and associated combat exposure.[10]

A patient's age at the time of trauma exposure may impact the development of TASD. In 1 report, avalanche survivors who were children (ages 2–12) at the time of trauma exposure were more likely to endorse DEB 16 years later (relative risk: 3.54), but those who were adults at the time of the exposure reported increased trauma-associated nightmares (relative risk: 2.69) without an increase in DEB.[12] These findings suggest that an immature brain may be susceptible to the development of trauma-related motor pathologies.[9]

An exemplary case of probable TASD has been reported in the literature[6]; a 53-year-old man, who had been previously diagnosed with PTSD following military service in the US Army, presented with DEB and complex motor behavior during sleep. After discharge, his wife observed frequent yelling and jerking during sleep with dream mentation reminiscent of traumatic military experiences. Polysomnography (**Fig. 1**) demonstrated REM sleep without atonia (RSWA) and severe obstructive sleep apnea treated with nasal continuous positive airway pressure (CPAP). DEB still persisted despite nasal CPAP and sequential fluoxetine, escitalopram, prazosin, and melatonin trials. The patient presented overlapping clinical features of

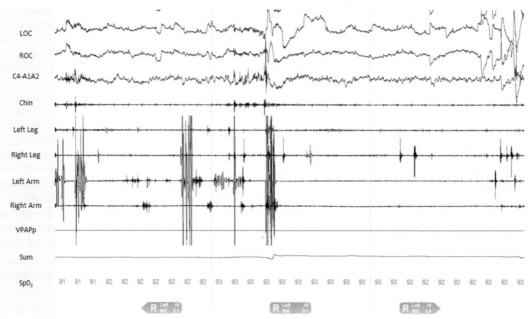

Fig. 1. 30-second epoch demonstrating a loss of normal REM sleep atonia in a 53-year-old man with probable TASD.[6]

PTSD and RBD with polysomnography features of RSWA supportive of idiopathic RBD without suggestion of underlying synucleinopathy.[6]

Given the overlap of TASD with symptoms of PTSD and with RBD, it is imperative that a review focusing on TASD includes a discussion on these other conditions insofar as delineating the similarities and differences between them.

POST-TRAUMATIC STRESS DISORDER

PTSD is a psychiatric condition resulting from experiencing, witnessing, or learning about an actual or threatened traumatic event[13,14] (**Box 2**). Insomnia and nightmares are common in patients with PTSD, and are associated with worse psychological and physical health, as well as worse treatment outcomes.

A patient must have symptoms from each of 5 criteria along with the presence of symptoms lasting for more than 1 month, creating distress or functional impairment, and that are not caused by medication, substance use, or other illness.

The primary nocturnal manifestation of PTSD is nightmares[16]; however, when nightmares include DEB, this transcends the established diagnostic criteria and thus merits consideration for TASD.[9,17] Trauma-associated nightmares commonly follow a traumatic experience, and those associated with PTSD may be more severe and distressing. The inciting experience is typically in the setting of extreme traumatic stress coupled with periods of sleep disruption and/or deprivation.[18] Some trauma survivors report trauma-associated nightmares accompanied by disruptive nocturnal behaviors.[10]

Those with PTSD have been demonstrated to have disturbances in sleep in general and REM sleep in particular,[19] including motor dysfunction,[20] increased activity in the REM-on and wake-promoting regions of the amygdala and medial prefrontal cortex, and corresponding decreased activity in the REM-off and anterior hypothalamic sleep-facilitating regions.[21] In 1 report of 27 US veterans with RBD, 20 subjects had suffered a previous major stressful life event; 15 of these also developed comorbid PTSD.[22] Considering that repeated traumas cause increased noradrenaline turnover, leading to its depletion in the locus coeruleus (LC), which in turn exerts an inhibitory action on the lateral dorsal tegmentum (LDT), the authors hypothesized that an LC dysfunction might underlie both these disorders.[22] Furthermore, 1 study found Vietnam combat veterans with PTSD had a higher percentage of REM-sleep epochs with at least 1 prolonged twitch burst.[20] PTSD may alter cortical thickness and regional brain volumes in structures involved in REM sleep control and dreaming, such as reduced amygdala and hippocampal volumes[23,24] (**Fig. 2**).

In 1 report, veterans with probable TASD were much more likely to have comorbid mental health disorders, particularly PTSD; there was also an increase in major depression, suicidal ideation, and self-reported trouble controlling violent behavior, compared to those without probable TASD.[10] A study of veteran suicidality demonstrated that the peak incidence of suicide occurs between 12 a.m. and 3 a.m.[26]; it was posited that this window may coincide with the causes of nocturnal distress and wakefulness resulting from sleep disorders (such as TASD).[10] Indeed, TASD should be considered a severe sleep disorder, and the associated

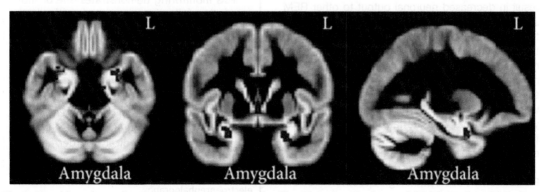

Fig. 2. Voxel-based morphometry analyses indicating significantly reduced volume of the bilateral anterior amygdala in the PTSD group compared with the control group (L: left).[25]

nocturnal distress and wakefulness highlight the need to determine appropriate treatment.[10]

In 1 recent paper,[10] it was demonstrated that 23% of veterans with TASD did not have PTSD, further supporting the notion that these are likely 2 distinct, but overlapping clinical disorders.[5] Although nightmares frequently occur in PTSD, the occurrence of disruptive nocturnal behaviors, such as DEB, are a symptom and objective finding that distinguishes TASD from PTSD.[2] It should also be mentioned that the criteria for TASD, in which there is a history of altered dream mentation related to a prior traumatic event, results in nearly every patient with PTSD potentially meeting the diagnostic criteria, prompting the need for further clarification.[18] Future studies will aid in determining if TASD is, in fact, a distinct disorder evolving from PTSD, or if it resides in a realm between PTSD and RBD, an interaction between PTSD symptoms in an individual harboring otherwise-silent pre-existing synuclein pathology.[6]

RAPID EYE MOVEMENT SLEEP BEHAVIOR DISORDER

RBD is a parasomnia consisting of elevated muscle tone during REM sleep (ie, RSWA) combined with a history of recurrent nocturnal DEB[27]. The proposed diagnostic criteria for TASD are clinical in nature and rely on symptoms that are self-reported and/ or provided by a bed partner, leading to possible overlap with RBD and/or misdiagnosis.[28] However, the preceding trauma helps to distinguish TASD from RBD, as RBD is not reported to develop after traumatic exposure.[29] Additionally, although disruptive nocturnal behaviors are present in both TASD and RBD, RBD lacks the autonomic hyperactivity (ie, tachycardia, tachypnea, diaphoresis) that has been noted in patients with TASD.[2,17]

The fundamental mechanisms of TASD and its overlapping symptoms with other parasomnias are poorly understood. As described earlier, the reduction in LC neurons following a traumatic event could result in decreased neuronal output to other REM sleep-modulating nuclei such as the pedunculopontine and magnocellularis nuclei,[30] in a manner similar to the pathophysiologic process underlying RBD, resulting in both loss of normal REM sleep atonia regulation and increased motor activity during REM sleep as seen in RBD.[22] Some have postulated whether TASD is similar to the cases of RBD in younger patients who are taking antidepressants, thus posing a completely different prognosis in terms of development of neurodegenerative disease.[6]

Ultimately, the possibility remains that TASD and RBD are on the same pathologic spectrum. However, individuals with TASD report having an inciting traumatic experience, as well as a history of dream mentation related to this prior traumatic experience and evidence of autonomic hyperarousal not caused by sleep-disordered breathing; these facts differentiate it from RBD. Additionally, capturing overt DEB in RBD can occur commonly, but this is somewhat rarer in TASD. Further prospective and longitudinal follow-up of this and other cases will be necessary to determine where TASD falls on this spectrum, and to determine the risk of phenoconversion.[6]

DIAGNOSTIC CRITERIA

As previously stated, TASD consists of features of trauma-related nightmares, disruptive nocturnal behaviors, and autonomic disturbances, and shares similarities with PTSD and RBD. However, the pathophysiology of TASD and how it relates to other parasomnias is not well understood, and only proposed diagnostic criteria exist (**Box 3**).

Box 3
Proposed criteria for trauma-associated sleep disorder[1,5,28]

A. Onset of symptoms after combat or other traumatic experience

B. A history of altered dream mentation that is related to prior traumatic experience

C. Self or witnessed reports of disruptive nocturnal behaviors to include at least 1 of the following:

  1. Abnormal vocalizations

    a. Moaning, screaming, or yelling

  2. Abnormal motor behaviors in sleep

    b. Tossing, turning, or thrashing

    c. Combative behaviors such as striking bed partner

D. Symptoms of autonomic hyperarousal or PSG monitoring demonstrates one or more of the following associated with dream mentation

  1. Tachycardia

  2. Tachypnea

  3. Diaphoresis

E. There is an absence of EEG epileptiform activity on PSG and the disturbance is not better explained by another sleep disorder, mental disorder, medical disorder, medication, or substance use

A patient must meet all Criteria A-E, EEG: electroencephalography.

Table 1
A selection of relevant literature

Mysliwiec V, et al. Trauma associated sleep disorder: a proposed parasomnia encompassing disruptive nocturnal behaviors, nightmares, and REM without atonia in trauma survivors. J Clin Sleep Med 2014;10(10):1143–8.	Characterization of the clinical, polysomnographic and treatment responses of patients with disruptive nocturnal behaviors and nightmares following traumatic experiences; utilizes a case series of 4 young male, active duty US Army soldiers; TASD is proposed as a unique sleep disorder[1]
Mysliwiec V, et al. Trauma associated sleep disorder: a parasomnia induced by trauma. Sleep Med Rev 2018;37:94–104.	Theoretic review: (1) summarizing the known cases and clinical findings supporting TASD, (2) differentiating TASD from clinical disorders with which it has overlapping features, (3) proposing criteria for the diagnosis of TASD, and 4) presenting a hypothetical neurobiological model for the pathophysiology of TASD[5]
Feemster JC, et al. Trauma-associated sleep disorder: a posttraumatic stress/rem sleep behavior disorder mash-up? J Clin Sleep Med 2019;15(2):345–349.	The authors report RSWA and other neurologic features in a patient with complex vocal and motor DEB following traumatic combat military exposure; the patient demonstrated overlapping clinical features of PTSD and RBD with PSG features of RSWA supportive of idiopathic RBD but not suggesting underlying synucleinopathy[6]
Brock MS, et al. Clinical and polysomnographic features of trauma associated sleep disorder. J Clin Sleep Med 2022;18(12):2775–2784.	Case series including clinical interview and detailed video-PSG review of 40 patients; clinical and video-polysomnography correlations are invaluable in assessing patients with TASD to document objective abnormalities; this case series provides a further basis for establishing TASD as a unique parasomnia[2]
Taylor DJ, et al; Consortium to Alleviate PTSD. Treatment of comorbid sleep disorders and posttraumatic stress disorder in U.S. active duty military personnel: a pilot randomized clinical trial. J Trauma Stress 2023 Jun 15.	This pilot study suggests that treating comorbid insomnia, nightmares, and PTSD symptoms results in clinically meaningful advantages in improvement for all 3 concerns compared with treating PTSD alone[31]
Taylor KA, et al. VA Mid-Atlantic MIRECC Registry Workgroup; Ulmer CS. Probable trauma associated sleep disorder in post-9/11 US veterans. Sleep Adv 2023 Jan 12;4(1):zpad001.	Used cross-sectional data from the postdeployment mental health study of post-9/11 veterans, including 3618 veterans (22.7% female); TASD prevalence was 12.1% and sex-stratified prevalence was similar for female and male veterans. Veterans with TASD had a much higher comorbid prevalence of PTSD and MDD; combat was the highest reported distressing traumatic experience among veterans with TASD (62.6%); supports the need for improved screening and evaluation for TASD in veterans, which is currently not performed in routine clinical practice[10]

Abbreviations: DEB, dream enactment behavior; MDD, major depressive disorder; PTSD; post-traumatic stress disorder; RBD, REM behavior disorder; RSWA, REM sleep without atonia, TASD, trauma-associated sleep disorder.

MANAGEMENT

The standard treatment approach for patients with PTSD includes cognitive behavioral therapy for insomnia (CBT-I) and cognitive processing therapy.[31] For patients with RBD, counseling on bed environment safety and use of melatonin and/or clonazepam are recommended.[32] Unfortunately, the treatment paradigm for TASD is plagued by a paucity of data, although there is speculation that prazosin may be efficacious.

Prazosin is a centrally active alpha-1-adrenergic receptor antagonist, and TASD symptoms have been shown to improve with its use (suggesting that TASD could be driven by hyper-adrenergic function).[6] In a recent paper, the primary pharmacologic treatment for TASD was prazosin, ranging in dosages from 1 mg to 8 mg, with most patients demonstrating improvement in their symptoms.[2] However, the question as whether to this pharmacologic treatment alone was the reason for improvement or was it some combination of their overall sleep management is a question that remains unanswered; these patients received positive airway pressure (PAP) therapy, CBT-I, and/or imagery rehearsal therapy.[2]

Once considered the standard treatment for PTSD-associated trauma nightmares,[33] several clinical trials, including a meta-analysis of placebo-controlled studies, showed prazosin to significantly improve nightmare frequency, PTSD severity, and sleep quality.[34] However, a large multicenter trial of prazosin in military veterans with chronic PTSD did not demonstrate beneficial outcomes.[35] Additionally, prazosin may not be effective in patients with chronic PTSD with obstructive sleep apnea because of interference of the drug's mechanism or masking of its beneficial effects.[35]

Although there has been a change in the clinical practice guidelines for treatment of nightmare disorder,[36] some have surmised that objective sleep testing via polysomnography could identify patients with disruptive nocturnal behaviors and/or autonomic hyperactivity (ie, TASD) that may better respond to this antiadrenergic therapy.[2] Further controlled studies of prazosin and other treatments typically effective for RBD (such as melatonin and clonazepam) are needed to clarify which treatment strategies are safe and effective for the management of TASD.[6]

SUMMARY

Clarification of the prevalence of TASD, its complete semiology, and associated comorbidities is of vital import; understanding this severe nocturnal disorder among veterans and victims of trauma is important for policymakers and funding organizations in allocating resources, especially given that misclassification of TASD cases may be likely. Future research should investigate the association between nightmares and disruptive nocturnal behaviors and the clinical diagnosis of TASD. Interested readers are directed to **Table 1** for a summary of the relevant literature.

CLINICS CARE POINTS

Pearls

- TASD is a proposed parasomnia that develops following a traumatic event, consisting of clinical features of trauma-related nightmares, disruptive nocturnal behaviors, and autonomic disturbances

- Treatment includes prazosin and management of comorbid sleep disorders, of which there may be several, including obstructive sleep apnea and insomnia

Pitfalls

- Although TASD shares similarities with PTSD and RBD, it is a distinct condition, and should be considered in situations in which trauma precedes the symptoms

DISCLOSURE

The authors have nothing to disclose.

REFERENCES

1. Mysliwiec V, O'Reilly B, Polchinski J, et al. Trauma associated sleep disorder: a proposed parasomnia encompassing disruptive nocturnal behaviors, nightmares, and REM without atonia in trauma survivors. J Clin Sleep Med 2014;10:1143–8.

2. Brock MS, Matsangas P, Creamer JL, et al. Clinical and polysomnographic features of trauma associated sleep disorder. J Clin Sleep Med 2022;18:2775–84.

3. Lavie P. Sleep disturbances in the wake of traumatic events. N Engl J Med 2001;345:1825–32.

4. Mellman TA, Pigeon WR, Nowell PD, et al. Relationships between REM sleep findings and PTSD symptoms during the early aftermath of trauma. J Trauma Stress 2007;20:893–901.

5. Mysliwiec V, Brock MS, Creamer JL, et al. Trauma associated sleep disorder: a parasomnia induced by trauma. Sleep Med Rev 2018;37:94–104.

6. Feemster JC, Smith KL, McCarter SJ, et al. Trauma-associated sleep disorder: a posttraumatic stress/REM sleep behavior disorder mash-up? J Clin Sleep Med 2019;15:345–9.

7. Khawaja ISB, Singh S. REM sleep behavior disorder. (FL): StatPearls Publishing; 2023 [Updated 2023 Apr 24]. In: StatPearls [Internet]. Treasure Island.

8. Elliott JE, Opel RA, Pleshakov D, et al. Posttraumatic stress disorder increases the odds of REM sleep behavior disorder and other parasomnias in

Veterans with and without comorbid traumatic brain injury. Sleep 2020;43(3):zsz237.

9. Brock MS, Powell TA, Creamer JL, et al. Trauma associated sleep disorder: clinical developments 5 years after discovery. Curr Psychiatr Rep 2019;21: 80.

10. Taylor KA, Mysliwiec V, Kimbrel NA, et al. Probable trauma associated sleep disorder in post-9/11 US veterans. Sleep Adv 2023;4:zpad001.

11. Caldwell JA, Knapik JJ, Shing TL, et al. The association of insomnia and sleep apnea with deployment and combat exposure in the entire population of US army soldiers from 1997 to 2011: a retrospective cohort investigation. Sleep 2019;42:zsz112.

12. Thordardottir EB, Hansdottir I, Valdimarsdottir UA, et al. The manifestations of sleep disturbances 16 years post-trauma. Sleep 2016;39:1551–4.

13. Rachakonda TD, Balba NM, Lim MM. Trauma-associated sleep disturbances: a distinct sleep disorder? Current Sleep Medicine Reports 2018;4:143–8.

14. Roepke S, Hansen ML, Peter A, et al. Nightmares that mislead to diagnosis of reactivation of PTSD. Eur J Psychotraumatol 2013;4.

15. American Psychiatric Association. Diagnostic and statistical manual of mental disorders. 5th edition. Washington, DC: American Psychiatric Publishing; 2013.

16. Germain A. Sleep disturbances as the hallmark of PTSD: where are we now? Am J Psychiatr 2013; 170:372–82.

17. American Academy of Sleep Medicine. International classification of sleep disorders. 3rd edition. Darien, IL: American Academy of Sleep Medicine; 2014.

18. Barone DA. Dream enactment behavior-a real nightmare: a review of post-traumatic stress disorder, REM sleep behavior disorder, and trauma-associated sleep disorder. J Clin Sleep Med 2020; 16:1943–8.

19. Ross RJ, Ball WA, Dinges DF, et al. Rapid eye movement sleep disturbance in posttraumatic stress disorder. Biol Psychiatry 1994;35:195–202.

20. Ross RJ, Ball WA, Dinges DF, et al. Motor dysfunction during sleep in posttraumatic stress disorder. Sleep 1994;17:723–32.

21. Germain A, Buysse DJ, Nofzinger E. Sleep-specific mechanisms underlying posttraumatic stress disorder: integrative review and neurobiological hypotheses. Sleep Med Rev 2008;12:185–95.

22. Husain AM, Miller PP, Carwile ST. REM sleep behavior disorder: potential relationship to post-traumatic stress disorder. J Clin Neurophysiol 2001;18:148–57.

23. Steven H, Woodward PD, Danny G, et al. Hippocampal volume, PTSD, and alcoholism in combat veterans. Am J Psychiatr 2006;163:674–81.

24. Kuo JR, Kaloupek DG, Woodward SH. Amygdala volume in combat-exposed veterans with and without posttraumatic stress disorder: a cross-sectional study. Arch Gen Psychiatr 2012;69: 1080–6.

25. Depue BE, Olson-Madden JH, Smolker HR, et al. Reduced amygdala volume is associated with deficits in inhibitory control: a voxel- and surface-based morphometric analysis of comorbid PTSD/Mild TBI. BioMed Res Int 2014;2014:691505.

26. McCarthy MS, Hoffmire C, Brenner LA, et al. Sleep and timing of death by suicide among US veterans 2006-2015: analysis of the american time use survey and the national violent death reporting system. Sleep 2019;42(8):zsz094.

27. Schenck CH, Bundlie SR, Ettinger MG, et al. Chronic behavioral disorders of human REM sleep: a new category of parasomnia. Sleep 1986;9:293–308.

28. Mysliwiec V, Brock MS. Time to recognize trauma associated sleep disorder as a distinct parasomnia. Sleep 2020;43(3):zsaa01.

29. Fernández-Arcos A, Iranzo A, Serradell M, et al. The clinical phenotype of idiopathic rapid eye movement sleep behavior disorder at presentation: a study in 203 consecutive patients. Sleep 2016;39:121–32.

30. Garcia-Rill E. Disorders of the reticular activating system. Med Hypotheses 1997;49:379–87.

31. Taylor DJ, Pruiksma KE, Mintz J, et al. Treatment of comorbid sleep disorders and posttraumatic stress disorder in US active duty military personnel: a pilot randomized clinical trial. J Trauma Stress 2023; 36(4):712–26.

32. Howell M, Avidan AY, Foldvary-Schaefer N, et al. Management of REM sleep behavior disorder: an American Academy of Sleep Medicine clinical practice guideline. J Clin Sleep Med 2023;19:759–68.

33. Raskind MA, Dobie DJ, Kanter ED, et al. The α1-adrenergic antagonist prazosin ameliorates combat trauma nightmares in veterans with posttraumatic stress disorder: a report of 4 cases. J Clin Psychiatr 2000;61:507.

34. Raskind MA, Peskind ER, Kanter ED, et al. Reduction of nightmares and other PTSD symptoms in combat veterans by prazosin: a placebo-controlled study. Am J Psychiatr 2003;160:371–3.

35. Raskind MA, Peskind ER, Chow B, et al. Trial of prazosin for post-traumatic stress disorder in military veterans. N Engl J Med 2018;378:507–17.

36. Morgenthaler TI, Auerbach S, Casey KR, et al. Position paper for the treatment of nightmare disorder in adults: an American Academy of Sleep Medicine position paper. J Clin Sleep Med 2018;14:1041–55.

Recurrent Isolated Sleep Paralysis

Ambra Stefani, MD PhD*, Qi Tang, MD

KEYWORDS

- REM parasomnia • REM sleep • Sleep paralysis • Dissociate state • Hallucinations

KEY POINTS

- Recurrent isolated sleep paralysis represents a dissociate state, with persistence of the muscle atonia typical of REM sleep in the waking state. Episodes are self-limiting and benign.
- The lifetime prevalence of at least 1 episode of sleep paralysis is 7.6% in the general population, with a wide variation (from 2% to 60%) in single studies.
- Irregular sleep-wake schedules, sleep deprivation, and jetlag are predisposing factors for the occurrence of sleep paralyses.
- The polysomnography electroencephalogram typically shows the intrusion of alpha EEG into REM sleep, followed by an arousal response, and then by the persistence of REM atonia into wakefulness.
- No drug treatment is required. Patients should be reassured and informed about sleep hygiene, adhering to regular sleep-wake schedules, and the necessity of obtaining sufficient sleep and striving to optimize sleep-wake schedule regularity. A specific cognitive behavioral therapy may be useful in cases of sleep paralyses accompanied by anxiety and frightening hallucinations.

DEFINITION AND DIAGNOSTIC CRITERIA

Recurrent isolated sleep paralysis is an rapid eye movement (REM) sleep parasomnia characterized by an inability to initiate voluntary movements either at sleep onset (hypnagogic or predormital form) or upon awakening (hypnopompic or postdormital form), in the absence of a diagnosis of narcolepsy.[1] During the episode, subjects are awake and aware of the environment. Episodes of sleep paralysis are fully recalled.

Hypnagogic or hypnopompic hallucinations can accompany a sleep paralysis[2,3] in 25% to 75% of cases. The hallucinations can be visual, auditory, or tactile, as well as take the form of a feeling that someone is in the room.

An episode of sleep paralysis lasts seconds to minutes and usually resolves spontaneously. Thus, recurrent isolated sleep paralysis is a benign phenomenon.

Diagnostic criteria[1] according to the American Academy of Sleep Medicine, International Classification of Sleep Disorders 3rd edition–text revisions (ICSD-3-TR) are reported in **Box 1**.

CLINICAL FEATURES

Sleep paralysis affects the somatic muscles under voluntary control,[4,5] with the exception of the external eye muscles. Involuntary muscles, including the diaphragm and the stapedius muscle, are not affected.[6] Thus, events consist in the inability to speak or move the limbs, trunk, and head, while eye movements are still possible. Respiration is only partially affected, as auxiliary respiratory muscles (such as the intercostal muscles) are paralyzed, but the diaphragm is not.

Sleep paralyses occur more often in the supine position. Some factors are able to abort sleep paralysis episodes, for example, sensory stimulation,

Department of Neurology, Sleep Disorders Clinic, Medical University of Innsbruck, Anichstrasse 35, 6020 Innsbruck, Austria
* Corresponding author. Department of Neurology, Sleep Disorders Clinic, Medical University of Innsbruck, Anichstrasse 35, 6020 Innsbruck, Austria
E-mail address: ambra.stefani@i-med.ac.at

Sleep Med Clin 19 (2024) 101–109
https://doi.org/10.1016/j.jsmc.2023.10.006

> **Box 1**
> **Recurrent isolated sleep paralysis diagnostic criteria according to the American Academy of Sleep Medicine (AASM), as reported in the International Classification of Sleep Disorders 3rd edition–text revision (ICSD-3-TR).[1]**
>
> Criteria A-D must be met
>
> A. A recurrent inability to move the trunk and all of the limbs at sleep onset or upon awakening from sleep.
>
> B. Each episode lasts seconds to a few minutes.
>
> C. The episodes cause clinically significant distress, including bedtime anxiety or fear of sleep.
>
> D. The disturbance is not better explained by another sleep disorder (especially narcolepsy), medical disorder, mental disorder, or medication/substance use.

such as being touched or spoken to, or an intense effort to move.[1]

Severe anxiety is usually present due to the mixture of wakefulness and complete inability to move, at least during the first episodes, as the experience is new to patients, and they may not be aware that episodes fully resolve spontaneously in seconds to a few minutes.

Despite a normal function of the diaphragm, affection of the auxiliary respiratory muscles (eg, intercostal muscles) may partially impact breathing and contribute to the commonly reported feeling of pressure on the chest. The frequent occurrence of hallucinations, in particular the feeling that someone is in the room, sometimes reported as the perception of the presence of an evil or a demon, and illusory perceptions of movement (ie, vestibular-motor hallucinations[7]) may contribute to anxiety during the episodes.

EPIDEMIOLOGY

Over a lifetime, the prevalence of at least 1 episode of sleep paralysis has been estimated to be 7.6% in the general population. However, there is a wide variation (from 2% to 60%) in single studies. Moreover, a higher frequency of sleep paralysis has been reported in student populations (up to 28.3%) and in psychiatric patients (31.9%, increasing to 34.6% in those having a history of panic disorder) compared to the general population.[8]

Ethnic differences have been described, with a slightly higher lifetime prevalence in people of African descent in the general population. Also in psychiatric samples a higher prevalence of sleep paralysis has been found in people of African

descent compared to other ethnicities. In student samples, the lifetime prevalence of sleep paralysis is higher in people of Asian descent.[8]

No consistent sex differences have emerged thus far, although a large systematic review reported a slightly higher lifetime prevalence of sleep paralysis among women (18.9%) compared to men (15.9%).[8]

The typical onset of recurrent isolated sleep paralysis is in adolescence, usually between 14 and 17 years, and most episodes occur in the second and third decades of age.

FOLKLORE, ART, AND LITERATURE

Sleep paralyses are frequent in the general population, may be associated to a feeling of pressure on the chest and the perception of the presence of a demon, and are frequently accompanied by anxiety, thus having a notable impact on people experiencing them. It is therefore not surprising that mentions of sleep paralysis in medieval Persia are reported,[9] and that folkloric terms to describe such episodes exist in more than 100 cultures. For example, sleep paralyses are known as "*the ghost oppression phenomenon*" in Hong Kong,[10] as "*Se me subio un muerto*" ("A cadaver climbed on me") in Mexico, or as *Guǐ yā chuáng* ("*to be oppressed by a spirit*") in China,[11] to mention a few examples.

Sleep paralysis fascinated also fine artists. The most known example is Johann Heinrich Füssli's painting *The Nightmare* (1781), depicting a sleep paralysis with hypnagogic hallucinations[12]: *The Nightmare* portrays a woman lying on her back on a divan, with her head and arms hanging over the edge. An incubus is sitting on her chest. Of note, Füssli created this work decades before the first scientific description of sleep paralysis (**Fig. 1**).

Sleep paralysis, classically perceived as an enigmatic and mysterious phenomenon, has been also described in classic literature by great novelists, including Guy de Maupassant in *The Horla*,[13,14] Herman Melville in *Moby Dick*, Charles Dickens in *Oliver Twist*, Fyodor Dostoyevsky in *The Brothers Karamazov*,[11] and Gogol in the tale *The Portrait*.[15]

An interesting but difficult to answer question is why has sleep paralysis been universally interpreted similarly, with an evil or demonic figure sitting on the chest? A study suggested that sleep paralysis occurring together with hypnagogic or hypnopompic hallucinations may be interpreted by specific evolutionary relevant scenarios, or micronarratives, to render these experiences meaningful.[7] The nightmare experience presents

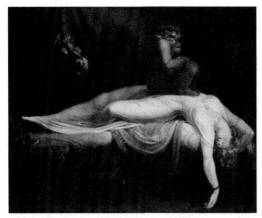

Fig. 1. Johann Heinrich Füssli's painting *The Nightmare* (1781). (From: https://archive.org/details/The_Nightmare.)

remarkably uniform interpretations across different cultures, consistent with the experiential-source hypothesis. According to this hypothesis, cultural accounts of supernatural and paranormal events are not made up as metaphysical allegories and metaphors, but are instead constructions generating a rational interpretation of concrete human experiences.[16] In line with the experiential-source hypothesis, the authors proposed and tested a 3-factor structural model (**Fig. 2**): (1) Intruder: consists of sensed presence, fear, auditory and visual hallucinations (which the authors suggest originating in a hypervigilant state initiated in the midbrain); (2) Incubus: comprises pressure on the chest,

breathing difficulties, and pain (attributed to effects of motoneurons' hyperpolarization on perceptions of respiration); (3) Unusual bodily experiences: consists of floating/flying sensations, out-of-body experiences, and feelings of bliss (generated by conflicts of endogenous and exogenous activation related to body position, orientation, and movement). Consistent with the universal consistency of these cultural accounts, the narratives are constrained by the raw experiences. Traditional narratives of demons, shades, spirits, and lost souls offer labels, narrative coherence, and explanations for sleep paralysis episodes.[7]

PREDISPOSING FACTORS AND ASSOCIATION WITH OTHER DISORDERS

Irregular sleep-wake schedules, sleep deprivation, obstructive sleep apnea, and jetlag have been identified as predisposing factors for the occurrence of sleep paralyses. Thus, sleep quality and insomnia symptoms should be investigated in patients with sleep paralysis.[17]

Episodes of sleep paralysis have been reported to be more common in the supine position.[1]

Sleep paralyses are more frequent in patients with post-traumatic stress disorder and anxiety disorder, compared to controls.[17] It has been reported that sleep paralysis may even be a symptom of post-traumatic stress disorder, with flashbacks of the trauma manifesting as hallucinations during a sleep paralysis.[17]

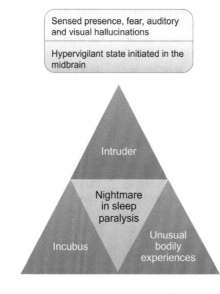

Sensed presence, fear, auditory and visual hallucinations

Hypervigilant state initiated in the midbrain

Intruder

Nightmare in sleep paralysis

Unusual bodily experiences

Incubus

Pressure on the chest, breathing difficulties, pain

Effects of motoneurons' hyperpolarization on perceptions of respiration

Floating/flying sensations, out-of-body experiences, feelings of bliss

Conflicts of endogenous and exogenous activation related to body position, orientation, and movement

Fig. 2. The 3-factor structural hypothesis of nightmares in sleep paralysis.

An increase prevalence of sleep paralysis has been reported also in some sleep disorders, such as insomnia, obstructive sleep apnea,[18] and nocturnal leg cramps.[17] This is not unexpected, as these disorders can lead to sleep disruption, which is a known predisposing factor for sleep paralysis.

A retrospective study found a positive association between lucid dreaming and sleep paralysis featuring intense vestibulo-motor hallucinations.[19]

Other factors reported to be associated with sleep paralysis include the use of anxiolytic medication, alcohol use, shift work, insufficient sleep syndrome, exploding head syndrome, bipolar disorder, hypertension, idiopathic hypersomnia, and Wilson's disease.[1]

PATHOPHYSIOLOGY

Sleep paralysis is an example of state dissociation,[20] with persistence of the muscle atonia typical of REM sleep in the waking state. One early study reported the occurrence of sleep paralysis after acute reversal of the sleep-wake-cycle.[21] Another study triggering sleep paralysis by sleep interruption demonstrated that sleep paralysis occurs in the transition between REM and wakefulness and during ambiguous REM sleep. In particular, a typical sequence in polysomnography electroencephalogram (EEG) was described, with the intrusion of alpha EEG into REM sleep, followed by an arousal response, and then by the persistence of REM atonia into wakefulness.[22] As sleep paralysis episodes occurred more frequently from sleep-onset REM periods after forced awakening, the authors suggested that conditions inducing sleep-onset REM periods, such as an interruption of the REM-non-rapid REM (NREM) cycle or a disruption of the circadian sleep-wake rhythm, might favor sleep paralysis.[22] Thus, it is hypothesized that sleep paralyses may more likely occur in individuals who are less tolerant to sleep disruption.[1] In line with this hypothesis, an association between sleep quality and the occurrence of sleep paralysis has been reported.[23]

Genetic factors play a role at least in some cases, as a few families with recurrent isolated sleep paralysis have been described,[1] A preclinical genetic analysis showed that variations in the circadian rhythm gene PER2 (single nucleotide polymorphism rs2304672) increase the odds of sleep paralysis.[23] PER2 is a member of the Period (PER) family of genes and plays an important role in the regulation of circadian rhythms. Thus, these findings are pointing to an impaired circadian rhythm in families with recurrent isolated sleep paralysis. However, genetic studies are sparse, and genome-wide association studies in recurrent isolated sleep paralysis are lacking.

NEUROPHYSIOLOGICAL FINDINGS

Polysomnography studies providing insights into the neurophysiology of sleep paralysis are scarce, and most of the knowledge about neurophysiological features of sleep paralysis derives from case reports and case series, narcolepsy patients presenting sleep paralysis.

In one study, four people with diagnosed (one subject) or suspected (three subjects) narcolepsy with cataplexy and unprovoked sleep paralysis were investigated. Polysomnography was conducted with four EEG channels, and electromyography of the chin and of a single lower limb. Sleep paralysis was documented here to occur in REM sleep.[24] This was however not confirmed in subsequent studies, which showed different neurophysiological features of sleep paralysis episodes. A case report documented via polysomnography an incomplete sleep paralysis in a patient with narcolepsy. REM sleep ended before the beginning of the sleep paralysis, EEG during the episode revealed alpha activity with low-voltage fast activity, and chin electromyography showed tonic and phasic muscle activity.[25]

Another case report in a patient with narcolepsy type 1 documented a sleep paralysis occurring upon awakening from a sleep onset REM period during the fourth multiple sleep latency test nap. The patient was unable to move his limbs, had bilateral myosis and slowed/slurred speech. The EEG showed alpha frequencies with low-voltage fast activity, bursts of rapid eye movements, and a chin electromyography pattern characterized by muscle atonia mixed with episodes of loss of atonia (ie, phasic muscle activity). Of note, the authors reported that the patient's recall of the episode was characterized by uncertainty between real and unreal, as well as uncertainty between dream and wakefulness. The authors performed EEG frequency domain analysis on 30-s EEG epochs during wake (with eyes closed), and during sleep onset REM periods before and during sleep paralysis on the occipital channel. They calculated fast Fourier transformed frequency spectra, which were then normalized to their integrals in the frequency domain. Wake activity peaked at 9.5 Hz, whereas REM activity peaked at 19 Hz. Of note, sleep paralysis episodes presented two peaks, one in the 9.5 Hz range and one in the 17 to 18.5 Hz range. A new spectrum was reconstructed summing up the amplitudes of the wake eyes-closed and the REM spectra, which matched very closely the spectrum of the paralysis episode. Based on the patient's recall and the EEG frequency analysis suggesting an intermediate state between wake and REM sleep during the episodes of sleep paralysis, the authors suggested that sleep paralyses are not pure motor phenomena, but instead a more complex dissociated state having a state of mind component in addition to the motor one.[26] This is in line with the theory of dissociated states of mind,[27] stating that wakefulness, REM and non-REM sleep are not necessarily mutually exclusive states and that under certain circumstances they may inappropriately overlap. This has been documented for example in confusional arousals.

A more recent study assessed in details REM sleep in a case-control study investigating 19 patients with recurrent isolated sleep paralysis. No differences were found in REM sleep macrostructure (ie, percentage of REM sleep and REM sleep latency), nor in REM sleep fragmentation (ie, REM sleep arousal index, percentage of wakefulness, and stage shifts within REM sleep). Power spectral analysis showed higher bifrontal beta activity during REM sleep in the recurrent isolated sleep paralysis group, compared to controls. The authors suggested that an underlying persistent trait of higher cortical activity may predispose patients with sleep paralysis to recurrent episodes.[28]

DIFFERENTIAL DIAGNOSIS

Usually, the diagnosis of recurrent isolated sleep paralysis is straight forward, in particular when hallucinations are absent, due to the typical clinical features of episodes of sleep paralysis. Cataplexies are similar dissociated states with presence of the muscle atonia typical of REM during wakefulness, but they occur during wakefulness (not upon awakening) and are triggered by emotions (**Table 1**). Atonic epileptic seizures also manifest in the waking state. They usually present as a loss of postural tone (such as a sudden decrease in partial or generalized muscle tone), resulting in a drop of the neck, mouth, limb ptosis, or fall with trunk dystonia, which also need to be distinguished from cataplexy in patients with narcolepsy. Atonic seizures can be either focal or generalized epileptic onset, and awareness is usually impaired. Abnormal interictal activity can be recorded. Nocturnal panic attacks are characterized by sudden awakening from NREM sleep in a state of panic, usually during transition from stage N2 to N3 within the first four hours after sleep onset, and are common in patients with panic disorder.[1]

Some other conditions need to be considered in the differential diagnosis of sleep paralysis, in particular when isolated recurrent sleep paralyses are associated with hallucinations. Those conditions include includes sleep terrors, nightmare disorder, lucid dreaming. However, sleep terrors is a disorder of arousal consisting of complex behaviors during NREM sleep, often accompanied by a cry or piercing scream, intense autonomic discharge, and increased muscle tone, and may be accompanied by incoherent vocalizations.[1] However, lucid dreaming occurs during unequivocal REM sleep.[22] Both lucid dreaming (LD) and recurrent isolated sleep paralysis are dissociated experiences related to REM sleep, and LD was thought to be positively correlated with sleep paralysis featuring intense vestibulo-motor hallucinations (as opposed to intruder and incubus hallucinations). The occurrence of sleep paralysis was associated with poorer quality sleep and higher levels of stress and anxiety, while lucid dreaming was usually related to positive constructive daydreaming and more vivid imagination, possibly reflecting increased insight, control, access to waking memories, and imaginative abilities.[19,29] Frequent nightmares can be distinguished from recurrent isolated sleep paralysis as they are associated with sleep disruption, insomnia, impaired daytime functioning, and other complaints.[30] Patients with nightmare disorder (ND) awaken completely, are quickly alert, and remember the dream content. ND can cause insomnia due to fear of falling asleep through dread of nightmare occurrence. ND is particularly frequent in psychiatric disorders and posttraumatic stress disorder. Frequent nightmares can be distinguished from recurrent isolated sleep paralysis as they are associated with sleep disruption, insomnia, impaired daytime functioning, and other complaints.[19,30]

Focal epileptic seizures should also be considered in the differential diagnosis of episodes of sleep paralysis.[31] In unclear cases, assessment should be extended to both video polysomnography and prolonged video-EEG-monitoring[32] to achieve a correct diagnosis. Focal seizures can be divided into motor seizures, non-motor seizures, with retained or impaired awareness for focal seizures.[33] The interictal epileptiform discharges and ictal patterns in focal seizures are variable. Patients with etiologically unclear complaints during daytime and night, especially those that are suspected to be seizures or sleep-related disorders, should use both video polysomnography and prolonged video-EEG-monitoring to achieve a correct diagnosis.[32]

In addition, other potential causes of paralysis arising from sleep need to be considered: any paralysis upon awakening should be differentiated from a wake-up stroke. Wake-up stroke (WUS) is

Table 1
Differential diagnosis of recurrent isolated sleep paralysis

Condition	Triggers	Timing	EEG/Neurophysiology	Consciousness/ Awareness
Recurrent isolated sleep paralysis	Irregular sleep-wake schedules, sleep deprivation, jetlag	At sleep onset or upon awakening	Intrusion of alpha EEG into REM sleep, followed by an arousal response, and then by the persistence of REM atonia into wakefulness	Preserved
Cataplexy	Emotions	Wakefulness	Transition state from wakefulness to REM sleep	Preserved
Atonic seizures	Hyperventilation, flashing lights	Wakefulness	Abnormal interictal activity	Impaired
Nocturnal panic attacks	None known	Awakening from NREM sleep, usually within the first 4 hours after sleep onset	Awakening from N2 or N3 sleep	Preserved
Sleep terrors	Fever, sleep deprivation, sleep schedule disruptions, extreme tiredness, periods of emotional tension, stress or conflict. Underlying conditions interfering with sleep (sleep-related breathing disorders, restless legs syndrome, medications, mood disorders, alcohol)	Disorder of arousal from NREM sleep	Intense autonomic discharge, increased muscle tone	Partially impaired
Lucid dreaming	External stimuli, for example, flashing lights	Mostly REM sleep	Unknown	Preserved
Nightmare disorder	Stress, anxiety, trauma, sleep deprivation, medications, substance misuse, psychiatric disorders	REM sleep	Increase in EEG alpha power, increased arousal-related phenomena in NREM-REM transitions, imbalance in sleep-promoting and arousing mechanisms. Increased sympathetic activity.	Heightened sense of awareness upon awakening
Focal epileptic seizures	Sleep disruption, hyperventilation, flashing lights	Wakefulness, NREM sleep	Variable ictal patterns and interictal epileptiform discharges	Preserved or impaired

(continued on next page)

Table 1
(*continued*)

Condition	Triggers	Timing	EEG/Neurophysiology	Consciousness/ Awareness
Wake-up stroke	Sleep-disordered breathing, overnight changes in autonomic tone affecting blood pressure with morning surges, morning increases in platelet aggregation	Sleep	Lateralized theta and/or delta activity in case of ipsilateral cortical infarction	Preserved or impaired
Familial periodic paralysis syndromes	Strenuous exercise, high carbohydrate meals, injection of insulin, glucose, or epinephrine (hypokalemic periodic paralysis); rest after exercise, fasting (hyperkalemic periodic paralysis)	At rest or upon awakening	EMG: positive sharp waves and myotonia (hyperkalemic periodic paralysis); In the long exercise test a focal attack of paralysis is induced by exercise of a single muscle.	Preserved

Abbreviations: EEG, electroencephalography; EMG, electromyography; NREM, non-rapid eye movement; REM, rapid eye movement.

a subtype of ischemic stroke in which patients wake up with neurologic deficits and without any abnormality before going to sleep.[34] Patients with WUS usually have 1 or more symptoms of neurologic deficits corresponding to ischemia lesions, such as numbness or weakness of the face, arm, or leg, especially on 1 side of the body. Unlike sleep paralysis, stroke-induced weakness or inability to move limbs or trunk cannot resolve spontaneously or disappear within a short time. Familial periodic paralysis syndromes, in particular hypokalemic periodic paralysis, can occur during day and night, but also upon awakening. The most common type is hypokalemic periodic paralysis, which can occur at rest, as well as upon awakening. However, those episodes usually last hours, may be associated with carbohydrate intake, and are usually accompanied by hypokalemia.[1] However, those episodes usually last hours, may be associated with carbohydrate intake, and are usually accompanied by hypokalemia (although there are also hyperkalemic and normokalemic periodic paralysis syndromes).[1]

MANAGEMENT

Recurrent isolated sleep paralysis is a benign condition, fully resolves spontaneously being usually self-limiting, and has no clinical consequences. Patients should thus be reassured, providing them information about the benignity of those episodes and their natural course (**Box 2**). It is also useful to make patients aware of factors able to resolve sleep paralysis episodes earlier, such as sensory stimuli (eg, being touched or spoken to).[1] If patients have bed partners, they may be instructed to touch the subject when low vocalizations occur in the morning before awakening.

As chronic sleep deprivation, fragmented sleep, or an irregular sleep-wake schedule facilitate sleep paralyses, it is important to inform patients about sleep hygiene, adhesion to regular sleep-wake schedules, and the necessity of obtaining sufficient sleep (ie, 7–9 hours) whenever possible, to reduce the probability of occurrence of sleep paralysis episodes.

Box 2
Management of recurrent isolated sleep paralysis

Management

- Factors such as sensory stimuli can resolve episodes earlier.
- Sleep hygiene, adhesion to regular sleep-wake schedules, and obtaining sufficient sleep (7–9 hours).
- Avoid the supine position.
- In cases of accompanying anxiety and frightening hallucinations, a specific cognitive behavioral therapy may be useful.
- Drug treatment is not indicated.

Avoidance of the supine position may be recommended, in particular when other predisposing factors are present (eg, during or after travels across multiple time zones), as it has been reported that sleep paralysis occur more frequently in the supine position. Despite an expected travel-related sleep disruption during long flights, the occurrence of sleep paralysis during sleep in sitting positions (such as in airplanes) has not been reported.

A specific cognitive behavioral therapy is available and may be useful in cases of sleep paralyses accompanied by anxiety and frightening hallucinations. It includes for example, ways to cope with frightening hallucinations, and imaginary repetition of successful resolution of sleep paralysis.

Drug treatment of sleep paralysis is not indicated. However, it has been reported that in patients with narcolepsy antidepressants (tricyclic or other[35]) may reduce the number of episodes of sleep paralysis, and one case of occurrence of recurrent isolated sleep paralysis following Bupropion cessation has been described.[36]

SUMMARY

Recurrent isolated sleep paralysis is a common condition, with a reported lifetime prevalence of at least 1 episode of 7.6% in the general population, although recurrence is less frequent. Very intense and vivid hallucinations can accompany the sleep paralysis episodes. Episodes are self-limiting and benign. It represents a dissociated state, with persistence of REM atonia into wakefulness. The polysomnography electroencephalogram typically shows the intrusion of alpha EEG into REM sleep, followed by an arousal response, and then by the persistence of REM atonia into wakefulness. Predisposing factors include sleep deprivation, irregular sleep-wake schedules, and jetlag. Avoiding these factors is the most effective therapy, and no drug treatment is required.

CLINICS CARE POINTS

- Sleep paralysis is a common benign phenomenon. Drug treatment is not indicated.
- Recurrent isolated sleep paralysis can be accompanied by hallucinations.
- Genetic factors have been described, pointing to an impaired circadian rhythm in families with recurrent isolated sleep paralysis.
- Irregular sleep–wake schedules, sleep deprivation, and jetlag are predisposing factors for the occurrence of sleep paralyses. It is important to inform patients about sleep hygiene,

- adhesion to regular sleep-wake schedules, and the necessity of obtaining sufficient sleep (ie, 7–9 hours) whenever possible.
- Patients should be aware of factors able to resolve sleep paralysis episodes earlier, such as sensory stimuli (eg, being touched or spoken to). If patients have bed partners, they may be instructed to touch the subject when low vocalizations occur in the morning before awakening.

FUNDING

Qi Tang was funded by the China Scholarship Council, China.

DISCLOSURE

Nothing to disclose.

REFERENCES

1. American Academy of Sleep Medicine. International classification of sleep disorders. 3rd edition. Darien, IL: American Academy of Sleep Medicine; 2023. text revision.
2. McCarty DE, Chesson AL Jr. A case of sleep paralysis with hypnopompic hallucinations. Recurrent isolated sleep paralysis associated with hypnopompic hallucinations, precipitated by behaviorally induced insufficient sleep syndrome. J Clin Sleep Med 2009; 5(1):83–4.
3. Hogl B, Iranzo A. Rapid eye movement sleep behavior disorder and other rapid eye movement sleep parasomnias. Continuum 2017;23(4): 1017–34. Sleep Neurology.
4. Chase MH, Francisco R. The control of motoneurons during sleep. In: Kryger MH, Roth T, Dement WC, editors. Principles and practice of sleep medicine. 2nd edition. Philadelphia: Saunders; 1994.
5. Nielsen TA, Zadra A. Dreaming disorders. In: Kryger MH, Roth T, Dement WC, editors. Principles and practice of sleep medicine. 3rd edition. Philadelphia: Saunders; 2000.
6. Kryger MH, Roth T, Dement WC. Principles and practice of sleep medicine. 2nd edition. Philadelphia: Sauderns; 1994.
7. Cheyne JA, Rueffer SD, Newby-Clark IR. Hypnagogic and hypnopompic hallucinations during sleep paralysis: neurological and cultural construction of the night-mare. Conscious Cogn 1999;8(3):319–37.
8. Sharpless BA, Barber JP. Lifetime prevalence rates of sleep paralysis: a systematic review. Sleep Med Rev 2011;15(5):311–5.
9. Golzari SE, Khodadoust K, Alakbarli F, et al. Sleep paralysis in medieval Persia - the hidayat of

akhawayni (?-983 AD). Neuropsychiatr Dis Treat 2012;8:229–34.

10. Wing YK, Lee ST, Chen CN. Sleep paralysis in Chinese: ghost oppression phenomenon in Hong Kong. Sleep 1994;17(7):609–13.

11. Stefani A, Iranzo A, Santamaria J, et al. Description of sleep paralysis in the Brothers Karamazov by dostoevsky. Sleep Med 2017;32:198–200.

12. Baumann C, Lentzsch F, Regard M, et al. The hallucinating art of Heinrich Fussli. Front Neurol Neurosci 2007;22:223–35.

13. Miranda M, Bustamante M. Depiction of parasomnia in the arts. Somnologie 2015;19:248–53.

14. Miranda M, Hogl B. Guy de Maupassant and his account of sleep paralysis in his tale, "The Horla". Sleep Med 2013;14(6):578–80.

15. Aguirre C, Miranda M, Stefani A. Nikolai Gogol's account of sleep paralysis in the tale "The Portrait". Sleep Med 2021;85:317–20.

16. Hufford DJ. The terror that comes in the night: an experience-centered study of supernatural assault traditions. Philadelphia: University of Pennsylvania Press; 1982.

17. Denis D. Relationships between sleep paralysis and sleep quality: current insights. Nat Sci Sleep 2018; 10:355–67.

18. Sharma A, Sakhamuri S, Giddings S. Recurrent fearful isolated sleep paralysis - a distressing co-morbid condition of obstructive sleep apnea. J Family Med Prim Care 2023;12(3):578–80.

19. Denis D, Poerio GL. Terror and bliss? Commonalities and distinctions between sleep paralysis, lucid dreaming, and their associations with waking life experiences. J Sleep Res 2017;26(1):38–47.

20. Mahowald MW, Schenck CH. Status dissociatus–a perspective on states of being. Sleep 1991;14(1): 69–79.

21. Weitzman ED, Kripke DF, Goldmacher D, et al. Acute reversal of the sleep-waking cycle in man. Effect on sleep stage patterns. Arch Neurol 1970; 22(6):483–9.

22. Takeuchi T, Miyasita A, Sasaki Y, et al. Isolated sleep paralysis elicited by sleep interruption. Sleep 1992; 15(3):217–25.

23. Denis D, French CC, Rowe R, et al. A twin and molecular genetics study of sleep paralysis and associated factors. J Sleep Res 2015;24(4):438–46.

24. Dyken ME, Yamada T, Lin-Dyken DC, et al. Diagnosing narcolepsy through the simultaneous clinical and electrophysiologic analysis of cataplexy. Arch Neurol 1996;53(5):456–60.

25. Buskova J, Pisko J, Dostalova S, et al. Incomplete sleep paralysis as the first symptom of narcolepsy. Sleep Med 2013;14(9):919–21.

26. Terzaghi M, Ratti PL, Manni F, et al. Sleep paralysis in narcolepsy: more than just a motor dissociative phenomenon? Neurol Sci 2012;33(1):169–72.

27. Mahowald MW, Schenck CH. Insights from studying human sleep disorders. Nature 2005;437(7063): 1279–85.

28. Kliková M, Piorecký M, Miletínová E, et al. Objective rapid eye movement sleep characteristics of recurrent isolated sleep paralysis: a case–control study. Sleep 2021;44(11):zsab153.

29. Voss U, Schermelleh-Engel K, Windt J, et al. Measuring consciousness in dreams: the lucidity and consciousness in dreams scale. Conscious. Cogn 2013;22:8–21 [PubMed] [Google Scholar].

30. Gieselmann A, Ait Aoudia M, Carr M, et al. Aetiology and treatment of nightmare disorder: state of the art and future perspectives. J Sleep Res 2019;28(4): e12820.

31. Galimberti CA, Ossola M, Colnaghi S, et al. Focal epileptic seizures mimicking sleep paralysis. Epilepsy Behav 2009;14(3):562–4.

32. Bergmann M, Brandauer E, Stefani A, et al. The additional diagnostic benefits of performing both video-polysomnography and prolonged video-EEG-monitoring: when and why. Clin Neurophysiol Pract 2022;7:98–102.

33. Fisher RS, Cross JH, French JA, et al. Operational classification of seizure types by the international league against epilepsy: position paper of the ILAE commission for classification and terminology. Epilepsia 2017;58(4):522–30.

34. Zhang YL, Zhang JF, Wang XX, et al. Wake-up stroke: imaging-based diagnosis and recanalization therapy. J Neurol 2021;268(11):4002–12.

35. Hintze JP, Gault D. Escitalopram for recurrent isolated sleep paralysis. J Sleep Res 2020;29(6): e13027.

36. Bieber ED, Bieber DA, Romanowicz M, et al. Recurrent isolated sleep paralysis following bupropion cessation: a case report. J Clin Psychopharmacol 2019;39(4):407–9.

Nightmare Disorder

Victoria R. Garriques, MPS, Deepali M. Dhruve, MS, Michael R. Nadorff, PhD*

KEYWORDS

- Nightmares • Nightmare disorder • Parasomnia • REM sleep • Dream • Sleep disturbances
- Sleep disorders

KEY POINTS

- Nightmares are a highly prevalent parasomnia that are associated with several negative outcomes such as psychopathology (eg, anxiety, post-traumatic stress, borderline personality disorder) and suicidal behavior.
- Strong treatments for nightmare disorder exist, with the leading interventions being Imagery Rehearsal Therapy (psychotherapy) and prazosin (pharmacotherapy).
- Novel treatments like NightWare or using service animals for nightmares require additional empirical support before they can be widely recommended.
- The nightmare treatment literature is still underdeveloped, with more work needed to best understand the order in which treatments should be prescribed and how they may interact.

INTRODUCTION, DEFINITION, AND BACKGROUND

Nightmares are a rapid eye movement (REM) parasomnia defined as disturbing or frightening dreams that evoke fear, sadness, despair, shame, and/or disgust through visuals and narratives.[1] Nightmares are most prominent in the second half of the night, most commonly happening during REM sleep, though rarely occurring during N2 sleep. Typically REM sleep is required due to the vividness of a nightmare.[2] There is ongoing debate about whether the dreamer must awaken from the dream for it to qualify as a nightmare and not simply a *bad dream*, which is defined as a negatively-valanced dream that does not lead to a startled awakening. Some researchers categorize a dream as a nightmare if it is well-remembered upon awakening, even if the dreamer is not awakened directly by it, as it is possible, if not likely, that both are merely different intensities of the same phenomenon.[3]

When one experiences recurrent nightmares and bad dreams that are associated with clinically significant distress or impairment in social, occupational, or other important areas of functioning,

and that cannot be attributed to a substance or coexisting mental or medical disorder, then nightmare disorder can be diagnosed.[4–6] These dreams can lead to significant distress, with patients demonstrating sleep resistance or avoidance in an attempt to not have the disturbing dreams.[6] One oddity with the diagnostic manuals is that unlike other disorders: a frequency is not specified for the diagnosis, just that the dreams are recurrent. That said, at least 1 nightmare per week is commonly thought of as the threshold for clinically significant nightmares, as this is the cutoff that is commonly used in treatment studies.[7]

Nightmares may be posttraumatic, depicting an experienced traumatic event or containing trauma-related emotions, or idiopathic, depicting imaginative stories that do not reflect a traumatic event.[1] Nightmares are commonly confused with night terrors, a non-REM parasomnia that also leads to a startled awakening. There are several notable differences that can be used to help differentiate these disorders (**Table 1**). After waking from a nightmare, patients are typically alert and oriented because REM is a much lighter stage of sleep, whereas, after awakening from a night

Department of Psychology, Mississippi State University, 110 Magruder Hall, P.O. Box 6161, Mississippi State, MS 39762, USA
* Corresponding author
E-mail address: mnadorff@psychology.msstate.edu

Sleep Med Clin 19 (2024) 111–119
https://doi.org/10.1016/j.jsmc.2023.10.011

Table 1
Nightmare disorder differential diagnoses

Differential Diagnosis	Overlap with Nightmare Disorder	Key Differences from Nightmare Disorder
Sleep Terror Disorder	• Awaken suddenly from sleep Feelings of fearfulness upon awakening	• No dream recall • Confusion and disorientation upon awakening • Typically occurs early in the night • Occurs during NREM sleep • May not remember event in the morning
RBD	• Possible frightening dreams • Takes place during REM sleep	• Dream enactments involving complex vocal and/or motor activity • May result in nocturnal injury
PTSD or acute stress disorder	• Nightmares	• High severity or frequency of nightmares may indicate a comorbid diagnosis and independent nightmare treatment may be necessary • Dreams are typically about a traumatic event the person experienced
Breathing-related sleep disorders	• Awaken from sleep with autonomic arousal	• Typically no dream recall

Abbreviation: NREM, non-rapid eye movement; RBD, REM sleep behavior disorder; PTSD, posttraumatic stress disorder

terror, patients are often confused, disoriented, and difficult to console due to coming out of deeper stages of non-REM sleep. Nightmares also commonly happen later in the sleep period, whereas night terrors are more common earlier in the sleep period. Nightmares also may need to be differentiated from REM sleep behavior disorder, which is characterized by complex motor activity during dreams and may be associated with more violent dreams as well as nocturnal injuries. Nightmares do not typically involve much re-enactment of the dream but may involve some movements, such as punching and kicking, depending on the dream experienced. Additionally, in REM sleep behavior disorder, the dream is not necessarily negative, and the movements are the primary feature instead of a smaller, secondary feature as they could be with bad dreams and nightmares.

It is estimated that 4 to 10% of the United States population is affected by nightmare disorder, though higher rates are commonly seen in children and young adults as well as those who have experienced trauma.[8] Frequent nightmares are often accompanied by further sleep disturbances, including insomnia, which can lead to daytime sleepiness, lack of energy, sleep anxiety, and difficulty concentrating.[1] Nightmares are also associated with many mental health complaints, including anxiety, depression, and maladaptive

personality functioning.[1] The burden of nightmares falls heavily on those with comorbid psychiatric illnesses, with a prevalence of 38.9%.[9] Up to 80% of patients with posttraumatic stress disorder (PTSD) endorse nightmares, and nightmare disorder is seen in 66.7% of PTSD patients.[9] Even if they do not meet the criteria for nightmare disorder, these nightmares are associated with more severe PTSD symptoms.[10,11] Even more disturbingly, nightmares have been shown to be associated with suicidal behavior, with longitudinal research showing that nightmares are associated with a more than 400% increase in future suicide attempts among those who have attempted before, even after statistically accounting for depression, anxiety, PTSD, and substance use.[12] In fact, nightmares are one of the few factors that can differentiate between those who attempt suicide once and those who attempt more than once,[13] and they prospectively predict death by suicide.[14]

Despite the interference nightmares cause to daily functioning, they are severely underreported and undertreated, with less than 30% of patients reporting weekly nightmares having ever reported them to a healthcare provider.[15] Many patients are unaware of treatment options for nightmares, and healthcare providers rarely screen for nightmares or nightmare disorder, so the vast majority of patients go untreated.

ASSESSMENT OF NIGHTMARES AND NIGHTMARE DISORDER

The most commonly used tools for assessing nightmare characteristics are self-reported retrospective questionnaires and prospective logs.[16] Although prospective nightmare logs are the gold standard for assessment, due to time limitations, self-report measures are commonly used. Self-report measures can also assess aspects of the nightmare phenomenon that are difficult to assess in a simple log, such as nightmare distress, so clinicians commonly utilize self-report measures in addition to dream logs.

Various instruments exist to assess nightmare frequency and the distress associated with nightmares. The Nightmare Frequency Questionnaire (NFQ)[17] is a self-report measure that assesses nightmare frequency continuously. The NFQ queries respondents about the frequency of nightmares experienced, including the number of nights with nightmares and the number of recalled nightmares within the past week, month, and year. Although the NFQ has good test-retest reliability and good validity in clinical populations,[17] it has demonstrated lower validity in nonclinical populations.[18] The Mannheim Dream Questionnaire[19] prompts for information about the frequency of nightmares experienced both currently and in childhood, as well as the proportion of recurring nightmares experienced by adults. Moreover, it demonstrates higher validity among non-clinical populations.[18]

To assess the extent of distress caused by nightmares, some authors utilize a single question to inquire if participants are experiencing any problems related to nightmares.[20] Other researchers have constructed psychometric instruments to evaluate overall worries regarding nightmares. The most frequently used distress instrument, the Nightmare Distress Questionnaire,[21] probes various nightmare-related problems, including their effect on sleep quality and their impact on beliefs and perceptions during the day. A subscale of the SLEEP-50 measures the degree of distress experienced as a result of nightmares as per the diagnostic and statistical manual of mental disorder-IV criteria.[22] There are other questionnaires that center on how nightmares affect aspects such as social life, sleep, health, psychic dysregulation, and somatization; these include the Nightmare Effects Survey,[23] the Trauma Related Nightmare Survey,[24] the Nightmare Quality of Life Questionnaire,[25] and the Nightmare Proneness Scale.[26] Other tools also assess internalizing and externalizing symptoms. For example, the Van Dream Anxiety Scale, developed by Agargün and colleagues,[27] focuses on anxiety symptoms related to nightmares. Conversely, the Nightmare Behavior Questionnaire[28] evaluates behavioral consequences of nightmares.

There also exist measures that combine assessment of nightmare frequency and distress. In adults, these measures include the Disturbing Dream and Nightmare Severity Index (DDNSI),[29] the Nightmare Experience Scale,[30] and the Nightmare Disorder Index.[31] The DDNSI is a widely used measure that is well-validated across differing races and ages.[7,32–35] Additionally, the Nightmare Effects Questionnaire[36] evaluates combined nightmare frequency with nightmare effects for adolescents between 14 to 18 years of age.

GUIDELINES AND CURRENT EVIDENCE

There are many effective treatments for nightmare disorder (**Table 2**), though for some, accessibility is a challenge, as we will outline below. The recommended treatment for nightmare disorder from the American Academy of Sleep Medicine (AASM) is Imagery Rehearsal Therapy (IRT).[37] IRT is a cognitive behavioral therapy (CBT) where a nightmare is rescripted into a new, positive dream that is rehearsed for 10 to 20 minutes per day.[37,38] In randomized controlled trial (RCT) studies, this treatment has been shown to reduce nightmare frequency for both PTSD-associated and idiopathic nightmares, as well as in those with comorbid psychiatric disorders.[39,40] Exposure, relaxation, and rescripting therapy (ERRT) is a variation of IRT developed to better fit patients who have nightmares associated with trauma that require exposure therapy. It includes sleep hygiene education, progressive muscle relaxation, and exposure to trauma in addition to nightmare rescripting. The rescripting in ERRT is also a bit different, with more of the original dream content being kept in the rescripted dream. ERRT does not have the same level of recommendation as IRT, though this is primarily due to it being a newer treatment with a smaller literature base. The literature examining ERRT is strong and growing. In 2 RCTs and a case series, ERRT was shown to reduce nightmare frequency as well as severity.[24,41,42] It should be noted that due to the trauma focus of ERRT, these studies did not include participants with idiopathic nightmares, so ERRT is best conceptualized as a posttraumatic nightmare-focused treatment. Lucid Dreaming Therapy (LDT) is a different approach to treating nightmares that is commonly confused with IRT. In Lucid Dreaming, the patient is taught how to identify when they are dreaming and is encouraged to actively change their dream *while*

Table 2
Nightmare disorder management

Treatment	Description	Advantages	Disadvantages
IRT	Cognitive behavioral therapy rescripting nightmares into new, positive dreams that are then rehearsed using visual imagery	• Recommended treatment for nightmare disorder • Patients can implement strategies on their own for future nightmares • May reduce PTSD severity • Well tolerated	• Trained therapists may be inaccessible
ERRT	Nightmare rescripting with additional sleep hygiene education, progressive muscle relaxation, and exposure to trauma	• Works to improve overall sleep health • May reduce symptoms of PTSD • Ideal for nightmares that do not respond to rescripting alone and require exposure	• Trained therapists may be inaccessible • Some patients may not want exposure to dream content • No research on effectiveness for idiopathic nightmares
LDT	Recognizing dreaming and being able to actively change the dream while in it	• Does not require exposure to nightmare content during wake	• Trained therapists may be inaccessible • Not every dreamer can reach lucid dreaming state
Prazosin	alpha-1 adrenergic receptor agonist often used to treat PTSD-related nightmares; reduces CNS sympathetic outflow through the brain	• Accessible • Well-tolerated by a majority of patients	• Nightmares return after medication cessation • Recent research on effectiveness is inconclusive

Abbreviation: IRT, Imagery Rehearsal Therapy; PTSD, Posttraumatic stress disorder; ERRT, Exposure, relaxation, and re-scripting therapy; LDT, Lucid Dreaming Therapy; CNS, Central nervous system

they are having it. This differs from IRT, in which rescription is done in advance and practiced while the individual is awake. Two randomized trials and 1 case study found that LDT decreased the frequency of nightmares, and this result was maintained at 12-week follow-ups.[43–45] In addition to IRT and its variates, multiple other forms of CBT have been shown to effectively target nightmares, though with weaker empirical support. These include cognitive behavioral therapy for insomnia (CBT-I), sleep dynamic therapy, and systematic desensitization.

Although the current recommendation is using IRT for nightmares where available, there is a shortage of clinicians trained in nightmare interventions, and because of this, many areas lack a provider for this treatment. For this reason, as well as some patients preferring pharmaceutical treatments, medications are commonly utilized in treating nightmares. The preferred pharmacologic treatment for nightmare disorder is prazosin. Prazosin is an alpha-1 adrenergic receptor agonist that is Food and Drug Administration (FDA)-approved for the treatment of hypertension but is often prescribed off-label for the treatment of PTSD-related nightmares. The distinction of PTSD-related nightmares is important, as there is no research to our knowledge that examines prazosin's effect on idiopathic nightmares, though it is still commonly used to treat these nightmares despite this gap. Prazosin was recently demoted by the AASM from "recommended" to "may be used" for the treatment of nightmare disorder.[1] This is following a large, well-controlled RCT that found no significant effect of prazosin on both sleep and PTSD-related measures when compared with placebo.[46] However, a meta-analysis of IRT and prazosin RCTs (including the one previously mentioned) found that the two treatments did not significantly differ in their efficacy in treating posttraumatic nightmares.[47] There are several other medications that have been examined as well (please see Morgenthaler and colleagues[37] for a review), but the evidence for other medications is weak and is surpassed by prazosin, which is clearly the leading pharmaceutical treatment for nightmare disorder.

CONSIDERATIONS
Medication Versus Psychotherapy

One of the primary considerations in relation to nightmare disorder is whether to treat it using pharmacotherapy or psychotherapy. In the recent position paper from the American Academy of Sleep Medicine published by Morgenthaler and colleagues[37] the recommendation was that IRT, a psychotherapy, is the treatment of choice for both PTSD and idiopathic nightmares. Although this is a sound recommendation based upon the literature, as mentioned previously, there is still a shortage of therapists trained in IRT, as well as the other nightmare-focused psychotherapies, in many places. If these therapies are not available, then pharmacotherapies such as prazosin are reasonable and should be considered. Prazosin is the preferred pharmacotherapy in the Morgenthaler and colleagues[37] position paper and is well-tolerated by a majority of patients. There are also self-help options based on IRT, such as the book *Turning Nightmares Into Dreams* by Barry Krakow, but research has yet to examine this. Thus, medication may be preferred over a self-help option, especially for trauma-related nightmares. There previously was a smartphone application created by the US Veteran's Administration and Department of Defense called Dream EZ, but it is no longer supported, though a new application is currently in development.

Prioritization of Treatment with Comorbidities

Given that nightmares are comorbid with so many psychological disorders, the question emerges of when to treat the nightmares and whether there should be any modifications to the treatment plan. Treating patients at risk of suicide is 1 of the more challenging areas due to adverse findings regarding prazosin. The literature is sparse, but there is evidence that IRT can be utilized in patients who are at risk of suicide concurrent with other treatments, including in inpatient settings.[48] However, in regard to prazosin, McCall and colleagues[49] found that nightmare sufferers with suicidal ideation on prazosin in addition to a Selective serotonin reuptake inhibitor (SSRI) had poorer outcomes than those who were on an SSRI and placebo. Thus, for patients with concurrent suicidal ideation, it is indicated to treat the suicidality first. To address nightmares, if available, IRT can be used at the same time as treating the suicidality, or prazosin can be used once the suicidal ideation has been treated, but it is not indicated to treat nightmares with prazosin with active suicidal ideation in light of the findings of McCall and colleagues.[49]

Another comorbidity that comes up frequently is PTSD. Although research has not yet compared the efficacy of treating nightmares vs. PTSD first, there is evidence suggesting that treating nightmares first may result in a notable improvement in PTSD symptoms. For instance, Krakow and colleagues[50] investigated IRT in a randomized trial of 168 nightmare sufferers who were victims of sexual assault, finding not only a notable reduction in nightmares but also PTSD symptoms. This finding is notable because IRT requires little to no exposure, and because of this, it is typically better tolerated than exposure-based PTSD treatments. Thus, although more research is needed, clinicians may wish to consider treating nightmares first before utilizing an exposure-based PTSD treatment in order to see whether the client experiences enough symptom relief that an exposure-based therapy may not be necessary. As far as pharmacologic therapy, there is little research examining the use of SSRI medications and IRT together simultaneously. That said, based upon the positive findings of Ellis, Rufino, and Nadorff[48] in an inpatient sample, there is no reason to believe that IRT could not be done at the same time as an SSRI to treat nightmares and PTSD simultaneously. Similarly, a provider could consider utilizing both prazosin and an SSRI to treat nightmares simultaneously with PTSD should IRT not be available in the area.

Anxiety is also commonly comorbid with nightmare disorder, and treating anxiety has been shown to significantly reduce bad dreams in a sample of older adults with Generalized Anxiety Disorder.[51] Given that reducing anxiety has been shown to reduce nightmares as well, it makes sense to either treat nightmares and anxiety concurrently if using IRT or to treat whichever is believed to be the primary diagnosis first. Although research has yet to test this, since IRT is not an exposure-based therapy, its efficacy should not be impacted by treating anxiety first, whereas exposure-based therapies may be affected. IRT should be able to be used in conjunction with either psychotherapies, such as CBT for anxiety, or pharmacotherapies, such as SSRI medications.[52] The use of benzodiazepines for anxiety is beyond the scope of this article, as their use is debated in the literature,[52] but it is worth mentioning that these medications would impact the efficacy of any exposure-based treatments and thus treatments that involve exposure should be conducted before the initiation of benzodiazepine medication.

Cultural Implications

Although there is very little research on cultural differences in nightmares, the existing literature suggests that there may be meaningful differences in both how nightmares are reported as well as viewed. For instance, Worley, Bolstad, and Nadorff[53] utilized data from the Collaborative Psychiatric Epidemiology Surveys study to examine whether there are different prevalence rates across cultures/ethnicities of dreams about trauma, dreams about the worst event one has experienced, and dreams about separation from a loved one, finding notable differences in all 3 of these dreams across groups. For dreams about trauma, the overall prevalence in the sample was 1.98%, but it ranged from 0.07% endorsement in Afro-Caribbean participants up to 4.24% in Puerto Rican participants and 4.58% in those who endorsed "Other" for their background. These differences illustrate the importance of not only assessing for bad dreams, but also potentially for asking about them in different ways, as endorsement differs by the prompt across cultures.

In addition, another cultural challenge is that many individuals attribute meaning to their dreams. This could be due to culture, or also is commonly found among individuals who have benefitted from psychodynamic therapies that involved some form of dream interpretation. In these groups, the client may be reluctant to change their dream, even if it is disturbing. Although there is no literature describing how best to handle this, in our practice, we discuss the dream with the client, whether there could be any additional meaning that could be obtained from it, the impact it is having on them, and any objections they have to change the content of the dream. In doing this, we help them examine the benefits and costs of potentially treating their nightmares in order to obtain informed consent before moving forward with treatment.

Use of Technology and Service Animals

There has been growing interest in using either technology or a service animal to identify when an individual is having a negative dream and to awaken them from that dream. Perhaps the best-known device like this is NightWare, which received FDA clearance in 2020,[54] and has recently begun publishing outcome data.[55] However, in those recently published data, the device failed to outperform a sham treatment in the primary analyses, only showing a couple of differences in post-hoc analyses on perceived sleep quality. This result is unsurprising as it has long been believed that an awakening is typically necessary to recall one's dream.[56] In a more recent study further demonstrating this, participants who were awoken during REM sleep remembered dreams 80% of the time, whereas young adults typically recalled their dreams only once or twice per week.[57] Thus, there is reason to believe that awakening an individual during their dream greatly increases their likelihood of remembering it. This is problematic for treatments like NightWare and service dogs, where the goal is to awaken the individual during the dream because, in doing so, one greatly increases the likelihood that one will remember the dream. However, if one can help an individual not wake up during a bad dream, then it is likely they will not recall the dream.[56] Despite these theoretic challenges, these interventions are worthy of further study, but based upon the current data on their efficacy and in light of what we know about awakenings and dream recall it is difficult to recommend them at this point in time despite their popularity.

CLINICAL OUTCOMES

When treating nightmares, it is important to determine how your treatment affects your patient's symptoms and quality of life. Commonly reported clinical outcomes of nightmare treatments include sleep quality, nightmare frequency, and nightmare distress. Many studies also measure recovery from other associated symptoms, such as PTSD symptoms.

IRT trials showed significant decreases in nightmare frequency, with multiple studies showing decreases of around 50%.[22,39,40,50,58–61] These improvements were maintained after treatment, with similar frequencies of nightmares being seen at 30- and 42-week follow-ups.[59,62] Adverse events were uncommon in these IRT trials.[37] The use of IRT to treat posttraumatic nightmares is also associated with improvements in other PTSD symptoms.[63,64] This effect is not limited to patients with PTSD; IRT can be used for patients with a variety of mental health diagnoses in both inpatient and outpatient settings. IRT was shown to have moderate effects on nightmare frequency and distress when added to outpatient treatment plans,[40] and when added to inpatient treatment plans, IRT increased reductions in suicidal ideation.[48]

The majority of RCTs on prazosin found it superior to placebo at reducing nightmare frequency and improving sleep quality.[1] Some RCTs reported returning nightmares after discontinuing the use of prazosin.[65] Prazosin has also been shown to significantly improve posttraumatic stress symptoms, though it is unclear if these improvements are sustained after treatment cessation.[63,65] However, as previously noted, a recent study of prazosin failed to find any significant effect of prazosin on sleep or PTSD-related outcomes.[46] These mixed results necessitate further study into prazosin as a nightmare treatment.

Using recommended treatments for nightmare disorder, it is possible to significantly decrease the frequency and intensity of nightmares, as well as improve symptoms for comorbid disorders. Although currently available nightmare treatments are highly efficacious, they may not be accessible to everyone. There are some less prominent but more accessible treatments available, such as self-help books,[22,62,66–68] that may also be worthy of consideration.

SUMMARY AND RECOMMENDATIONS

Nightmares are not only a sleep parasomnia, but also a psychological disorder that is highly prevalent. Although it is estimated that only 2% to 6% of the population meet criteria for nightmare disorder,[4] we have found that over 9% of adults report having disturbing dreams,[53] with rates far higher in those with anxiety, histories of trauma, or other psychopathology. Thus, nightmares are prevalent, though they are also under-reported, with only roughly one-third of nightmare sufferers reporting having nightmares to a healthcare professional.[69] Given their high prevalence and clinical importance, it is important for clinicians to assess for nightmares and, when they are reported, to either treat them or refer the patient for treatment. IRT is currently the recommended treatment for nightmare disorder,[37] but it is not available in all locations. When not available, prazosin, the recommended pharmaceutical intervention, may be considered. Regardless of which treatment is chosen, nightmares should be treated, as without intervention, they can be prevalent into late-life,[51] and the longer one suffers from nightmares, the more strongly they have been shown to be associated with negative outcomes such as suicidal behavior.[13,70]

CLINICS CARE POINTS

- Nightmares are a highly prevalent parasomnia that is associated with several adverse outcomes, such as psychopathology (eg, anxiety, post-traumatic stress, borderline personality disorder) and suicidal behavior.
- Strong treatments for nightmare disorder exist, with the leading interventions being Imagery Rehearsal Therapy (psychotherapy) and prazosin (pharmacotherapy).

- Novel treatments like NightWare or using service animals for nightmares require additional empirical support before they can be widely recommended.
- The nightmare treatment literature is still underdeveloped, with more work needed to best understand the order in which treatments should be prescribed and how they may interact.

DISCLOSURE

The authors have no conflicts of interest to disclose.

REFERENCES

1. Gieselmann A, Ait Aoudia M, Carr M, et al. Aetiology and treatment of nightmare disorder: state of the art and future perspectives. J Sleep Res 2019;28(4): e12820.
2. Phelps AJ, Kanaan RAA, Worsnop C, et al. An ambulatory polysomnography study of the post-traumatic nightmares of post-traumatic stress disorder. Sleep 2018;41(1):zsx188.
3. Köthe M, Pietrowsky R. Behavioral effects of nightmares and their correlations to personality patterns. Dreaming 2001;11(1):43–52.
4. American Psychiatric Association, American Psychiatric Association. In: Diagnostic and statistical manual of mental disorders: DSM-5. 5th ed. Washington, DC: American Psychiatric Association; 2013.
5. World Health Organization, editor. International statistical classification of diseases and related health problems. 10th revision, 2nd edition. Geneva: World Health Organization; 2004.
6. American Academy of Sleep Medicine. International classification of sleep disorders. 3rd edition. Darien, IL: American Academy of Sleep Medicine; 2014.
7. Bolstad CJ, Szkody E, Nadorff MR. Factor analysis and validation of the disturbing dreams and nightmare severity index. Dreaming 2021;31(4):329–41.
8. Levin R, Nielsen T. Nightmares, bad dreams, and emotion dysregulation: a review and new neurocognitive model of dreaming. Curr Dir Psychol Sci 2009; 18(2):84–8.
9. Stefani A, Högl B. Nightmare disorder and isolated sleep paralysis. Neurotherapeutics 2021;18(1):100–6.
10. Gerhart JI, Hall BJ, Russ EU, et al. Sleep disturbances predict later trauma-related distress: cross-panel investigation amidst violent turmoil. Health Psychol 2014;33(4):365–72.
11. Pigeon WR, Campbell CE, Possemato K, et al. Longitudinal relationships of insomnia, nightmares, and PTSD severity in recent combat veterans. J Psychosom Res 2013;75(6):546–50.

12. Sjöström N, Hetta J, Waern M. Persistent nightmares are associated with repeat suicide attempt: a prospective study. Psychiatr Res 2009;170(2–3):208–11.

13. Speed KJ, Drapeau CW, Nadorff MR. Differentiating single and multiple suicide attempters: what nightmares can tell us that other predictors cannot. J Clin Sleep Med 2018;14(05):829–34.

14. Tanskanen A, Tuomilehto J, Viinamäki H, et al. Nightmares as predictors of suicide. Sleep 2001;24(7):844–7.

15. Thünker J, Norpoth M, Von Aspern M, et al. Nightmares: knowledge and attitudes in health care providers and nightmare sufferers. J Public Health Epidemiol 2014;6(7):223–8.

16. Standards of Practice Committee, Aurora RN, Zak RS, et al. Best practice guide for the treatment of nightmare disorder in adults. J Clin Sleep Med 2010;06(04):389–401.

17. Krakow B, Schrader R, Tandberg D, et al. Nightmare frequency in sexual assault survivors with PTSD. J Anxiety Disord 2002;16(2):175–90.

18. Kelly WE, Mathe JR. Comparison of single- and multiple-item nightmare frequency measures. Int J Dream Res 2020;28:136–42.

19. Schredl M, Berres S, Klingauf A, et al. The Mannheim Dream questionnaire (MADRE): retest reliability, age and gender effects. Int J Dream Res 2014;7(2):141–7.

20. Wood JM, Bootzin RR. The prevalence of nightmares and their independence from anxiety. J Abnorm Psychol 1990;99(1):64–8.

21. Belicki K. Nightmare frequency versus nightmare distress: relations to psychopathology and cognitive style. J Abnorm Psychol 1992;101(3):592–7.

22. Lancee J, Spoormaker VI, van den Bout J. Cognitive-behavioral self-help treatment for nightmares: a randomized controlled trial. Psychother Psychosom 2010;79(6):371–7.

23. Krakow B, Lowry C, Germain A, et al. A retrospective study on improvements in nightmares and post-traumatic stress disorder following treatment for co-morbid sleep-disordered breathing. J Psychosom Res 2000;49(5):291–8.

24. Davis JL, Wright DC. Randomized clinical trial for treatment of chronic nightmares in trauma-exposed adults. J Trauma Stress 2007;20(2):123–33.

25. El-Solh AA, Lawson Y, Wilding GE. The nightmare quality of life questionnaire. Behav Sleep Med 2022;20(6):774–86.

26. Kelly WE. The Nightmare Proneness Scale: a proposed measure for the tendency to experience nightmares. Sleep Hypn - Int J 2017. https://doi.org/10.5350/Sleep.Hypn.2017.19.0143.

27. Ağargün MY, Kara H, Bilici M, et al. The van dream anxiety scale: a subjective measure of dream anxiety in nightmare sufferers. Sleep Hypn 1999;1(4):204–11.

28. Pietrowsky R, Köthe M. Personal boundaries and nightmare consequences in frequent nightmare sufferers. Dreaming 2003;13(4):245–54.

29. Krakow B. Nightmare complaints in treatment-seeking patients in clinical sleep medicine settings: diagnostic and treatment implications. Sleep 2006;29(10):1313–9.

30. Kelly WE, Mathe JR. A brief self-report measure for frequent distressing nightmares: the Nightmare Experience Scale (NExS). Dreaming 2019;29(2):180–95.

31. Dietch JR, Taylor DJ, Pruiksma K, et al. The nightmare disorder index: development and initial validation in a sample of nurses. Sleep 2021;44(5):zsaa254.

32. Allen SF, Gardani M, Akram A, et al. Examining the factor structure, reliability, and validity of the disturbing dreams and nightmare severity Index (DDNSI) consequences sub-component. Behav Sleep Med 2021;19(6):783–94.

33. Lee R, Krakow B, Suh S. Psychometric properties of the disturbing dream and nightmare severity index–Korean version. J Clin Sleep Med 2021;17(3):471–7.

34. Park D, Kim S, Shin C, et al. Prevalence of and factors associated with nightmares in the elderly in a population based cohort study. Sleep Med 2021;78:15–23.

35. Suh S. Development and validation of a semi-structured clinical interview for nightmare disorder. J Sleep Med 2021;18(1):37–45.

36. Schlarb AA, Zschoche M, Schredl M. Der nightmare effects questionnaire (NEQ). Somnologie 2016;20(4):251–7.

37. Morgenthaler TI, Auerbach S, Casey KR, et al. Position paper for the treatment of nightmare disorder in adults: an American Academy of Sleep Medicine position paper. J Clin Sleep Med 2018;14(06):1041–55.

38. Abueg F. A Brief Guide to Imagery Rehearsal Therapy (IRT) for Nightmare Disorders for Clinicians and Patients. PsychCentral. Available at: https://psychcentral.com/blog/a-brief-guide-to-imagery-rehearsal-therapy-irt-for-nightmare-disordersfor-clinicians-and-patients/. Accessed October 25, 2023.

39. Thünker J, Pietrowsky R. Effectiveness of a manualized imagery rehearsal therapy for patients suffering from nightmare disorders with and without a comorbidity of depression or PTSD. Behav Res Ther 2012;50(9):558–64.

40. van Schagen AM, Lancee J, de Groot IW, et al. Imagery rehearsal therapy in addition to treatment as usual for patients with diverse psychiatric diagnoses suffering from nightmares: a randomized controlled trial. J Clin Psychiatry 2015;76(9):8490.

41. Davis JL, Rhudy JL, Pruiksma KE, et al. Physiological predictors of response to exposure, relaxation, and rescripting therapy for chronic nightmares in a randomized clinical trial. J Clin Sleep Med 2011;07(06):622–31.

42. Davis JL, Wright DC. Case series utilizing exposure, relaxation, and rescripting therapy: impact on nightmares, sleep quality, and psychological distress. Behav Sleep Med 2005;3(3):151–7.

43. Spoormaker VI, van den Bout J. Lucid dreaming treatment for nightmares: a pilot study. Psychother Psychosom 2006;75(6):389–94.

44. Zadra AL, Pihl RO. Lucid dreaming as a treatment for recurrent nightmares. Psychother Psychosom 2010;66(1):50–5.

45. Holzinger B, Klösch G, Saletu B. Studies with lucid dreaming as add-on therapy to Gestalt therapy. Acta Neurol Scand 2015;131(6):355–63.

46. Raskind MA, Peskind ER, Chow B, et al. Trial of prazosin for post-traumatic stress disorder in military veterans. N Engl J Med 2018;378(6):507–17.

47. Yücel DE, van Emmerik AAP, Souama C, et al. Comparative efficacy of imagery rehearsal therapy and prazosin in the treatment of trauma-related nightmares in adults: a meta-analysis of randomized controlled trials. Sleep Med Rev 2020;50:101248.

48. Ellis TE, Rufino KA, Nadorff MR. Treatment of nightmares in psychiatric inpatients with imagery rehearsal therapy: an open trial and case series. Behav Sleep Med 2019;17(2):112–23.

49. McCall WV, Pillai A, Case D, et al. A pilot, randomized clinical trial of bedtime doses of prazosin versus placebo in suicidal posttraumatic stress disorder patients with nightmares. J Clin Psychopharmacol 2018;38(6):618.

50. Krakow B, Hollifield M, Johnston L, et al. Imagery rehearsal therapy for chronic nightmares in sexual assault survivors with posttraumatic stress disorder: a randomized controlled trial. JAMA 2001;286(5):537–45.

51. Nadorff MR, Porter B, Rhoades HM, et al. Bad dream frequency in older adults with generalized anxiety disorder: prevalence, correlates, and effect of cognitive behavioral treatment for anxiety. Behav Sleep Med 2014;12(1). https://doi.org/10.1080/15402002.2012.755125.

52. Garakani A, Murrough JW, Freire RC, et al. Pharmacotherapy of anxiety disorders: current and emerging treatment options. Front Psychiatry 2020;11. Available at: https://www.frontiersin.org/articles/10.3389/fpsyt.2020.595584. Accessed July 31, 2023.

53. Worley CB, Bolstad CJ, Nadorff MR. Epidemiology of disturbing dreams in a diverse US sample. Sleep Med 2021;83:5–12.

54. NightWare prescribing information. NightWare U.S. product information. Minneapolis, MN: NightWare; 2020.

55. Davenport ND, Werner JK. A randomized sham-controlled clinical trial of a novel wearable intervention for trauma-related nightmares in military veterans. J Clin Sleep Med 2023. https://doi.org/10.5664/jcsm.10338.

56. Koulack D, Goodenough DR. Dream recall and dream recall failure: an arousal-retrieval model. Psychol Bull 1976;83(5):975–84.

57. Dal Sacco D. Dream recall frequency and psychosomatics. Acta Bio Medica Atenei Parm 2022;93(2). https://doi.org/10.23750/abm.v93i2.11218.

58. Krakow B, Kellner R, Pathak D, et al. Long term reduction of nightmares with imagery rehearsal treatment. Behav Cogn Psychother 1996;24(2):135–48.

59. Krakow B, Kellner R, Neidhardt J, et al. Imagery rehearsal treatment of chronic nightmares: with a thirty month follow-up. J Behav Ther Exp Psychiatry 1993;24(4):325–30.

60. Kellner R, Neidhardt J, Krakow B, et al. Changes in chronic nightmares after one session of desensitization or rehearsal instructions. Am J Psychiatr 1992;149(5):659–63.

61. Ulmer CS, Edinger JD, Calhoun PS. A multi-component cognitive-behavioral intervention for sleep disturbance in veterans with PTSD: a pilot study. J Clin Sleep Med 2011;07(01):57–68.

62. Lancee J, Spoormaker VI, Van Den Bout J. Long-term effectiveness of cognitive–behavioural self-help intervention for nightmares. J Sleep Res 2011;20(3):454–9.

63. Seda G, Sanchez -Ortuno Maria M, Welsh CH, et al. Comparative meta-analysis of prazosin and imagery rehearsal therapy for nightmare frequency, sleep quality, and posttraumatic stress. J Clin Sleep Med 2015;11(01):11–22.

64. Nappi CM, Drummond SPA, Thorp SR, et al. Effectiveness of imagery rehearsal therapy for the treatment of combat-related nightmares in veterans. Behav Ther 2010;41(2):237–44.

65. Kung S, Espinel Z, Lapid MI. Treatment of nightmares with prazosin: a systematic review. Mayo Clin Proc 2012;87(9):890–900.

66. Krakow B. Turning nightmares into dreams. Albuquerque, NM: The New Sleepy Times; 2002.

67. Gieselmann A, Böckermann M, Sorbi M, et al. The effects of an internet-based imagery rehearsal intervention: a randomized controlled trial. Psychother Psychosom 2017;86(4):231–40.

68. Burgess M, Marks IM, Gill M. Postal self-exposure treatment of recurrent nightmares: randomised controlled trial. Br J Psychiatry 1998;172(3):257–62.

69. Nadorff MR, Nadorff DK, Germain A. Nightmares: under-reported, undetected, and therefore untreated. J Clin Sleep Med JCSM 2015;11(7):747–50.

70. Nadorff MR, Nazem S, Fiske A. Insomnia symptoms, nightmares, and suicide risk: duration of sleep disturbance matters. Suicide Life Threat Behav 2013;43(2):139–49.

Exploding Head Syndrome
A Systematic Scoping Review

Dónal G. Fortune, ClinPsyD, PhD[a,b,c,*], Helen L. Richards, ClinPsyD, PhD[a,d]

KEYWORDS

- Exploding head syndrome • Parasomnias • Sleep disorders • Scoping review

KEY POINTS

- Exploding Head Syndrome (EHS) has historically been viewed as a disorder predominantly affecting older people and being more common in females.
- Through a comprehensive review of data since 2005, this scoping review provides updated evidence from 4082 participants reporting EHS across a variety of study designs on: how EHS presents; key information on comorbidity and correlates of EHS; how EHS is experienced in terms of symptoms and beliefs; causal theories arising from the research reviewed; and evidence-based information on how research has reported on the management of EHS.
- Since 2005, EHS has attracted increasing research interest; however, there are significant gaps in the research that are hindering a better understanding of EHS that might be helpful for clinicians.

BACKGROUND

Exploding head syndrome (EHS) is generally understood as a benign sensory parasomnia typified by the perception of a loud noise, bang, or explosion inside the head during the transition from sleep-to-wake or wake-to-sleep states.

EHS has a long past but a relatively short history. The earliest written reference to EHS was reported to have been made by Descartes in November 1619, where he described experiencing a loud noise or thunder sound in his head accompanied by a flash of light on wakening.[1] The first known medical description was from the Neurologist Silas Weir Mitchell in 1876, where he described one of his patients who reported the experience of a *"pistol shot"* within his head as he slept.[2] Mitchell used the term *"sensory shock'"* as a description of the disorder in a later paper,[3] while Armstrong-Jones[4] described the condition as a *"snapping of the brain"* in 1920. Despite these early descriptions of its phenomenology, EHS gained its current nomenclature in 1989[5] and it only entered the International Classification of Sleep Disorders (ICSD) in 2005.[6] In this context,

the literature in this area is likely to be significantly underdeveloped.

- ICSD third edition patients must meet criteria A-C as follows[7];
  - A. There is a complaint of sudden loud noise or sense of explosion in the head either at the wake-sleep transition or upon waking during the night.
  - B. The individual experiences abrupt arousal following the event, often with a sense of fright.
  - C. The experience is not associated with significant complaints of pain.

There is a clear need to systematically map the available current literature on EHS in relation to its prevalence and presentation, theories of causation, correlates/comorbidity, and experience of patients, including outcomes and management of the condition. The authors therefore aim to provide a systematic scoping review of the available published and gray literature in this area since EHS entered the ICSD in 2005. The authors aim to ask the following questions of the available

[a] Department of Psychology, University of Limerick, Ireland; [b] Health Service Executive, CHO3, Mid West Region, Ireland; [c] Health Research Institute, University of Limerick, Ireland; [d] Mercy University Hospital, Grenville Place, Cork, Ireland
* Corresponding author. University of Limerick, V94 T9PX Ireland.
E-mail address: donal.fortune@ul.ie

Sleep Med Clin 19 (2024) 121–142
https://doi.org/10.1016/j.jsmc.2023.10.007
1556-407X/24/© 2023 Elsevier Inc. All rights reserved.

literature which should be helpful for clinicians to increase understanding of EHS.

(1) How does EHS present clinically?
(2) What are the underlying comorbidities and correlates of EHS?
(3) What are the subjective complaints and beliefs associated with EHS and how do patients with EHS interpret symptoms?
(4) What are the current evidence-based causal theories of EHS?
(5) How is EHS currently managed?

METHODOLOGY

The protocol for this study was developed using the Preferred Reporting Items for Systematic Reviews and Meta-Analyses Extension for Scoping Reviews (PRISMA-ScR) Checklist.[8] The final protocol was registered in open science framework on 06/30/2023 and is available at: https://osf.io/vye68/.

DATA SOURCES AND SEARCH STRATEGY

The authors undertook a systematic search of English language articles published from 1st January 2005 to 1st July 2023. The authors chose 2005 as their inception date as EHS was entered into the ICSD during this year. The authors used the established scoping review framework[9] and the methods outlined in the JBI reviewers manual for scoping reviews.[10] The key databases searched were *cumulative Index to Nursing and Allied Health Literature* (CINAHL), Embase, Medline, Psych Info, Scopus, Web of Science, and the Cochrane Library. The authors searched the reference lists of all included papers for other relevant sources of data. They also undertook a search for gray literature on "Google," open access theses, and dissertations (oatd.org) and pre-print servers (BioRxiv, MedRxiv, and OSF Preprints). They anticipated that the literature on EHS was going to be sparse, so they kept their search terms as broad as possible to limit the possibilities of excluding relevant papers. The key search term used for all databases and gray literature searches was "Exploding head syndrome." No restrictions were made in relation to publication type. Studies were excluded if they were not published in English, if they did not contain reference to EHS, did not contain new data (eg, editorials, commentaries), were conference abstracts, if the full text of the article was not available, and if they were published before 2005, as a number of narrative reviews have been published that included this earlier work.

SELECTION OF SOURCES OF EVIDENCE

The de-duplicated bibliographic database citations were uploaded into Rayyan. The 2 authors independently screened titles and abstracts for full text review. In the event of disagreement, these were resolved through discussion and consensus. The authors aimed to include papers for full-text review if there were concerns raised by either author that relevant data may be contained within the full text. They subsequently performed full text review of the selected articles and were blinded to each other's decision. Titles and full texts of gray literature were also screened.

DATA EXTRACTION

An excel file was developed to record the data extracted from each of the included articles and data sources. The following data were extracted: author (s), country, study design, aim/purpose of the study, sample characteristics and size, and main outcomes of the study as they related to the research questions, how EHS presents, evidence-based etiologic theories, co-morbidities/correlates reported, nature of symptoms and beliefs reported by participants, and management issues. DGF extracted the data which were reviewed by HLR.

RESULTS
Selection of Sources of Evidence and Characteristics

Three hundred ninety six records in total were identified via the bibliographic database searches, with 142 articles remaining after de-duplication. Following initial screening of abstract and titles, 32 records remained which were sought for full-text review, with 30 articles being included in this review. See **Fig. 1** for PRISMA flow diagram of search results.

The characteristics of the 30 studies included in the synthesis are illustrated in **Table 1**. There were 2 sets of data which were used twice across articles.[11–14] The total number of participants with EHS extracted from these studies was 4082, with an age range from 13 to 93 year old. The majority of studies were case reports or case series (18 studies), and 12 studies were cross-sectional studies including 1 small retrospective case-controlled study. EHS samples sizes in case-control and cross-sectional studies ranged from N = 5 to 3286. In terms of diversity, 13 studies originated from Europe, 7 studies from Asia, 8 studies from North America, 1 study from South America (Mexico), and 1 study from the Middle east/western Asia (Saudi Arabia). Two international samples were also utilized. There were no

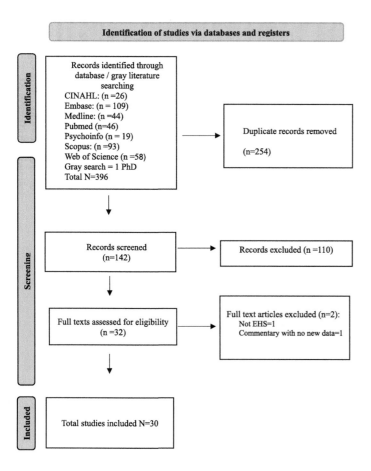

Fig. 1. PRISMA 2020 flow diagram of search results.

HOW DOES EHS PRESENT?
How Common Is EHS?

In community samples examined through survey methods, lifetime prevalence of EHS varied significantly. In a study of participants on a national sleep registry, EHS was reported by between 2.6% (n = 35/1333) in a control group and 6.8% (n = 60/877) in a probable insomnia sample.[15] In the development sample of the Munich Parasomnia Screening measure (MUPS),[16] the proportion of sleep-disordered patients reporting EHS (10%, 5/50) was not appreciably different to controls (10.8% 7/65), which were both somewhat lower than psychiatric patients (13.8% 9/65). A study of consecutive patients attending a tinnitus and hyperacusis clinic (n = 148) found 8% of patients reporting at least 1 episode of EHS.[17]

In college students, lifetime prevalence rates were very similar in 2 studies: 20% in an Irish sample[18] using the EHS screening questions from the MUPS, and 18% in a US sample[19] using a clinical interview protocol. A study in the UK reported higher rates at between 29% and 37%[20] despite using the same MUPS screening question.[18]

In the largest survey of EHS to date, 52.7% (n = 3286) of an international survey sample reported experiencing at least 1 episode of EHS in their lifetime.[13,14] EHS was assessed by clinical interview items in a questionnaire format. The authors acknowledge the very high rate of EHS reports may be related to the method of advertisement of the study.

The rates of EHS found across studies show wide variability depending on the nature of the samples and the way EHS is assessed (ie, questionnaire vs interview). The reported method of diagnosis of EHS varied among case reports. Clinical history, neurologic examination, routine laboratory tests alongside a variety of the following were generally employed: collateral history,[21] structured clinical interview of patients and their bed partners,[22] ICSD criteria,[23,24] electroencephalogram (EEG),[24–32] ambulatory EEG,[21] video-telemetry EEG,[21] video EEG,[33] computed tomography (CT),[31] MRI,[21,24,25,28,30–36] magnetic resonance (MR) angiogram,[30,31] "neuroimaging,"[25,26]

studies that met inclusion criteria that specified African or Australian participants.

Table 1
Characteristics of Studies Included in this Systematic Scoping Review

Study Authors	Country	Design	Overall Aim	Sample	Main Outcome Related to EHS
Aazh et al,[17] 2023	The United Kingdom	Retrospective cross-sectional survey	To assess prevalence of EHS and its related factors among patients referred to specialist tinnitus and hyperacusis clinic.	Patients attending tinnitus and hyperacusis clinic N = 148 EHS n = 12 (8.1%) Age 59[14] 50% female (n = 6)	No significant relationships between individuals with and without EHS on demographic (age, gender), audiological, sleep difficulties, or psychological distress (anxiety and depression).
Ariza-Serrano et al,[40] 2023	Mexico	Cross-sectional Survey	To compare sleep features and the number of non-rapid eye movement (NREM) and rapid eye movement (REM) parasomnias among medical residents with and without Shift Work Disorder (SWD).	First year medical/ surgical residents N = 84 (non SWD); N = 15 (SWD)	Significant difference ($P < .05$) between residents with and without SWD who experienced EHS; 3% (n = 3) nonSWD vs 33% (n = 5) SWD.
Blanken et al,[15] 2019	Netherlands	On-line survey	To investigate whether insomnia disorder presents as different subtypes that are reflected in a multivariate pattern of stable characteristics, such as life history, trait positive and negative affect, and personality.	EHS n = 35 (2.6%) of 1333 in the control group N = 60 of 877 participants in an insomnia disorder subtype classification (6.84%).	n = 17/162 (10.5%) = highly distressed; n = 16/267 (6%) = moderately distressed–reward sensitive; 6/134 (4.5%) = moderate distressed–reward insensitive; 13/184 (7.1%) = Slightly distressed–high reactive; 8/130 (6.2%) = Slightly distressed–low reactive.
Chakravarty,[33] 2008	India	Case report	To report 2 cases of EHS 1 of which occurred during daytime naps only (case 2)	Case 1 = 48-yrs-old male Case 2 = 65-yrs-old male	Case 1. Several month history of wake to sleep EHS with increasing frequency over past 3 mo. Improved following initiation of flunarazine 10 mg daily. Case 2. EHS every 2–3 wk for 4 mo during d time naps. EHS resolved at 4 mo follow-up following initiation of flunarazine 10 mg daily.

Study	Country	Study design	Aim	Sample	Results
Denis et al,[20] 2019	Study 1: the United Kingdom Study 2: International sample	Cross-sectional survey	To examine prevalence rates, whether sleep, unusual sleep experiences, and well-being are associated with EHS.	Study 1: 199 female university students (18–50 y, mean 20 years) Study 2: 1673 participants via advertisements on university mailing list and sleep paralysis websites and forums (18–82 years, 53% female)	Study 1: Lifetime prevalence EHS 37.19% (n = 74) 6.5% EHS more than once/month. Multiple logistic regression-illustrated symptoms of insomnia and sleep paralysis frequency significantly associated with EHS. Study 2: Lifetime prevalence EHS 29.5% (n = 496); 64.24% female (n = 318); 18–82 y. 3.89% EHS once/month. Replicated findings of study 1. Additionally, multiple logistic regression showed dissociative experiences during wakefulness and other sleep experiences including nightmares, associated with EHS.
Evans,[38] 2006	The United States of America	Case report	To describe case report of unusual migraine aura of EHS followed by brief episode of sleep paralysis.	26-year-old female 8 y history of 1–2 episodes a year.	EHS followed by sleep paralysis (6 s duration) and migraine. Normal neurologic findings. Authors suggest that auras of EHS and sleep paralysis due to brainstem dysfunction and this triggers the trigeminal vascular system via an unknown mechanism resulting in migraine.
Fotis Sakellariou et al,[11] 2020*	The United Kingdom	Retrospective case review with matched controls	To explore biomarkers of EHS by performing macrostructural and event-related dynamic spectral analysis of the whole-night electroencephalogram. (EEG)	Five EHS patients Females n = 3 Age 53–69 y (mean age ± SEM: 58.2 ± 5) 10 control subjects Mean age 58.1 (SEM ± 4)	EHS patients demonstrated additional oscillatory activity during wakefulness and at sleep/wake periods. The activity was different in terms of its frequency, topography, and source from the alpha rhythm that it accompanied.

(continued on next page)

Table 1
(continued)

Study Authors	Country	Design	Overall Aim	Sample	Main Outcome Related to EHS
Frese et al,[31] 2014	Germany	Case series	To extend the understanding of the clinical experience of EHS	N = 6 2 males, 4 females Age range 57–75 y	Patients experience on average 1 × daily–1 × weekly episodes with varying chronicity. Most frequent experience accompanying noise was flashes of light and fear. Polysomnography (PSG) did not identify any particular sleep pattern associated with EHS.
Fulda et al,[16] 2008	Germany	Questionnaire development	To develop a screening questionnaire, to assess the lifetime prevalence and current frequency of parasomnias and unusual nocturnal behaviors in adults.	65 psychiatric patients (33 females, mean age 47 ± 15) 50 sleep-disordered patients (26 females, mean age 51 ± 18) 65 healthy controls (37 females, mean age 35, ± 10) Validation sample n = 36 of above samples	Psychiatric patients lifetime prevalence EHS: 13.8% Sleep-disordered patients lifetime prevalence EHS:10% Healthy controls lifetime prevalence EHS: 10% Validation sample lifetime prevalence EHS: 11.1%
Ganguly et al,[30] 2013	The United States of America	Case report	To describe case report	57-year-old male	Flashing sound on the right side of the head, 4 occasions over 2 y. All investigations unremarkable. Reassurance provided. No recurrence of EHS in that time

Study	Country	Study design	Objective	Patient	Key findings
Gillis & Ng,[21] 2017	Canada	Case report	To report on EHS diagnosed in a patient with epilepsy.	81-year-old male	New nocturnal events "rushing" through head, awakening from sleep, which increased in frequency after stress. Unremarkable investigations. Video EEG arousal out of NREM sleep, with posterior dominant rhythm immediately after arousal.
Hayreh,[29] 2020	The United States of America	Self-case report	To explore personal observations about the experience of EHS	93-year-old male	1-3 times/week only in bed during the transition from wakefulness to sleep. Concurrent diagnosis of sick sinus syndrome. Following pacemaker implantation, EHS resolved.
Ji,[28] 2022	Korea	Case report	To examine the association between EHS and sleep-breathing event with polysomnography	67-year-old male	Flash of visual lightning, 2 y duration. PSG showed a hypopnea event during N2 sleep preceding EHS. Symptoms of EHS decreased following weight reduction and positional therapy.
Kallweit et al,[37] 2008	Switzerland	Case report	To examine a case reporting an exacerbation of migraine following EHS event	54-year-old male	Reported 3 y history "attacks of an exploding head," occurring every 2 h in daytime and twice nightly. Migraine exacerbated after each attack. Video PSG and multiple sleep latency test, EHS attacks occurred at the wake to sleep transition and from NREM2. Suggest EHS is a rare acoustic and/or visual migraine aura.

(continued on next page)

Table 1
(continued)

Study Authors	Country	Design	Overall Aim	Sample	Main Outcome Related to EHS
Kaneko et al,[36] 2020	Japan	Case report	To report on a case of EHS with panic attacks (PA)	62-year-old female	14 mo history, loud noise inside the head, like a guitar string and honking bus horn. Increasing in frequency from once monthly to > once nightly. Fear of going to sleep triggered PA. Unremarkable investigations. Treated with education and clonazepam 0.25 mg. EHS and PA improved.
Kirwan & Fortune,[18] 2021	Ireland	Cross sectional study	To examine the relationship between EHS, sleep quality, unusual sleep experiences, psychological distress, and chronotype	N = 135 60% female Mean age = 21.77 ± SD = 2.08 y; 91.9% undergraduate	Lifetime prevalence of EHS 20% (n = 27). Current or frequent EHS 15.6%. Those with a lifetime prevalence of EHS experienced more symptoms of anxiety and poorer sleep quality. Logistic regression analysis demonstrated that parasomnias and action-related sleep disorders were associated with lifetime experience of EHS. Chronotype was unrelated to presence of EHS.
Kitagawa et al,[24] 2023	Japan	Case report	To describe a case of EHS preceding onset of mild cognitive impairment with Lewy Bodies.	68-year-old male	Once a month for 2 y history of EHS during wake/sleep, sleep/wake transition. Mild cognitive impairment—LB also diagnosed following assessment/investigations. EHS resolved following education/sleep hygiene.

Nakayama et al,[27] 2021	Japan	Case report	To report 2 cases of EHS documented by PSG and treatment.	A 71-year-old female with tinnitus and Meniere's disease 55-year-old woman with psychiatric history and current depression	Following confirmation of EHS via PSG, Case 1 treated with rotigotine 2.25 mg/daily which did not impact symptoms but treatment of obstructive sleep apnea(OSA) with oral appliance was reported to resolve symptoms of EHS. Case 2 EHS is reported as improving symptoms of EHS with oral appliance for OSA and resolving EHS following electroconvulsive therapy(ECT) for severe depression.
Nesbitt,[12] 2020*	The United Kingdom	Retrospective case review with matched controls	To undertake a quantitative analysis of the whole-night sleep EEG of patients referred for evaluation of their EHS and to examine any trait-specific neurophysiological markers	EHS = 5; 3 female. Mean Age 58.2; SEM = 5.0 53–69 y)	EHS patients demonstrated additional oscillatory activity during wakefulness and at sleep/wake periods. The activity was different in terms of its frequency, topography, and source from the alpha rhythm that it accompanied.
Palikh & Vaughn,[26], 2010	The United States of America	Case report	To report on a case treatment of EHS with topiramate	A 39-year-old female, 3 y duration of EHS	Video confirmation of patient hearing a loud bang sound correlating with the transition from NREM stage 1 sleep to wake 200 mg topiramate, frequency of EHS did not change but intensity of sound became a low buzzing noise, and no longer impacted sleep.
Pirzada et al,[22] 2020	Saudi Arabia	Case series		EHS = 6. 4 men and 2 women of a mean age of 44.2 y (between 13 and 77 y)	Amitriptyline (50 mg) remission of EHS in a 46-year-old female with MS, experiencing EHS >1/wk over 2 y, supine sleeping position

(continued on next page)

Table 1
(continued)

Study Authors	Country	Design	Overall Aim	Sample	Main Outcome Related to EHS
					Sleep hygiene and cognitive behavioural therapy(CBT) improved insomnia and EHS is remission for 3 y in a 46-year-old male experiencing EHS 1–2/month over 12 y. Supine sleeping position.
					Sleep behavior education, EHS in remission for 2 y in a 13-year-old boy, experiencing EHS 2–3/month, not related to sleeping position.
					Amitriptyline (10 mg) remission of EHS in a 38-year-old male, experiencing EHS 1–2 times/week, over 4 y (2 psychiatric diagnoses).
					Ten mg amitriptyline complete remission at follow-up. A 77-year-old male experiencing EHS 3–4 times/month over 30 y (diabetes and hypertension) more frequent in supine sleeping position.
					Gabapentin (200 mg, later stopped after 6 mo) EHS in remission in a 45-year-old woman, experiencing EHS 2–3/month (restless legs syndrome). Prone sleeping position.

Author, year	Country	Study type	Aim	Sample	Findings
Puledda et al,[23] 2021	The United Kingdom	Case report	To report the case of a patient with EHS and outcome following treatment by single-pulse transcranial magnetic stimulation (sTMS)	A 62-year-old male experiencing EHS 10 times/night, also could occur during daytime naps. 30 y history of migraine without aura.	sTMS (2–3 pulses, twice to four times daily) EHS frequency reduced >50%, with minimal headache improvement. On cessation of sTMS, frequency of EHS increased again to baseline after 3 d
Rauf et al,[14] 2023#	The United Kingdom and International	Cross-sectional online study	Aimed to examine the associations between a wide range of paranormal beliefs and sleep variables	A total of 3286 individuals with and 2954 without lifetime EHS episodes (Mean age 47 y SD 15.3; 18–89 y). 66% female.	A total of 2.8% endorsed the belief that their EHS was the result of non-biological, supernatural causes. 2.3% believed it to be due to electronic devices The belief that aliens have visited Earth or interacted with humans was more common in people reporting EHS than non EHS participants (small effect size).
Salih et al,[34] 2008	Germany	Case report	To report a case of EHS in the context of a brainstem lesion	A 64-year-old female, up to 15 times/night; 12 y history. Pontomesencephalic lesion around the periaquaductal gray reaching into the tegmentum.	Clonazepam (0.5 mg at night) associated with undisturbed sleep at 8 mo follow-up. Removal of treatment associated with immediate relapse
Sharpless,[19] 2015	The United States of America	Cross-sectional study	To examine prevalence and psychological correlates of EHS in a sample of undergraduate students.	A total of 18% lifetime EHS n = 38. A total of 16.6% recurrent episodes.	EHS more common in fearful isolated sleep paralysis. Moderate fear was common. Mild distress and interference, although 2.8% reported clinically significant levels of distress.

(continued on next page)

Table 1
(continued)

Study Authors	Country	Design	Overall Aim	Sample	Main Outcome Related to EHS
Sharpless,[39] 2018	The United States of America	Cross-sectional study	To catalog sounds and their reported location experienced during EHS and report the frequency and relative fear/severity levels of symptoms	N = 49; 33 females, 15 males, and 1 transgender individual.	Median of 9.6 lifetime episodes. A total of 83% reported EHS during wake-sleep transitions and 43% during sleep-wake transitions. Volume of sounds 100%, Tachycardia 83%, Fear 81%, Muscle jerks 68%, Sweating 34%, Something seriously wrong 30%, Light 27%. A total of 11% reported to professionals. No diagnostic label or specific treatment provided. A total of 8% of participants attempted to prevent EHS.
Sharpless et al,[13] 2020[#]	The United States of America and the United Kingdom	Cross-sectional online study	Assess for differences in EHS prevalence; Determine frequency, fear level, and overall clinical distress and interference associated with EHS episodes; Replicate associations between sleep disturbances and EHS; Catalog the perceived etiologies of EHS; Catalog attempts taken to prevent EHS episodes and their perceived effectiveness.	Internationally sourced. Online survey 3286 individuals with and 2954 without lifetime EHS episodes.	EHS had shorter sleep durations, longer sleep onset latencies, poorer sleep quality, and less sleep efficiency, but effect sizes for these differences were small. Females were slightly more likely than males to endorse EHS. A total of 44.4% experienced significant fear during episodes; 25% clinically significant distress; 10.1% EHS interference. Something in the brain 60.6%; Stress 34.7%; Medication side effects 7.2%; Supernatural 2.8%; electronics 2.3%.

					Five prevention strategies with >50% reported effectiveness were identified: Using/refraining from substances; Changing sleep position, adjusting sleep patterns; relaxation/mindfulness/breathing techniques; wake up or rouse oneself; adjust sleep environment.
Sumi et al,[35] 2021	Japan	Case report	Report a case of an individual with kappa rhythm transition before every EHS attack.	A 57-year-old female, 2 mo history, during sleep onset (d or night) REM sleep behavior disorder Low-tone semineural hearing loss and tinnitus, anxiety, nervousness.	A total of 0.5 mg clonazepam, sound intensity decreased "to some extent."
Swingle et al,[32] 2023	The United States of America	Case report	To examine a possible case of EHS associated with hypoxic central hypoventilation probably engendered by opioid use.	A 36-year-old male 5 y history, nightly occurrence of EHS NREM1 or during transitions between wake and NREM1 State-dependent chronic hypoventilation accompanied by mild OSA.	Chronic methadone use may have led to elevation at the Pa_{CO} threshold causing hypoventilation which may trigger arousals.

(continued on next page)

Table 1
(continued)

Study Authors	Country	Design	Overall Aim	Sample	Main Outcome Related to EHS
Wang et al,[25] 2019	China	Case report	To report on 2 cases in the context of stress	26-year-old male 9 y history; "several" times during the night. Comorbid GAD. A 30-year-old male, 2 mo history, with 3 EHS episodes.	Stress reported as a cause and exacerbation of EHS in both cases. Reassurance did not lead to improvement in case 1. An serotonin and norepinephrine reuptake inhibitors (SNRI) was prescribed (duloxetine hydrochloride) which was reported to be associated with a significant decrease in the frequency and duration of episodes at 6 mo. Case 2 received reassurance and sleep education, outcome is unknown.

Abbreviations: LB, lewy bodies; MS, multiple sclerosis.
* both of these studies use the samm sample.
# both of these studies use the same sample.

polysomnography   (PSG),[28,30–32,34–36]   video PSG,[22,25,27,37] PSG with transcutaneous CO_2 (TCO$_2$) monitoring[32] and multiple sleep latency test.[22,35,37] As the EHS sometimes presented in the context of other possible conditions, additional structured assessments of mood,[24,25] cognitive function,[24] and insomnia[28,31,36] were also reported.

How Long do People Report the Duration of Their EHS?

Duration of EHS across case reports ranged from 2 months to 30 years, with the median duration of 2 years. Duration of EHS across surveys was not routinely provided within articles.

How Frequently do Sufferers Experience EHS Symptoms?

Case study data suggested a high frequency of EHS as might be expected with episodes more than once a night (n = 7),[23,25,31,34,36,37] nightly (n = 6),[26,31–33,35] weekly (n = 8),[22,24,27–29] monthly (n = 5),[22,25,33] and yearly (n = 4)[30,31,38] reported. In survey studies, the most common frequency of presentation was once or several times per year ranging from 7.4% in a university sample[20] to 34.9% of EHS participants in a large international sample.[13] The least common frequency of EHS was a high-frequency presentation where people were experiencing EHS on a weekly basis ranging from less than 2% in a university sample[20] and 10% in a large international survey.[13] A monthly presentation was endorsed by between 3%[20] and almost 10%.[13]; In a sample of patients referred to specialist audiology, two-thirds of the sample (n = 8/12) with EHS experienced an episode every 1 to 2 months.[17] In a student sample, where EHS was reported by 20% of the sample, no participant reported experiencing EHS frequently or very frequently.[18] While there was significant variation in EHS frequency reported across studies, within study frequencies were also subject to wide variation where frequencies ranged from 1 to 150 episodes, with a median of 9.6 lifetime episodes.[39] The self-reported duration of episodes was brief, with most EHS episodes lasting 1 second or less.[39]

Is EHS More Common in Older People?

In case study data (n = 31 cases), clinic sample,[17] and retrospective case-control data,[11] the age of patients with EHS ranged from 13 to 93 years. The mean and median for these 3 clinical samples fell within the 55 to 60 year old age range.

Only 1 survey study reported a statistically significant difference in the age of people reporting EHS[13] suggesting that, on average EHS participants were 2 years younger than non EHS participants (46.0 years vs 48.1 years). The age of EHS sufferers in student surveys was of course understandably younger.[20] There were no significant differences in studies that examined age and the presence of EHS in student or clinic samples, and the statistically significant finding in a very large online sample that EHS participants were on average 2 years younger than non-EHS participants is not likely to be meaningful.[13]

Are Women More Likely to Experience EHS?

Case report, case series, and a small retrospective case-control study reported data from 55.6% (n = 20) male and 44.4% (n = 16) female participants. Unfortunately, some of the larger survey and cross-sectional studies provided their data in such a way as to make abstraction of the actual number of males and females who reported EHS in their final sample/analyses not practicable. Where studies examined gender-related differences in prevalence of EHS, no gender differences were reported in most of these studies.[17–20] In 1 large study,[13] women were statistically more likely to report the presence of EHS than men; however, the difference between the overall sample of females versus the overall sample of males was less than 3% (53.5% females vs 50.7% males who endorsed EHS), again representing a very small effect size and would not be a meaningful result.

When Does EHS Occur—Wake to Sleep or Sleep to Wake?

The majority of the case report data suggest that it is more common for EHS to be experienced at the wake to sleep transition or early stages of sleep. Of the 18 case reports or case series reports, 23 patients reported wake to sleep, 5 patients reported sleep to wake, and 3 patients were reported as experiencing both. This in echoed in the larger studies. Nine out of 12 patients with EHS referred to a specialist audiology clinic reported a wake to sleep presentation, while 2/12 experienced EHS in the middle of the night.[17] Eighty-three percent (n = 41/49 participants) reported EHS during wake-sleep transitions and 43% (n = 21/49) during sleep-wake transitions.[39]

While self-report of EHS phenomena can be helpful, there are clearly limitations in relying solely on such reports to elucidate a sleep disorder. A number of case report polysomnography studies have shown arousal from non-rapid eye movement (NREM1) sleep,[26,27,37] and cases of arousal from NREM 2 sleep.[21,25,28,37] One case report showed EHS in transition from REM sleep to wakefulness.[27] Interestingly, in the only case-controlled study, all EHS patients (N = 5) demonstrated alpha coactivation oscillatory activity during pre-sleep wake or wake after sleep onset (WASO) periods,[11,12] which was not observed in the non-EHS controls. This result requires replication of course but is a very interesting observation.

WHAT ARE THE CO-MORBIDITIES AND CORRELATES OF EHS?

Many of the case report data reported on patients with EHS in the context of another (often related) condition see **Fig. 2** below. Sleep medicine and neurologic complaints were the most common co-morbidities reported.

What is the Emotional Impact of EHS?

A number of case studies reported distress arising from the experience of EHS including finding the experience unpleasant,[31] frightening,[23,28] embarrassing,[28] fearful and distressing,[22,23] and often accompanied by anxiety and nervousness.[25,26,35] One study reported EHS being associated with panic attacks and fear of falling asleep.[36]

The cross-sectional studies echoed this trend with reports of 10.5% of participants being highly distressed (n = 33) with a further 10.5% moderately distressed.[15] In a study of 12 patients under care of a tinnitus and hyperacusis service with EHS, fear and worry was reported in just under half this sample;[17] however, they were not more likely to experience higher levels of distress or mood compared with other patients accessing the service. In an EHS sample of 49 college students who were clinically assessed as meeting criteria for EHS, fear was reported by 81% of the sample as a result of EHS,[39] while 2.8% of a student sample reported clinically significant levels

of distress. EHS was also significantly more common in fearful isolated sleep paralysis.[19]

In a large study of 3286 international participants, 44.4% reported significant fear during episodes, 25% clinically significant distress, and 10.1% EHS interference.[13] Some studies have not found EHS to be consistently associated with validated questionnaire measures of depression or mood,[17,18,20] although mixed results have been reported (20; study 2). EHS has been shown to be associated with higher anxiety scores[18,20] and sleep variables,[18,20] with increased frequency of EHS episodes being associated with higher distress[13,20] and greater impairment resulting from episodes.[13] However, in a number of these studies, the relationship between EHS and measures of stress or anxiety substantially weaken or become non-significant when other sleep-related experiences are included in the statistical model.[18,20]

Does EHS Impact Sleep?

Of 18 case reports (n = 31 patients), there were 3 case reports of EHS associated with insomnia,[22,28,36] 2 reports of EHS with insomnia/sleep disorder,[24,31] 1 case of EHS and narcolepsy,[22] 1 case of EHS and rapid eye movement (REM) sleep behavior disorder,[35] and 3 reports of restless leg syndrome.[22,27,31] EHS and sleep apnea were reported in 6 individual cases.[22,27,28,31] Larger survey studies have demonstrated that insomnia and poor sleep quality are an important correlate of EHS and well-being,[13,15,18,20] and indeed 1 study has suggested that insomnia and other sleep experiences may serve to mediate the relationship between well-being and EHS.[20] People with EHS have been shown to be more likely to experience other parasomnias than people without EHS.[18,20] In insomnia disorder, 5.7% (N = 60/1046) of patients also reported EHS and of this number 21% of EHS patients

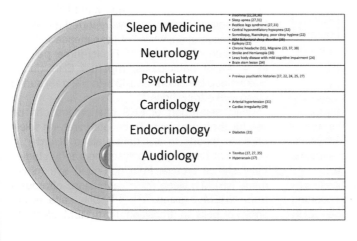

Fig. 2. Presence and nature of co-morbidities in EHS studies reviewed.

were reported to have a moderately distressed to severely distressed insomnia subtype.[15] A study on first year medical/surgical residents reported that residents with shift work disorder were also significantly more likely to experience EHS.[40] There is only 1 study to date to examine Chronotype and EHS, which did not find a relationship with self-report of EHS.[18]

Sleep Position

Data on sleeping position were provided in 3 case report studies on 7 patients.[22,28,30] EHS was observed in a supine position in 5 patients, 1 patient experienced EHS in the prone position, and no relationship was reported in relation to 1 patient. In a study on 49 college students assessed as meeting criteria for EHS,[39] almost half of the sample (47%) reported experiencing EHS while in a supine position, 17% in a prone sleeping position, and 30% in a lateral recumbent position. Only 6% of the sample reported EHS occurring in multiple positions. While care must be exercised in use of self-report in this context, the observational case report data of a predominance of EHS in a supine position are supportive of this cross-sectional self-report data.

WHAT ARE THE SUBJECTIVE COMPLAINTS AND BELIEFS ASSOCIATED WITH EHS AND HOW DO PATIENTS WITH EHS INTERPERET SYMPTOMS?

In all cases, the location of sound was perceived within the body–the head or brain. There was no identifiable right-sided or left-sided sound asymmetry or dominance in reported experience of EHS. Left versus right EHS lateralization was not regularly reported in cases or in larger scale studies and there were only 2 studies[30,39] that reported data on EHS lateralization. One case study reported a right lateralized EHS.[30] In a study on students, 26% experienced EHS on the right side, with 19% reporting the experience on the left. Most people (55% n = 27/49) experienced EHS bilaterally.[39]

While the predominant experience of EHS was an explosion or was described as a sound that could reasonably be understood as falling within the category of an "explosion, gunshot, or loud bang," there were other idiosyncratic sounds that were described or diagnosed as EHS including a "high pitched noise," "a guitar string and honking bus horn," "a loud beep," a "ding dong," or "white noise" (**Table 2**). There was also a case of a non-auditory "sudden rushing sensation moving up from the feet and up throughout the head."[21] The sound was accompanied by a flash of light in 9

studies, and with other behaviors or experiences were observed or reported, including jerking limbs,[26,28,33] brief frontal headache,[29] and a case of brief sleep paralysis.[38] The phenomenology of the experience of EHS suggests it is not solely limited to an explosive sound; however, caution must be exercised given the self-report nature of EHS in many of the survey studies, and in some case data, poor clarity on how EHS diagnosis was arrived at. There is also very high comorbidity in case reports or case series data.

Causal Beliefs Held by Sufferers About EHS

Only 3 case report studies reported the beliefs of patients as to the cause of EHS.[25,26,36] In all cases, patients believed that the symptoms represented something serious. In a large community sample study,[13] the perception that EHS was caused by something in the brain (60%) or represented something serious (30%) was echoed by the 3 case reports, where perceived causes relating to "Brain disease,"[36] or that "something serious was responsible"[25,26] were reported. Reports of EHS in the context of stress following a loss,[21] or beliefs held about EHS being caused by stress (34.7%), medication side effects (7.2%), supernatural events (2.8%), or electronic devices (2.3%) were endorsed in a large international survey.[13] When compared to people without EHS, participants reporting EHS were significantly more likely to believe that aliens have visited Earth or interacted with humans; however, the effect size in this very large study was small.[14]

WHAT ARE THE CURRENT EVIDENCE-BASED CAUSAL THEORIES OF EHS?

Nine studies used their results to provide evidence for a theory or model of the occurrence of EHS. Some studies, particularly case reports, reported comorbidity as a trigger, including obstructive sleep apnea,[28] cardiac asystole,[29] or that EHS might rarely present as a visual and/or acoustic migraine aura.[37]

The remaining studies also proposed a biological mechanism from observing outcomes in their case reports, including involvement of the serotonin system[36]; overactive or aberrant activity in the occipital network[25]; compromised gamma-aminobutyric acid(GABA)ergic transmission to the dorsal raphe nucleus[34]; modulation by brainstem neurons[23]; and delay in the reduction of activity in selected areas of the brainstem reticular formation as the person transitions from wakefulness to sleep.[38] The retrospective case-controlled study offered the hypothesis that at times of sleep-wake transition, aberrant

Table 2
Phenomenology of EHS experiences

	Nature of the Sound/Sensation	Study
Sounds	Explosion (n = 13)	23, 25, 27, 29, 30, 33, 39
	Loud bang (n = 14)	22, 25, 26, 31, 39
	Dropping an object from a height (n = 11)	39
	Gunshot (n = 3)	22, 39
	Cracking sound (n = 3)	22, 34
	Snapping sound (n = 2)	22
	Something hitting a tin roof (n = 1)	22
	Popping of a balloon (n = 1)	27
	Something hitting a wall (n = 3)	39
	Thud (n = 2)	39
	Fireworks (n = 2)	39
	Car Crash (n = 2)	39
	Breaking glass (n = 2)	39
	Metallic sounds, metal pans banging (n = 2)	24, 39
	Like a flying jet (n = 2)	22, 29
	High-pitched noise (n = 3)	39
	High-pitched whooshing sound like a car engine blowing (n = 1)	35
	Loud noise, like a guitar string and honking bus horn (n = 1)	36
	"Ding dong," drums, electrical explosion, music, scream, things being broken apart, train noise, white noise (all n = 1).	39
	Loud beep in both ears (n = 1)	38
Non auditory	Sudden rushing sensation (non-auditory) moving up from the feet and up throughout the head (n = 1)	21
	Accompanied by	
Visual Other	With short flash of light or lightning or electricity (n = 10)	23, 25, 28–31
		26
	Buzzing noise	31
	Mild jab-like pain	33
	Jerky elevation of right arm and "queer feeling" in the right chest	26, 28
		29
	Brief jerking movement of head leg or arm	38
	Frontal headache	
	Brief sleep paralysis	

attentional processing may lead to amplification and modulation of sensory stimuli.[11,12]

HOW HAS RESEARCH REPORTED ON THE MANAGEMENT OF EHS?

Management of EHS has included case reports of pharmacotherapy, use of *continuous positive airway pressure*, single-pulse transcranial magnetic stimulation, and a range of education and behavioral approaches with varying levels of outcome reported (**Table 3**). Again the majority of the data are from case report or case series studies.

DISCUSSION

The current systematic scoping review sought to provide a transparent evidence-based update of EHS based upon peer-reviewed studies and gray literature available since the condition entered the ICSD in 2005. The available data consisted of data from 4082 participants reporting EHS, and study designs comprised individual case report

Table 3
Management of EHS reported in the literature

Study	Management Strategy	Outcomes
Frese et al,[31] 2014	Calcium channel blocker (flunarizine 10 mg daily), 2 cases	• Reduction of daily EHS to twice in 6 mo. • Reduction from every 2–3 wk to zero at 4 mo follow-up
Frese et al,[31] 2014 Pirzada et al,[22] 2020 2 cases	10 mg amitriptyline, 1 case 25 mg amitriptyline, 1 case 25 mg amitriptyline, 1 case 50 mg amitriptyline, 2 cases	• Complete remission of EHS in 1 case.[31] • Substantial improvement in 1 case but patient was lost to follow-up.[31] • No positive effect.[31] • Case 1 (co-morbid MS) complete removal of EHS symptoms[22] • Case 2 initial improvement but discontinued due to unwanted side effects.[22]
Wang et al,[25] 2019	SNRI (Duloxetine) 1 case	• "Positive effect" at 6 mo follow-up[25]
Gillis & Ng,[21] 2017	clobazam (20 mg)[21] 1 case.	• Remission of EHS in a case with comorbid epilepsy[21]
Pirzada et al,[22] 2020	Gabapentin and control of serum ferritin level[22] 1 case.	• Unclear outcome[22]
Palikh & Vaughn,[26] 2010	topiramate (200 mg)[26] 1 case.	• Reduction in intensity of EHS, however, frequency of EHS did not change.[26]
Nakayama et al,[27] 2021	Dopamine agonist rotigotine (2.25 mg)[27] 1 case.	• Not effective[27]
Kaneko et al,[36] 2021,	25 mg clonazepam and reassurance[36] 1 case.	• Reduction from more than once every night to once every week at 6 mo[36]
Nakayama et al,[27] 2021 Ji,[28] 2022	Continuous positive airway pressure (CPAP) (sleep apnea) CPAP (sleep apnea)	• Two cases reported positive reductions in EHS frequency.[27,28] • Two cases where sleep apnea was reduced without any effect on EHS.[27,28]
Puledda et al,[23] 2021	Single-pulse transcranial magnetic stimulation (sTMS) 1 case.	• EHS frequency was reported to have reduced >50%. On cessation of sTMS, frequency of EHS increased again to baseline after 3 d.
Education and Behavioral Approaches		
Kitigawa,[24] 2023	psychoeducation, sleep hygiene instructions, cognitive behavioral approaches	• EHS symptoms reported to have become unnoticeable
Pirzada et al,[22] 2022	psychoeducation, sleep hygiene instructions, cognitive behavioral approaches	• EHS had resolved at 2 y, and 3 y follow-up
Sharpless,[39] 2018	Managing hypnotics Increasing levels of sleep	• 100% effective in 1 case • 80% and 100% effective–2 cases

(continued on next page)

Table 3 (continued)		
Study	**Management Strategy**	**Outcomes**
Sharpless et al,[13] 2020	5 prevention strategies were most helpful (n = 218): (1). More appropriately using substances or refraining from substances, (2). Changing sleep position, or adjusting sleep patterns, (3). Mindfulness/breathing techniques/relaxation, (4). Waking up or rousing oneself and (5). Adjusting the sleep environment, for example, increasing comfort in bed	• >50% effective

and case series data, small-scale retrospective case-control design, and cross-sectional survey studies.

Despite a number of larger survey studies having been published recently, it remains very challenging to abstract compelling data on EHS. Studies have tended to use uncontrolled case studies, convenience samples including students, small-scale clinic attendees, or surveys supported through the media. While these studies provide indicative data relevant to EHS, there are potential problems either with how EHS is assessed, with co-morbidity, or with the potential for bias in sample selection. However, a synthesis of the evidence reviewed in this scoping review suggests the following clinics care points.

CLINICS CARE POINTS

- While there are some interesting data suggesting the possibility of an interictal biomarker for EHS in the form of alpha coactivation, there is currently no objective test for EHS and most studies rely on self-report.
- EHS is most commonly reported at the transition from wake to sleep. However, it has also been observed in NREM2 sleep.
- Patients and study participants provide a variety of descriptions of EHS, where EHS may not necessarily be experienced as an explosion or bang.
- In most cases, patients have normal sleep architecture.
- The data currently available do not suggest significant gender differences in EHS.

- The majority of EHS events have been reported and clinically observed to occur in the supine sleeping position.
- EHS may be associated with distress in some cases and with poor self-reported sleep.
- Patients may hold unhelpful beliefs about the cause of EHS which may contribute to distress about EHS symptoms.
- There is no compelling evidence that medication should be a first-line treatment for the majority of patients, and EHS may be more responsive to low-intensity approaches such as education and reassurance.
- A number of prevention and management approaches have been reported by patients to be helpful including changing sleep position, adjusting sleep patterns, adjusting the sleep environment, waking up or rousing oneself, better management of medication/drugs, and engaging in relaxation practices.

FUTURE RESEARCH

There is a compelling need to broaden and deepen research into EHS. Specifically, there is a need for better prevalence studies using appropriate EHS criteria and standardized assessment protocols. Longitudinal and prospective studies with appropriate follow-up and with cleaner samples would be helpful to more accurately understand the course of the condition. There is a need for more adequately controlled studies on the potential biomarkers of EHS, and finally better studies on the management of EHS are required, especially controlled trials of brief and low-intensity interventions, which may include simple education and information provision, relaxation, and behavioral sleep management.

DISCLOSURE

The authors have no conflicts of interest to disclose.

REFERENCES

1. Otaiku AI. Did René Descartes have exploding head syndrome? J Clin Sleep Med 2018;14(4):675–8.
2. Mitchell SW. On some of the disorders of sleep. Va Med Mon 1876;11:769–81.
3. Mitchell SW. Some disorders of sleep. Am J Med Sci 1890;100:109–27.
4. Armstrong-Jones R. Snapping of the brain. Lancet 1920;193:720.
5. Pearce JMS. Clinical features of the exploding head syndrome. Journal ofNeurology, Neurosurgery, and Psychiatry 1989;52(7):907–10.
6. ICSD-2. International Classification of sleep disorders: Diagnostic and Coding manual. 2nd ed. Westchester, Illinois: American Academy of Sleep Medicine; 2005.
7. ICSD-3_TR. International Classification of sleep disorders. Darien, IL: American Academy of Sleep Medicine; 2023.
8. Tricco AC, Lillie E, Zarin W, et al. PRISMA extension for scoping reviews (PRISMA-ScR): checklist and explanation. Ann Intern Med 2018;169(7):467–73.
9. Arksey H, O'Malley L. Scoping studies: towards a methodological framework. Int J Soc Res Methodol 2005;2:19–32.
10. Peters M, Godfrey C, McInerney P, et al. Best practice guidance and reporting items for the development of scoping review protocols. JBI Evidence Synthesis 2002;20:953–68.
11. Fotis Sakollariou D, Nesbitt AD, Higgins S, et al. Co-activation of rhythms during alpha band oscillations as an interictal biomarker of exploding head syndrome. Cephalalgia 2020;40(9):949–58.
12. Nesbitt A. Sleep, biological rhythms & headache, 2020, PhD Submitted to Kings College London; University of London.
13. Sharpless BA, Denis D, Perach R, et al. Exploding head syndrome: clinical features, theories about etiology, and prevention strategies in a large international sample. Sleep Med 2020;75:251–5.
14. Rauf B, Perach R, Madrid-Valero JJ, et al. The associations between paranormal beliefs and sleep variables. J Sleep Res 2023;e13810.
15. Blanken TF, Benjamins JS, Borsboom D, et al. Insomnia disorder subtypes derived from life history and traits of affect and personality. Lancet Psychiatr 2019;6(2):151–63.
16. Fulda S, Hornyak M, Müller K, et al. Development and validation of the Munich parasomnia screening (MUPS). Somnologie - Schlafforschung und Schlafmedizin 2008;12(1):56–65.
17. Aazh H, Stevens J, Jacquemin L. Exploding Head Syndrome among patients seeking help for tinnitus and/or hyperacusis at an Audiology Department in the UK: a preliminary study. J Am Acad Audiol 2023. https://doi.org/10.1055/a-2084-4808.
18. Kirwan E, Fortune DG. Exploding head syndrome, chronotype, parasomnias and mental health in young adults. J Sleep Res 2021;30(2):e13044.
19. Sharpless BA. Exploding head syndrome is common in college students. J Sleep Res 2015;24(4):447–9.
20. Denis D, Poerio GL, Derveeuw S, et al. Associations between exploding head syndrome and measures of sleep quality and experiences, dissociation, and well-being. Sleep 2019;42(2).
21. Gillis K, Ng MC. Exploding head syndrome in the epilepsy monitoring unit: case report and literature review. Neurodiagn J 2017;57(2):133–8.
22. Pirzada AR, Almeneessier AS, Bahammam AS. Exploding head syndrome: a case series of underdiagnosed hypnic parasomnia. Case Rep Neurol 2020; 12(3):348–58.
23. Puledda F, Moreno-Ajona D, Goadsby PJ. Exploding head syndrome (a.k.a. episodic cranial sensory shock) responds to single-pulse transcranial magnetic stimulation. Eur J Neurol 2021;28(4):1432–3.
24. Kitagawa S, Okamoto N, Ikenouchi A, et al. A case of exploding head syndrome preceding the onset of mild cognitive impairment with Lewy bodies. Psychogeriatrics 2023;23(2):368–70.
25. Wang X, Zhang W, Yuan N, et al. Characteristic symptoms of exploding head syndrome in two male patients. Sleep Med 2019;57:94–6.
26. Palikh GM, Vaughn BV. Topiramate responsive exploding head syndrome. J Clin Sleep Med 2010;6(4):382–3.
27. Nakayama M, Nakano N, Mihara T, et al. Two cases of exploding head syndrome documented by polysomnography that improved after treatment. J Clin Sleep Med 2021;17(1):103–6.
28. Ji KH. Exploding head syndrome associated with severe obstructive sleep apnea. Sleep Medicine Research 2022;13(3):176–8.
29. Hayreh SS. Exploding head syndrome: new observations. Eur J Neurol 2020;27(11):2333–5.
30. Ganguly G, Mridha B, Khan A, et al. Exploding head syndrome: a case report. Case Rep Neurol 2013;5(1): 14–7.
31. Frese A, Summ O, Evers S. Exploding head syndrome: six new cases and review of the literature. Cephalalgia 2014;34(10):823–7.
32. Swingle N, Davis EM, Quigg M. Exploding head syndrome associated with central hypoventilatory hypopnea. Ann Am Thorac Soc 2023;20(7):1061–5.
33. Chakravarty A. Exploding head syndrome: report of two new cases. Cephalalgia 2008;28(4):399–400.
34. Salih F, Klingebiel R, Zschenderlein R, et al. Acoustic sleep starts with sleep-onset insomnia related to a brainstem lesion. Neurology 2008;70(20):1935–7.

35. Sumi Y, Miyamoto T, Sudo S, et al. Explosive sound without external stimuli following electroencephalography kappa rhythm fluctuation: a case report. Cephalalgia 2021;41(13):1396–401.
36. Kaneko Y, Kawae A, Saitoh K, et al. Exploding head syndrome accompanied by repeating panic attacks: a case report. Front Psychiatr 2021;11.
37. Kallweit U, Khatami R, Bassetti CL. Exploding head syndrome - more than "snapping of the brain"? Sleep Med 2008;9(5):589.
38. Evans RW. Exploding head syndrome followed by sleep paralysis: a rare migraine aura. Headache 2006;46(4):682–3.
39. Sharpless BA. Characteristic symptoms and associated features of exploding head syndrome in undergraduates. Cephalalgia 2018;38(3):595–9.
40. Ariza-Serrano J, Santana-Vargas D, Millan-Rosas G, et al. Parasomnias related to shift work disorder among medical residents during the first year of training in Mexico. Sleep Biol Rhythm 2023;21(1):105–11.

Sleep-Related Hallucinations

Flavie Waters, MSc, MPsych, PhD[a,b,*], Ivan Ling, MBBS, FRACP[c,d], Somayyeh Azimi, PhD[a,e], Jan Dirk Blom, MD, PhD[f,g,h]

KEYWORDS

- Classification • Hallucinations • Dream-like experiences • Hypnagogic • Hypnopompic
- Hypnagogia

KEY POINTS

- Sleep-related hallucinations (SRH) refer to a diagnostic category within the ICSD-3 group of "Other Parasomnias" that comprises two symptoms: hypnagogic and hypnopompic hallucinations (HHH) and complex nocturnal visual hallucinations (CNVH).
- Some individuals may also experience clinical hallucinations during the day that are unassociated with SRS.
- HHH are extremely common and generally benign in the general population. They are also a nonspecific symptom for any sleep disorders, or psychiatric, medical, and neurologic conditions.
- Little information exists about CNVH, though their resemblance to visual hallucinations in Charles Bonnet syndrome and other neurologic conditions suggest that they reflect a marker for psychopathology.
- A categorical approach to assessment reliant solely on the presence of SRH is not helpful as a diagnostic aid as SRH frequently co-occur with other sleep disorders and medical conditions.

INTRODUCTION

There has been a long-standing historical interest in the relationship between sleep and hallucinations. The American psychiatrist William Charles Dement (1928–2020) went so far as to suggest that "there can be little question that dreams qualify as hallucinations."[1] This notion contrasts with the engrained distinction between sleep and waking states, but many researchers are intrigued by the possibility of a continuum.[2–4] In the second and third editions of the International Classification of Sleep Disorders (ICSD, 2005[5]; 2014;[6] 2023[7]), hallucinatory phenomena that occur in the context of sleep are included as a diagnostic group called sleep-related hallucinations (SRH). SRH refer to a class of hallucinations that occur at sleep onset or on awakening from sleep and are reported on after the transition to a waking state has occurred.

In the ICSD,[5] SRH are classed within the broader group of parasomnia disorders. They solely include two hallucinatory events, comprising (1) hypnagogic and hypnopompic hallucinations ("HHH," also referred to collectively as hypnagogia) occurring in the drowsy state at the time of falling asleep or waking in the morning, respectively and (2) complex

[a] Clinical Research Centre, Graylands Hospital, North Metropolitan Health Service Mental Health, Brockway Road, John XXIII Avenue, Mount Claremont, Perth, Western Australia 6009, Australia; [b] School of Psychological Science, The University of Western Australia, Crawley, Western Australia, Australia; [c] West Australian Sleep Disorders Research Institute, Perth, Australia; [d] Department of Pulmonary Physiology & Sleep Medicine, Sir Charles Gairdner Hospital, 5th Floor, G-block, Nedlands, Western Australia 6009, Australia; [e] School of Human Sciences, University of Western Australia, Crawley, Western Australia, Australia; [f] Parnassia Psychiatric Institute, Kiwistraat 43, The Hague 2552 DH, the Netherlands; [g] Faculty of Social and Behavioural Sciences, Leiden University, Leiden, the Netherlands; [h] Department of Psychiatry, University Medical Center Groningen, Groningen, the Netherlands
* Corresponding author.
E-mail addresses: flavie.waters@health.wa.gov.au; Flavie.waters@uwa.edu.au

Sleep Med Clin 19 (2024) 143–157
https://doi.org/10.1016/j.jsmc.2023.10.008
1556-407X/24/© 2023 Elsevier Inc. All rights reserved.

nocturnal visual hallucinations (CNVH), following a sudden awakening during the night. The latter occurs mostly in the setting of visual and neurologic disorders. Some individuals may have hallucinations during the day, which are not associated with these sleep-related events.

The similarities between sleep-related events and "daytime" hallucinations have received much scrutiny, but a lot remains unknown about this new relatively category called "SRH." In any case, they can reveal fascinating insights into the activities of the sleeping brain that are not readily available to our conscious awareness. In addition, they can shed light on other types of hallucination, notably visual hallucinations occurring in the context of Charles Bonnet syndrome (deafferentation phenomena) and release phenomena.

The objective of this review is to facilitate an understanding of SRH. To achieve this, it will address the history, background, and descriptions of SRH and discuss the continuity between SRH and other conditions. Similarities and differences to daytime clinical hallucinations are outside of our scope (for a detailed discussion, see Ref[3]).

HISTORY AND BACKGROUND

Although sleep has been a topic of philosophic and prescientific investigation since the time of Aristotle (384–322 BC) and beyond (Aristotle, 1984), the modern study of sleep only truly began with the application of the electroencephalogram (EEG) and eye movement detection techniques to the sleeping brain. These techniques revealed that human consciousness commutes between three naturally occurring and reversible neurophysiological and behavioral states called wakefulness, rapid eye movement (REM) sleep, and non-rapid eye movement (NREM) sleep.[2] These states are continuous and cyclical and quantifiable by the degree of complexity in which neurons interact within the central nervous system.[8] Far from being passive, these states of consciousness all involve active brain functions, although connectivity with prefrontal cortex and executive functions distinguishes wakefulness from NREM and REM.

Mental events occurring during sleep have a physiologic basis that can be recorded. For example, dreaming during sleep coincides with cyclically recurring periods of EEG-recorded sleep states and eye movements.[9] Although sleep electrophysiology progresses in a relatively uniform way across individuals, elements of REM and NREM sleep are not mutually exclusive. In some individuals, REM and NREM may dissociate and/or recombine to create undesirable experiences during sleep, which are termed "parasomnias."[10–12]

The first reference to hallucinations in sleep diagnostic manuals can be traced back to the initial edition of the ICSD (1990[13]) and its subsequent revision, the ICSD-R (2001[14]), under the category of Terrifying Hypnagogic Hallucinations. These were described as intensely frightening hallucinatory phenomena occurring only at sleep onset and a type of nightmare that interrupts the process of falling asleep and leads to a sudden return to full wakefulness.[15] These phenomena may be accompanied by a realistic awareness of the presence of someone or something, often causing a profound sense of fear or dread (**Table 1**). In these earlier versions of the ICSD,[13,14] they were described as extremely rare, and their clinical significance was rated using criteria based on severity (mild, moderate, severe) and duration (acute, subacute, chronic).

Subsequent versions of ICSD (−2,[5] −3,[6] and 3 TR[7]) featured the newly identified group of SRH within the broader diagnostic cluster of the parasomnias. Thus, from 2005 onward, SRH have been defined as "Hallucinatory experiences that occur at sleep onset or on awakening from sleep," thereby expanding on the previous diagnostic category of Terrifying Hypnagogic Hallucinations. They can occur in the absence of other symptoms or disorders ("idiopathic type") or as a symptom of another sleep disorder. The specification for clinical significance states that this experience must be recurrent and that infrequent hallucinations of this type may be within the limits of normal sleep–wake transition.

DESCRIPTION AND CLASSIFICATION

ICSD-3 criteria of SRH include (1) a complaint of recurrent hallucinations that are experienced just before sleep onset or on awakening; (2) prominently in the visual modality, and (3) the disturbance is not better explained by another sleep, mental, or medical disorder, medication, or substance use.[6,7]

SRH refer to two separate experiences: HHH and CNVH.

The first published descriptions of hypnagogic hallucinations in the general population can be traced back to almost 180 years ago to French neurologist and psychiatrist Jules-Gabriel Francois Baillarger (1809–1890).[16] By contrast, descriptions of CNVH are very recent.[17,18]

Since Alfred Maury's (1817–1892) observation in 1865[4] of a continuum in form and content with daytime hallucinations, the classification systems for all clinical and clinical subtypes of hallucinations have sought to chart their sensory modality, contents, form, and duration.[19,20]

Table 1
Characteristics of sleep-related hallucinations in different sleep disorders categories and other conditions

	Time of the Night	Content that is Intense, Vivid and with an Array of Simple and Complex Forms	Negative Affective Content (Fright, Anxiety, Dread, Threatening)	Detailed Memory Recall	Type of Wakening	Clear Separation of Sleep and Wake States	Co-occurs with Other Parasomnias
Hallucinations in sleep disorders within the "Other Parasomnia" category							
Hypnagogic hallucinations[30]	Sleep onset, usually first third of the night (from NREM sleep, or from sleep onset REM period)	Sometimes. Gradual progression from simple to complex multimodal with auditory component as sleep approaches REM	Rarely	Immediate recall if awoken but rapidly forgotten	Brief arousal from sleep may be followed by a return to sleep or progression to wake	Sometimes difficult to differentiate from sleep-onset dreams	Yes
Hypnopompic hallucinations[30]	On waking, usually in the 2nd half (out of a period of REM)	Sometimes complex, especially if occurring out of period of REM	Rarely	Immediate recall if awoken but rapidly forgotten	Brief arousal from sleep may be followed by a return to sleep or progression to wake	Sometimes difficult to differentiate from dreams	Yes
Terrifying hypnagogic hallucinations	Sleep onset Sudden awakening	Yes, similar to nightmares	Yes	Yes: immediate recall, and prominently remembered	Sudden and abrupt arousal With autonomic hyperactivity	No separation: Persist into wake state "Double consciousness" simultaneous recall of dreams and external environment	Yes
Complex nocturnal visual hallucinations[49]	During the night: Sudden awakening	Yes, complex visual images, sometimes superimposed on the environment	Yes	Yes: immediate recall, and prominently remembered	Sudden and abrupt arousal With autonomic hyperactivity	No separation: Persist into wake state Identified as separate from dreams	Yes

(continued on next page)

Table 1
(*continued*)

	Time of the Night	Content that is Intense, Vivid and with an Array of Simple and Complex Forms	Negative Affective Content (Fright, Anxiety, Dread, Threatening)	Detailed Memory Recall	Type of Wakening	Clear Separation of Sleep and Wake States	Co-occurs with Other Parasomnias
Exploding head syndrome (other parasomnias)[88]	Sleep onset or when waking up	Simple auditory hallucination of an abrupt loud noise, sometimes accompanied by a simple visual hallucination (noise, light)	Yes	Yes	Abrupt arousal	Recognized as dreams	n/a
Hallucinations in REM-related parasomnias and NREM disorders of arousal							
Nightmare Disorders (REM-related parasomnias)	Anytime during the night, often in the 2nd half and REM sleep	Yes: as vivid but less intense than sleep terrors	Yes	Yes	Full awakening With autonomic hyperactivity	Recognized as dreams Do not persist into wake state	Yes
Recurrent sleep paralysis (REM-related parasomnias)[47]	Anytime, but often early in the night, from sleep-onset REM	Multisensory with auditory, somatic, olfactory senses. Feelings suffocation	Yes	Yes	Awakening with feeling of suffocation	Recognized as dreams	n/a
Sleep terrors (NREM disorders of arousal)	SWS, often in the early hours	Yes	Yes	Poorly recalled unless awakened during the episode	Sudden and abrupt arousal from NREM (fearful and with high autonomic hyporeactivity)	Recognized as dreams	n/a
Hallucinations in narcolepsy							
Hypnopompic and hypnagogic hallucinations in the setting of narcolepsy[76]	Can occur at any time during the night.	Intense, vivid, brief, and dream-like. Multisensory, visual, auditory and tactile, vivid	Yes	Yes	No awakening (hypnagogic) Normal awakening (hypnopompic)	Hallucinations may intrude into wakefulness and may be experienced in semiconscious state.	n/a

Sleep disorders associated with a medical condition

Sleep-related epilepsy	Any, often during N2	Multisensory; may involve somaesthetic (all sensory and somatic dimensions), auditory or visual depends on the localization of the epilepsy. Usually brief, simple, but may be complex if parietal and temporal association areas are involved.	Sometimes	Unusual	Yes	Yes	Yes	n/a

Other neurologic and psychiatric disorders encountered in the differential diagnosis of sleep disorders

Visual hallucinations in the setting of alpha synucleinopathies (Lewy body disease and Parkinson's disease)	Often in the evenings or at night, with darkness or reduced vigilance.	Primarily visual unimodal hallucinations of formed hallucinations. People, animal, varying in intensity.	Sometimes	Yes			Yes	Yes
Hallucinations due to a psychotic disorder	n/a	Primarily auditory-verbal, but visual, tactile hallucinations also occur in 30% of cases	Yes	Yes	n/a		Yes	Yes
Hallucinations due to CNS injury (Peduncular Hallucinations, Charles Bonnet syndrome)	May occur at night. Vivid dreams. Occur with eyes open or closed	Primarily visual unimodal, simple or complex; Complex include detailed, complex and colourful images of people, objects or animals. Sometimes bizarre, deformed or panoramic	No	Yes	n/a		Yes	Yes

(continued on next page)

Table 1
(*continued*)

	Time of the Night	Content that is Intense, Vivid and with an Array of Simple and Complex Forms	Negative Affective Content (Fright, Anxiety, Dread, Threatening)	Detailed Memory Recall	Type of Wakening	Clear Separation of Sleep and Wake States	Co-occurs with Other Parasomnias
Delirium	May occur at night. Vivid dreams.	Visual hallucinations are typical, but multimodal hallucinations are also common. Prolonged duration, and involving complex formed images.	Yes	Reduced insight, confusion, and altered consciousness			
Other hallucinations encountered in the differential diagnosis of sleep disorders							
Medications and substances	Increased abnormal dreams and nightmares	Dopaminergic medication; Anticholinergic therapy; Also psychostimulants; dissociative anaesthetics and psychedelics. Contents are usually complex and varied and depends on psychoactive contents and context	Sometimes	Reduced insight, confusion, and altered consciousness	n/a	Yes	Yes
Lucid dreams	n/a	Often visual, tactile, proprioceptive; complex; sometimes superimposed on the environment	No	Yes	n/a dynamic and voluntary; switch with conscious awareness	Sometimes, strategies include the use of cues to distinguish wake from lucid dream episodes	

Methodological Approaches

Daytime hallucinations and SRH are assessed using similar methods involving subjective reports.[21,22] In contrast to daytime experiences, however, SRH require individuals to think back retrospectively to an experience that occurred in a different state of consciousness. A common approach for assessing SRH includes epidemiologic and psychological methods such as surveys or interviews.[22]

In sleep medicine, subjective reports are combined with objective methods to examine the sleep stages in which SRH occur. Study participants are typically allowed to fall asleep according to their regular sleep schedule and then awoken at a predetermined interval coinciding with the sleep stage of interest. Sleep stages can be identified by real-time EEG recordings and/or eye movement detection and using analyses of EEG patterns, power, cortical distribution, and eye/head movements.[19,23,24] Participants are asked to report on their most recent experience before awakening. Multiple experimental sessions across one or multiple nights allow for repeated measurements for each individual.[19,25]

Self-reports are an essential conduit to human subjective experiences. However, mental processes in the sleeping brain are locked in a different state of consciousness, and the limited interactions between the sleep and wake states call for caution. As we fall asleep, mental functions gradually shut down, and memory transfers are interrupted contributing to anterograde amnesia on awakening.[26] Other factors compromising recall include the time elapsed between awakening due to memory interference and degradation.[27] In people with medical and neurologic conditions—who have elevated rates of HHH and especially CNVH—confusion, cognitive impairment, and memory difficulties may also affect the reliability of descriptions.

Of note, it has been suggested that some sleep stages may be more directly accessible to conscious memory than others. For example, the distinct neurophysiological features of REM sleep, in which the sleeper may experience vivid dreams, are closest to the waking state so that REM dreams may be better recalled.[22] Regardless, the interpretation of SRH studies should take into account the quality and accessibility of events that happened during sleep.

Hypnagogic and Hypnopompic Hallucinations

Hypnagogic hallucinations

Hypnagogic hallucinations are fleeting perceptual phenomena that occur around the moment of falling asleep (see **Table 1**). They are extremely common, usually non-pathological, and perhaps universal experiences. Lifetime prevalence rates range between 2% and 75% in the general population,[28,29] although these rates may be skewed due to differences in study design and the methodological limitations mentioned above. Results from epidemiologic surveys suggest that the prevalence follows a U-curve and is more likely to occur in younger people and older people,[30] whereas observations about gender effects are mixed.[31] Reportedly, hypnagogic hallucinations occur at elevated rates in people with psychiatric disorders, such as anxiety disorders, post-traumatic stress disorder (PTSD), psychotic disorders, and mood disorders (50%–80%[30]), and in those taking psychotropic medications.[30,32] However, the nature of the association with mental illness and medications is poorly understood, and poor sleep quality and frequent awakening may well contribute to more opportunities for the recall of sleep-related experiences rather than truly elevated rates.

Hypnagogic hallucinations are defined as occurring at sleep onset, although precise definitions of sleep onset vary.[33–35] Definitions typically include light sleep ("N1"), but may also refer to the second stage of NREM ("N2"),[19,36–38] or any other sleep stage immediately preceding REM.[17]

Studies describe a progression in the form and content of sleep mentation as sleep progresses from N1 toward REM sleep.[9,19,20,23] When awoken during N1, people typically provide vague and fragmentary reports of imagery, with primarily visual contents.[19,25] As sleep progresses, thought-like imagery acquires perceptual features (auditory–somatosensory components) and unusual contents that blend into dream features. The loss of reality monitoring and voluntary control resembles the characteristics of clinical hallucinations.[23] The affective intensity and complex narrative structure of some hypnagogic events can also be difficult to differentiate from the onset of REM dreams.[6,19]

The visual component is the most commonly emphasized and is possibly related to spontaneous activity that occurs in the occipital cortex in the transition to sleep.[39–41] Visual images comprise 55% to 86% of hypnagogic reports[35,42,43] and are described as kaleidoscopically changing (some of them possibly entoptic) phenomena such as geometric patterns, shapes, and light flashes.[3] Other visual images may involve a broad array of events ranging from simple (lights, patterns, designs, written text, formless shapes) to complex phenomena (human faces or figures, animals or objects, scenes involving landscapes and/or people).[20]

Hypnagogic hallucinations often feature sensations in multiple modalities, either concurrently or sequentially.[23] Auditory impressions, in 8% to 35% of hypnagogic events, can include sounds (radio, phone, doorbell, music) or voices.[35,44–46] Bodily sensations are also frequent occurrences (in 25% to 50% of reports)[19,29,42] and are described as a sense of touch and bodily distortions, or feelings of weightlessness, flying, or falling into an abyss. Affective contents occur in a minority of events (<5%), and examples include being caught in a fire, or being involved in an attack.[30] A final phenomenon is a sense of presence in the room, although this is associated more commonly with sleep paralysis.[47]

Hypnopompic hallucination

Hypnopompic hallucinations accompany the departure from sleep for the duration of a few seconds to minutes[15] (see **Table 1**). They typically occur in the morning, although this is not always the case. They are reported to occur less frequently than hypnagogic hallucinations (7%–13%).[29] Here too, frequency rates are reportedly higher in people with psychiatric disorders (15%–36%) compared with the general population.[30]

They can arise from a period of REM sleep, with their features more closely resembling the continuation of a dream sequence than sleep-onset hypnagogic hallucinations. They are described as vividly real and intense, and sometimes involving a narrative, albeit rarely frightening (30% of cases). Individuals may be uncertain whether they represent waking or dream-related experiences (ICSD-3). A typical example is a person with whom we were conversing in a dream, who is still being seen and heard when the eyes are open and perceived as actually present in the bedroom. Examples may include relatives or acquaintances, children, and varied animals.[17] The dreamer may be in the middle of a conversation, although the hallucinated people

rarely reply and disappear with the transition of awakening. Forgetting appears less rapid than with hypnagogic hallucinations, and they can linger in the mind after awakening.

Complex Nocturnal Visual Hallucinations

CNVH are differentiated from hypnagogia as occurring during the night and representing a distinct form of SRH.[5,6] The mental imagery and perceptual forms of CNVH closely resemble normal dreams. However, the episodes are distinguished from dreams because they occur during a state resembling an intermediate state of consciousness, and they are associated with behavioral acting out. The episode also terminates with a sudden waking[6,7] (see **Table 1**) associated with the recollection the vivid "dream like" imageries.[18,48,49] The eyes may be open and visually tracking the object's change across space.[48] One case study describes the patient as sitting up on the bed yellow, looking around mumbling unintelligible words and/or pointing to nonexisting objects.[49] The presence of emotional content within a narrative structure may cause fright or alarm. **Fig. 1** shows a patient sitting up in bed, acting out on the hallucination by pointing and displaying facial emotional.

CNVH have so far only been reported in small case series,[17,49] small cohorts,[18] and in patients with documented sleep disorders,[48] rather than at the population level. Descriptions include complex contents such as small animals (insects, rodents), persons, or distorted forms,[17,18] which may be superimposed on the perceptual word and disappear when the ambient illumination is increased. The contents may take varied and multicolored forms of vivid, intricate, relatively immobile images sometimes distorted in shape or size and superimposed on veridical perceptions similar to the daytime hallucinations typical of Charles Bonnet

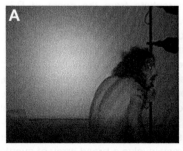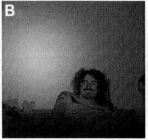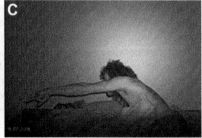

Fig. 1. (*A*) During this episode, the patient sat on the bed staring at a nonexistent presence or object with a scared expression. (*B*) During this episode, the patient laughed and displayed positive emotions. (*C*) During this episode, the patient stared and pointed toward an invisible object in the room with his finger, as if hallucinating. (*From* Castelnovo A, Loddo G, Provini F and Manconi M. Frequent, complex and vivid dream-like/hallucinatory experiences during NREM sleep parasomnia episodes. Sleep medicine 2021; 82: 61–64.)

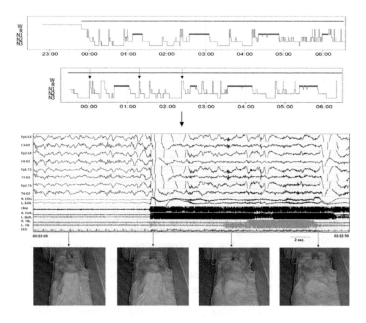

Fig. 2. Upper panel: Hypnograms of the first and second polysomnography (PSG) nights. Black arrows indicate minor NREM sleep parasomnia episodes. Sleep architecture was preserved on both nights (N1 proportion 12% and 10%, N2 = 39% and 39%, N3 = 26% and 26%, REM = 23% and 25%, sleep efficiency = 94% and 93%, REM sleep latency = 70 and 69 minute—in the first and night, respectively), but characterized by several abrupt awakenings out of NREM sleep (21 and 12 awakenings—with and arousal index (AI) of 13.6 and 11.5—in the first and second night, respectively). Central panel: 30 s-epoch of the v-PSG during a Type 1B episode, illustrating the dissociated sleep–wake state. The PSG montage included eight EEG bipolar traces from fronto-polar (Fp), temporal (T), central (C), occipital (O) leads, two electrooculograms (EOG), electromyograms from the chin, left and right deltoids (L and R Delt), and left and right tibialis anterior muscles (L and R Tib). The EEG shows diffuse slow wave activity (N3 stage) before the activation of EMG, then a movement artifact, followed by slow waves of small amplitude in the frontal leads, mixed with higher mixed and largely artifactual frequencies in the central, temporal, and occipital leads. Lower panel: The black vertical line indicates the time of the picture shown in the bottom-right corner. In the first picture, the subject was still sleeping, and in the second picture, he opened his eyes and flexed his neck, his arms, and extended his fingers, and stared perplexedly at his hands. In the third picture, he turned his head and partially his trunk to the left and in the last picture he went back lying in the bed. The episode lasted about 20 s and the patient gradually woke up soon after it. He described having had a dream but could remember only brief sketches of it. (*Adapted from* Castelnovo A, Loddo G, Provini F and Manconi M. Frequent, complex and vivid dream-like/hallucinatory experiences during NREM sleep parasomnia episodes. Sleep medicine 2021; 82: 61–64.)

syndrome.[17] CNVH have been described as rare with a frequency that can average four times a week in affected individuals.[18,29]

Some individuals may report both HHH and CNVH at different times.[17] Descriptions point to differences between CNVH and HHH in the timing during sleep and electrophysiological features. Their epidemiologic and clinical profiles also point to important differences:

- CNVH interrupt sleep, which differs from HHH which occur in the borderlands between sleep and wake.
- CNVH are characterized by a distinct EEG and behavioral patterns consisting of low-voltage, mixed-frequency signals[48] during NREM sleep[18,50] (**Fig. 2**, showing CNVH during NREM REM).
- CNVH have a mean onset age of 40 years and are associated with increased age,[18] whereas HHH can occur in healthy and unmedicated people in the context of normal sleep and in both younger and older people.[29,31]
- CNVH are commonly associated with neurologic conditions and visual disorders[18,51,52]

(although they have also been described in groups of people without diagnosed pathology[51]).

There are striking similarities between CNVH and daytime visual hallucinations in disorders associated with visual pathways or brain stem lesions. These include visual hallucinations in Charles Bonnet syndrome.[17] Both types include visual percepts (highly detailed, colorful, and at times grotesque images of people or animals) and rapid transformations of images, although an affective component is often lacking in CBS, but not for CNVH.[53,54] Explanations of CNVH involving visual release overlap with those of Charles Bonnet syndrome, which is attributed to lesions of the afferent visual pathway,[53–55] both resulting in the visual cortex generating aberrant images.

CNVH also resemble visual hallucinations associated with brainstem or thalamic lesions, such as neurodegenerative disorders associated with alpha-synucleinopathies pathologies, such as Lewy body disease and Parkinson's disease,[56–58] in which oculo-visual problems are common.[59–61]

Visual hallucinations in Parkinson's disease also change with darkness or illumination.[62]

Peduncular hallucinosis in brainstem disorders with midbrain and diencephalic pathology also resemble CNVH[63,64] where the hallucinations are described as complex, vivid, and colorful and are sometimes associated with auditory content and retention of insight.[63]

The resemblance of CNVH to the typical complex visual hallucinations of these disorders has led to suggestions of common neurophysiological substrates, with separate neural system involvement.[52,56,65]

Although previous studies have linked complex hallucinations to "REM" dysfunctions or intrusions[17,66–69] NREM sleep.[50] In an attempt to reconcile these mixed findings, Gnoni and colleagues[48] suggested that CNVH may involve multiple coexisting states of consciousness (wake, NREM, and REM) which have been decoupled and reassembled. It is proposed that the unique combination of co-occurring wake, NREM, and REM elements manifests as hallucinatory experiences in CNVH. Other evidence of parallel processing of multiple states includes neurobiological evidence of nighttime EEG microstates of alpha band activity that are indistinguishable from waking conscious states.[70] Micro-wake "fragments" activity, recorded during slow-wake sleep (SWS) and REM,[71,72] are localized in the midbrain regions including the pedunculopontine nucleus[64,73] which is a region of interest given that virtually every sensory system projects onto the brain stem. Furthermore, lesions in this area produce visual hallucinations that closely resemble CNVH.[63] In the next decades, technological advances can hopefully further build on this new knowledge about biological explanations of SRH.

Association with Other Sleep Disorders

Within the parasomnia cluster of ICSD-3, SRH are grouped under "Other Parasomnias." This residual category encompasses a range of unusual sleep-related conditions with diverse presentations, loose boundaries, and assorted pathophysiological bases for which there is insufficient or inadequate information to substantiate their unequivocal existence.

Other parasomnias are distinguished from NREM- and REM-related parasomnias (the two main categories of this classification), although they frequently co-occur with these other parasomnias and other sleep disorders. HHH and CNVH can occur either at the same time or on different nights as other behavioral symptoms of sleep disorders, making them difficult to identify and isolate.

Narcolepsy

SRH commonly occur in individuals with narcolepsy, which is a disorder of somnolence, with frequency rates of approximately 33% to 80%.[74,75] Unlike CNVH which intrude on nighttime sleep, narcolepsy comprises sleep episodes intruding on daytime functions. Narcolepsy typically begins in youth between the ages of 10 to 20 years, unlike CNVH which is associated with older age.[76] In addition, narcolepsy is associated with a paralysis of the skeletal muscles, whereas CNVH is associated with sitting up or sudden movements.

Rapid eye movement-related parasomnias

Among all parasomnias, this category of parasomnias is the most commonly associated with vivid and prominent perceptual events, although their symptom presentation differs somewhat from SRH descriptions.

- In REM sleep behavior disorders, where the patient acts out dreams during REM sleep, the event ceases when the person is awoken, while CNVH tend to persist into wakefulness.[77]
- Nightmares share features with both hypnagogic hallucinations and CNVH. The emotive and frightening contents resemble hypnagogic hallucinations, but nightmares are recognized as dreams and are vividly remembered. One point of difference between CNVH and nightmares is that the individual is usually fully orientated when awakened during the nightmare.[6] The person with nightmares also usually remembers the dream content in vivid detail. Finally, nightmares also generally occur out of REM-sleep stage, whereas SRH are commonly associated with NREM.
- Sleep paralysis commonly co-occurs with SRH, especially in the context of hypersomnia or insufficient sleep (4% to 40%).[6,47] Sleep paralysis involves the disturbing temporary inability to move voluntary muscles at sleep–wake transitions. It can be accompanied by hallucinations (25%–75% of patients, ICSD-3), including the incubus phenomenon (ie, a hallucinated figure that presses down on one's chest).[78] Apart from the visual and tactile components of this phenomenon, hallucinations in the context of sleep paralysis may have auditory, visual, and kinesthetic components, or involve the sense of a presence in the room, either concurrently or at separate times from episodes of paralysis. They have strong dream-like surreal contents, with auditory and bodily elements that are perceived to be real and ominous.[79–81] In contrast to simple hypnagogic experiences,

the person feels awake and conscious but unable to move. Episodes of sleep paralysis elicited by awakening patients from nocturnal sleep seem to arise from REM sleep, but almost always correspond with mixed REM and waking EEG.[82,83]

Non-rapid eye movement-related parasomnias

Disorders of arousal from NREM (eg, confusional arousals, sleepwalking, and sleep terrors)[50] can also be associated with SRH, but those events are frequently recognized as dreams which do not persist into wakefulness.

Sleep terrors commonly feature SRH, too. Sleep terrors are characterized by sudden arousal, intense fear, or panic and accompanied by autonomic and behavioral manifestations including piercing screams or cries, sitting up in bed, and attempts to "escape" from terrifying dream-like contents. The patient is usually unresponsive to external stimuli, and, if awakened, is confused and disoriented. Amnesia for the episode occurs frequently, although sometimes there are reports of fragments or very brief vivid dream images or hallucinations. They occur out of N2, often at the beginning of the night, or in slow wave sleep (SWS, N3) at any time during the night. Studies of CNVH also suggest a contribution of NREM sleep.[48,50]

Other parasomnias

Finally, there is some overlap with other categories within the cluster of other parasomnias. Exploding head syndrome consists of a sudden loud bang, usually at sleep onset and sometimes accompanied by a flash of light. A point of difference with SRH is that it does not involve complex visual imagery and lasts only a fraction of a second. Also, exploding head syndrome has a lower prevalence than hypnagogic states.[84]

SUMMARY AND DISCUSSION

Our current state of knowledge is that SRH is a diagnostic category that features in ICSD alone and solely comprises HHH and CNVH. These phenomena are thought to represent a single symptom cluster with distinctive presentations, but it is not yet clear whether they have a single underlying mechanism or perhaps different ones.

There has been an evolution in the conceptualization of SRH over time. Although SRH are interesting to study in their individual forms, there are a number of distinctive questions that remain to be answered.

1. What is the link between CNVH and Terrifying Hypnagogic Hallucination described in the ICSD-R?

CNVH closely resembles THH, except in the timing of sleep. THH occur at sleep onset, whereas CNVH can occur at any time during sleep.

Similarities between CNVH and THH are that: their contents resemble nightmares, and the accompanying emotional effect includes fear, foreboding, and threatening contents; both are associated with body movements (vocalization and screaming for THH; sitting up and eyes open with CNVH); both are associated with intact recall and may in fact represent a continuation into wakefulness; and THH have sometimes been described as a "double consciousness" simultaneous recall of dreams and external environment, which resemble descriptions of CNVH. Another common and distinctive feature of both is that they terminate with sudden awakening, and they persist into awakenening. This separates them from other SRS that are associated with a brief arousal and a subsequent return to sleep.

2. Do HHH and CNVH represent the same or distinct phenomena within the SRH category:

HHH are extremely common and, mostly benign, in the normal population. The upgrading of their clinical significance from benign phenomena to the status of sleep disorders across successive ICSD versions raises questions about unsubstantiated pathologization. HHH are now labeled as sleep disorders, although they are not identified as symptoms with substantial clinical merit. Their clinical significance is identified if they are "recurrent," and because they are common symptoms of other sleep disorders, especially parasomnias and other psychiatric conditions.

By contrast, evidence for CNVH comes from descriptions of patients with sleep disorders or medical conditions, in whom they may be a symptom of a clinical condition. CNVH are also differentiated from HHH (and other different parasomnia-related events) by the timing, complex visual contents, sudden arousal, affective contents, and good memory recall of events.

There are therefore questions about whether they represent the same or different phenomena, and they should be combined under the same category of SRH. A commonality is that many EEG studies link both to NREM.[85] However, other evidence links them to all states of consciousness, including waking, sleep onset, sleep offset, and REM sleep, and it is not clear whether they have distinct neurophysiological basis or polysomnography (PSG) features.

One possibility is that SRH can be represented along a continuum of severity, with normal variants of HHH at one end, and CNVH as a pathologic entity at the other. If this is the case, a better explication of the threshold of clinical significance would be useful to clinicians. A continuum of presentation, however, does not necessarily imply a continuous of mechanisms. Notwithstanding their similarity, evidence from their demographic profile and clinical course suggests different mechanisms between HHH and CNVH. CNVH are a common feature of neurologic disorders, whereas HHH occur in a non-pathological form in the majority of cases. Many questions remain about their association with other sleep disorders. Their lack of specificity to any that one sleep disorder or a specific somatic or psychiatric condition should remain at the forefront of all clinical assessments.

SUMMARY

In conclusion, perceptual phenomena which occur around and during sleep represent a fascinating topic for study as they reveal a world that is not easily accessible to our waking state. One suggestion is that they are a mirror image of each other, with the dreaming brain being an "offline" virtual reality simulation of the "online" waking world.[86] However, our knowledge of sleep states and associated perceptual phenomena is still rather limited. Methodological issues are important barriers that constrain our understanding of the nature, causes, and significance of SRH. Advances in the conceptualization of the wake versus sleep dichotomy may also help to facilitate direct comparisons between phenomena with similar clinical features.

CLINICS CARE POINTS

- Sleep-related hallucinations (SRH) have been documented in all stages of sleep (non-rapid eye movement [NREM] and rapid eye movement [REM]), in healthy individuals, and in people with a variety of general medical, neurologic, and psychiatric disorders.

- Not all hallucinations require interventions. Infrequent hallucinations may be within the limits of normal sleep–wake transitions.

- SRH can occur independently from, but are frequently associated with, other sleep disorders. The presence of other symptoms that occur concurrently with SRH may therefore be indicative of narcolepsy or other disorders.

- SRH cannot be understood in isolation, and it is inadvisable to give excessive weight to individual features of SRH.[87] The combination of features accompanying complex nocturnal visual hallucinations is an important factor that

can assist in diagnosis and help to determine whether treatment is needed.

- Future research should focus on the development of reliable assessment tools that can differentiate between different features of daytime and SRH outside of the simple wake–sleep dichotomy.

DISCLOSURE

The authors have nothing to disclose.

REFERENCES

1. Dement WC. Recent studies on the biological role of rapid eye movement sleep. Am J Psychiatr 1965; 122:404–8.
2. Windt JM. How deep is the rift between conscious states in sleep and wakefulness? Spontaneous experience over the sleep–wake cycle. Philosophical Transactions of the Royal Society B 2021;376: 20190696.
3. Waters F, Blom JD, Dang-Vu TT, et al. What is the link between hallucinations, dreams, and hypnagogic–hypnopompic experiences? Schizophr Bull 2016; 42:1098–109.
4. Maury A. Le sommeil et les rêves: études psychologiques sur ces phénomènes et les divers états qui s'y rattachent. Paris: Didier; 1878.
5. Medicine AAoS. International classification of sleep disorders. Diagnostic and coding manual 2005; 148–52.
6. American Academy of Sleep M. International classification of sleep disorders. 3rd edition. Darien, IL: American Academy of Sleep Medicine Darien, IL; 2014.
7. American Academy of Sleep M. International classification of sleep disorders ICSD-3-Text revision. 3. uberarbeitete Auflage ed. Darien, Ill. Ill: American Acad. of Sleep Medicine Darien; 2023.
8. Walter N, Hinterberger T. Determining states of consciousness in the electroencephalogram based on spectral, complexity, and criticality features. Neuroscience of Consciousness 2022;2022:niac008.
9. Dement W, Kleitman N. The relation of eye movements during sleep to dream activity: an objective method for the study of dreaming. J Exp Psychol 1957;53:339.
10. Mahowald MW, Schenck CH. NREM sleep parasomnias. Neurol Clin 1996;14:675–96.
11. Schenck CH, Cramer Bornemann M, Kaplish N, et al. Sleep-related (psychogenic) dissociative disorders as parasomnias associated with a psychiatric disorder: update on reported cases. J Clin Sleep Med 2021;17:803–10.

12. Schenck CH, Mahowald MW. REM sleep parasomnias. Neurol Clin 1996;14:697–720.

13. Thorpy MJ. Classification of sleep disorders. J Clin Neurophysiol 1990;7:67–82.

14. American Academy of Sleep M. The international classification of sleep disorders, revised : diagnostic and coding manual. Westchester (Illinois): American Academy of Sleep Medicine Westchester (Illinois); 2001.

15. Blom JD. A dictionary of hallucinations. 3rd edition. London, UK: Springer; 2023.

16. Baillarger JGF. Extrait d'un mémoire intitulé: des hallucinations, des causes qui les produisent, et des maladies qu'elles caractérisent. Paris, France: Baillière; 1846.

17. Takata K, Inoue Y, Hazama H, et al. Night-time hypnopompic visual hallucinations related to REM sleep disorder. Psychiatr Clin Neurosci 1998;52:207–9.

18. Silber MH, Hansen MR, Girish M. Complex nocturnal visual hallucinations. Sleep Med 2005;6:363–6.

19. Foulkes D, Vogel G. Mental activity at sleep onset. J Abnorm Psychol 1965;70:231.

20. Mavromatis A. On shared states of consciousness and objective imagery. J Ment Imagery 1987; 102(1):28–41.

21. Murphy DB, Myers TI. Occurrence, measurement and experimental manipulation of visual "hallucinations". Percept Mot Skills 1962;15:47–54.

22. Strauch I, Meier B. In search of dreams: results of experimental dream research. Paris, France: SUNY Press; 1996.

23. Rowley JT, Stickgold R, Hobson JA. Eyelid movements and mental activity at sleep onset. Conscious Cognit 1998;7:67–84.

24. Diezig S, Denzer S, Achermann P, et al. EEG microstate dynamics associated with dream-like experiences during the transition to sleep. Brain Topogr 2022;1–13. https://doi.org/10.1007/s10548-022-00923-y.

25. Foulkes D, Spear PS, Symonds JD. Individual differences in mental activity at sleep onset. J Abnorm Psychol 1966;71:280.

26. Tivadar RI, Knight RT, Tzovara A. Automatic sensory predictions: a review of predictive mechanisms in the brain and their link to conscious processing. Frontiers in human neuroscience 2021;15:702520.

27. Wyatt JK, Bootzin RR, Anthony J, et al. Sleep onset is associated with retrograde and anterograde amnesia. Sleep 1994;17:502–11.

28. Honig A, Romme MA, Ensink BJ, et al. Auditory hallucinations: a comparison between patients and nonpatients. J Nerv Ment Dis 1998;186:646–51.

29. Ohayon MM. Prevalence of hallucinations and their pathological associations in the general population. Psychiatr Res 2000;97:153–64.

30. Ohayon MM, Priest RG, Caulet M, et al. Hypnagogic and hypnopompic hallucinations: pathological phenomena? Br J Psychiatry 1996;169:459–67.

31. Bless JJ, Hugdahl K, Kråkvik B, et al. In The twilight zone: an epidemiological study of sleep-related hallucinations. Compr Psychiatr 2021; 108:152247.

32. Pandi-Perumal SR, Kramer M. Sleep and mental illness. London, UK: Cambridge University Press; 2010.

33. Berry RB, Brooks R, Gamaldo CE, et al. The AASM manual for the scoring of sleep and associated events. rules, terminology and technical specifications, Darien, Illinois. American Academy of Sleep Medicine 2012; 176:2012.

34. Guo D, Thomas RJ, Liu Y, et al. Slow wave synchronization and sleep state transitions. Sci Rep 2022; 12:7467.

35. Yang C-M, Han H-Y, Yang M-H, et al. What subjective experiences determine the perception of falling asleep during sleep onset period? Conscious Cognit 2010; 19:1084–92.

36. Agnew H, Webb W. Measurement of sleep onset by EEG criteria. Am J EEG Technol 1972;12:127–34.

37. Davis H, Davis PA, Loomis A, et al. Human brain potentials during the onset of sleep. J Neurophysiol 1938;1: 24–38.

38. Carskadon MA, Dement WC. Normal human sleep: an overview. Principles and practice of sleep medicine 2005;4:13–23.

39. Goupil L, Bekinschtein T. Cognitive processing during the transition to sleep. Arch Ital Biol 2012;150: 140–54.

40. Horovitz SG, Fukunaga M, de Zwart JA, et al. Low frequency BOLD fluctuations during resting wakefulness and light sleep: a simultaneous EEG-fMRI study. Hum Brain Mapp 2008;29:671–82.

41. Kjaer TW, Law I, Wiltschiøtz G, et al. Regional cerebral blood flow during light sleep–a H215O-PET study. J Sleep Res 2002;11:201–7.

42. Sidgwick H. Report on the census of hallucinations. In: Proceedings of the society for psychical researchXXVI. London, UK: Kegan Paul, Trench, Trübner & Co: Cambridge University Press Cambridge; 1894. p. 25–422. Part X.

43. Leaning F. An introductory study of hypnagogic phenomena. In: Paper presented at: proceedings of the society for psychical research 1925, Society for Psychical Research; Nottingham, UK.

44. Jones SR, Fernyhough C, Larøi F. A phenomenological survey of auditory verbal hallucinations in the hypnagogic and hypnopompic states. Phenomenol Cognitive Sci 2010;9:213–24.

45. Leroy E-B. Les visions du demi-sommeil: hallucinations hypnagogiques. Paris; 1933.

46. Hori T, Hayashi M, Morikawa T. Topographical EEG changes and the hypnagogic experience. In: Ogilvie RD, Harsh JR, editors. Sleep onset: Normal and abnormal processes. American Psychological Association; 1994. p. 237–53.

47. Cheyne JA, Rueffer SD, Newby-Clark IR. Hypnagogic and hypnopompic hallucinations during sleep paralysis: neurological and cultural construction of the night-mare. Conscious Cognit 1999;8:319–37.

48. Gnoni V, Duncan I, Wasserman D, et al. Nocturnal visual hallucinations in patients with disorders of arousal: a novel behavioral and EEG pattern. Croat Med J 2022;63:438.

49. Castelnovo A, Loddo G, Provini F, et al. Frequent, complex and vivid dream-like/hallucinatory experiences during NREM sleep parasomnia episodes. Sleep Med 2021;82:61–4.

50. Diaz-Abad M, Sanchez AM, Kabir A, et al. A case of complex and abnormal behaviors at night: the role of the epilepsy monitoring unit in diagnosis. Case Rep Neurol 2020;12:18–23.

51. Lysenko L, Bhat S. Melatonin-responsive complex nocturnal visual hallucinations. J Clin Sleep Med 2018;14:687–91.

52. Manford M, Andermann F. Complex visual hallucinations. Clinical and neurobiological insights. Brain 1998;121:1819–40.

53. Madill S, Ffytche D. Charles Bonnet syndrome in patients with glaucoma and good acuity. Br J Ophthalmol 2005;89:785–6.

54. Santhouse A, Howard R, Ffytche D. Visual hallucinatory syndromes and the anatomy of the visual brain. Brain 2000;123:2055–64.

55. Ffytche DH, Catani M. Beyond localization: from hodology to function. Phil Trans Biol Sci 2005;360:767–79.

56. Barnes J, David A. Visual hallucinations in Parkinson's disease: a review and phenomenological survey. J Neurol Neurosurg Psychiatr 2001;70:727–33.

57. Eversfield CL, Orton LD. Auditory and visual hallucination prevalence in Parkinson's disease and dementia with Lewy bodies: a systematic review and meta-analysis. Psychol Med 2019;49:2342–53.

58. UP Mosimann, Rowan EN, Partington CE, et al. Characteristics of visual hallucinations in Parkinson disease dementia and dementia with Lewy bodies. Am J Geriatr Psychiatr 2006;14:153–60.

59. Armstrong R. Oculo-visual dysfunction in Parkinson's disease. J Parkinsons Dis 2015;5:715–26.

60. Hinkle JT, Pontone GM. Lewy body degenerations as neuropsychiatric disorders. Psychiatr Clin 2020;43:361–81.

61. Pang L. Hallucinations experienced by visually impaired: Charles Bonnet syndrome. Optom Vis Sci 2016;93:1466.

62. Fénelon G, Mahieux F, Huon R, et al. Hallucinations in Parkinson's disease: prevalence, phenomenology and risk factors. Brain 2000;123:733–45.

63. Benke T. Peduncular hallucinosis: a syndrome of impaired reality monitoring. J Neurol 2006;253:1561–71.

64. Vita MG, Batocchi AP, Dittoni S, et al. Visual hallucinations and pontine demyelination in a child: possible REM dissociation? J Clin Sleep Med 2008;4:588–90.

65. Bertram K, Williams DR. Visual hallucinations in the differential diagnosis of parkinsonism. J Neurol Neurosurg Psychiatr 2012;83:448–52.

66. Gottesmann C. The dreaming sleep stage: a new neurobiological model of schizophrenia? Neuroscience 2006;140:1105–15.

67. Kelly PH. Defective inhibition of dream event memory formation: a hypothesized mechanism in the onset and progression of symptoms of schizophrenia. Brain Res Bull 1998;46:189–97.

68. Arnulf I, Bonnet A-M, Damier P, et al. Hallucinations, REM sleep, and Parkinson's disease: a medical hypothesis. Neurology 2000;55:281–8.

69. Manni R, Terzaghi M, Ratti P-L, et al. Hallucinations and REM sleep behaviour disorder in Parkinson's disease: dream imagery intrusions and other hypotheses. Conscious Cognit 2011;20:1021–6.

70. Bréchet L, Brunet D, Perogamvros L, et al. EEG microstates of dreams. Sci Rep 2020;10:17069.

71. Eschenko O, Magri C, Panzeri S, et al. Noradrenergic neurons of the locus coeruleus are phase locked to cortical up-down states during sleep. Cerebr Cortex 2012;22:426–35.

72. Destexhe A, Hughes SW, Rudolph M, et al. Are corticothalamic 'up'states fragments of wakefulness? Trends Neurosci 2007;30:334–42.

73. Smith DM, Terhune DB. Pedunculopontine-induced cortical decoupling as the neurophysiological locus of dissociation. Psychol Rev 2023;130:183.

74. Szűcs A, Janszky J, Hollo A, et al. Misleading hallucinations in unrecognized narcolepsy. Acta Psychiatr Scand 2003;108:314–7.

75. Leu-Semenescu S, DeCock VC, Le Masson VD, et al. Hallucinations in narcolepsy with and without cataplexy: contrasts with Parkinson's disease. Sleep Med 2011;12:497–504.

76. Scammell TE. Narcolepsy. N Engl J Med 2015;373:2654–62.

77. Atassi MDS, Atassi PhD K, Sandberg MSM. Rem behavior disorder and sleep related hallucinations, a case study. Marshall Journal of Medicine 2021;7:4.

78. Kompanje EJO. 'The devil lay upon her and held her down'Hypnagogic hallucinations and sleep paralysis described by the Dutch physician Isbrand van Diemerbroeck (1609–1674) in 1664. J Sleep Res 2008;17:464–7.

79. Cheyne JA, Newby-Clark IR, Rueffer SD. Relations among hypnagogic and hypnopompic experiences associated with sleep paralysis. J Sleep Res 1999;8:313–7.

80. Molendijk ML, Bouachmir O, Montagne H, et al. The incubus phenomenon: prevalence, frequency and

risk factors in psychiatric inpatients and university undergraduates. Front Psychiatr 2022;13:1040769.

81. Cheyne JA, Pennycook G. Sleep paralysis postepisode distress: modeling potential effects of episode characteristics, general psychological distress, beliefs, and cognitive style. Clin Psychol Sci 2013;1:135–48.

82. Takeuchi T, Miyasita A, Inugami M, et al. Laboratory-documented hallucination during sleep-onset REM period in a normal subject. Percept Mot Skills 1994;78:979–85.

83. Takeuchi T, Miyasita A, Sasaki Y, et al. Isolated sleep paralysis elicited by sleep interruption. Sleep 1992;15:217–25.

84. Sharpless BA. Exploding head syndrome. Sleep Med Rev 2014;18:489–93.

85. Hurwitz TD, Schenck CH, Parasomnias. Foundations of Psychiatric Sleep Medicine 2010;160:85–9.

86. Hobson JA, Friston KJ. Waking and dreaming consciousness: neurobiological and functional considerations. Progress In Neurobiology 2012;98:82–98.

87. Waters F, Fernyhough C. Hallucinations: a systematic review of points of similarity and difference across diagnostic classes. Schizophr Bull 2017;43:32–43.

88. Sharpless BA. Exploding head syndrome is common in college students. J Sleep Res 2015;24:447–9.

Sleep-Related Dissociative Disorders

Alan S. Eiser, PhD

KEYWORDS

- Dissociative disorder • Nocturnal dissociative disorder • Parasomnia • Non-REM parasomnia
- Somnambulism • Sleep-related injury • Childhood abuse • Trauma

KEY POINTS

- In sleep-related dissociative disorders (SRDDs), phenomena of the psychiatrically defined dissociative disorders emerge in the sleep period, occurring during sustained electroencephalographic wakefulness either in the transition to sleep or following awakening from sleep.
- Patients are predominantly female; typically have daytime dissociative episodes, histories of trauma, and often major coexisting psychopathology; and may suffer injury or cause injuries to others during episodes.
- Behavioral manifestations are widely varied but are united by the core mechanism of dissociation, which entails the separating off from mainstream consciousness of significant mental functions and contents in order to avoid overwhelming experiences with insupportable affects, typically related to trauma.
- After the diagnosis of SRDD was included in the *International Classification of Sleep Disorders*, Second *Edition (ICSD-2)*, it was omitted from the ICSD-3 and ICSD-3-TR., to the detriment of the clinician faced with patients with these disorders or other disorders for which SRDD is a key element in the differential diagnosis.
- Information about effective treatment is limited; in a few reported cases, psychological treatments were effective. Clinicians skilled in psychotherapy and medication management of patients with histories of trauma and dissociation should be involved.

INTRODUCTION

Sleep-related dissociative disorders (SRDDs) are clinical conditions of considerable importance for the practitioner of sleep medicine. Patients with these disorders present to the sleep clinic and require careful investigation, accurate diagnosis, and informed referral for treatment. These conditions are also an important element in the differential diagnosis for many other sleep disorders, particularly parasomnias involving complex behavior arising out of sleep. Although the question of their proper place in the diagnostic nomenclature is currently unsettled, there is no disputing the importance of familiarity with these disorders for the sleep medicine clinician.

HISTORY AND NOMENCLATURE

The term 'sleep-related dissociative disorders' refers to clinical entities in which phenomena of the dissociative disorders, a psychiatric diagnostic category, emerge during the major sleep period or periods of napping. They are understood to occur out of sustained, unambiguous electroencephalographic (EEG) wakefulness, either during the period of transition to sleep or following awakening from stages N1, N2, or rapid eye movement (REM) sleep. An increasing but still relatively small number of cases have been studied polysomnographically and reported in the literature, and knowledge and understanding are accordingly somewhat limited and tentative. An initial case of

Department of Psychiatry, University of Michigan Sleep Disorders Center, University of Michigan, C728 Med Inn Building, SPC 5845, 1500 East Medical Center Drive, Ann Arbor, MI 48109, USA
E-mail address: aeiser@med.umich.edu

Sleep Med Clin 19 (2024) 159–167
https://doi.org/10.1016/j.jsmc.2023.10.003
1556-407X/24/© 2023 Elsevier Inc. All rights reserved.

fugue states emerging out of sleep was described by Rice and Fisher in 1976,[1] and the first case series, composed of 8 cases accompanied by a careful delineation of the syndrome, was published by Schenck and colleagues in 1989[2]; at that time the term "nocturnal dissociative disorders" was used. An updated review and summary of the literature was published in 2021,[3] followed by a further series of 8 cases in 2022.[4]

It was only in 2005, in the second edition of the American Academy of Sleep Medicine's official nosology, the *International Classification of Sleep Disorders, Second Edition* (ICSD-2), that the diagnosis of SRDD was included, under the heading "Other Parasomnias".[5] The diagnosis was subsequently omitted from the *International Classification of Sleep Disorders, Third Edition* (ICSD-3),[6] and this omission was carried forward in the recent *International Classification of Sleep Disorders, Third Edition, Text Revision* (ICSD-3-TR).[7] As discussed in the "Formal Status of the Diagnosis" section, the proper status of this diagnosis is currently a matter of controversy.

To date, fewer than 60 cases of SRDDs have been reported in the literature, in some instances with only limited data or summarized in aggregate form in an abstract. However, cases of SRDD may be more frequently found in populations other than general sleep medicine patients, for example in psychiatric patients with backgrounds of trauma and/or with daytime dissociative disorders. It is also possible that the omission of SRDD from official recognition in the ICSD-3 may have acted to dampen reporting of new cases.

Background Considerations from Psychiatry

Within psychiatry, dissociative phenomena were first emphasized by the French psychologist, physician, and philosopher Pierre Janet in the late nineteenth and early twentieth centuries.[8] Janet explained clinical symptoms such as amnesia and fugue on the basis of memories of traumatic experiences being separated, or dissociated, from ordinary consciousness. In recent decades, increasing interest in dissociative phenomena has been spurred by work on understanding the effects of trauma and posttraumatic stress disorder (PTSD), and by the growing awareness that childhood trauma, especially sexual and physical abuse, is more common than was previously appreciated. Childhood abuse is frequently present in the backgrounds of patients with dissociative disorders.

The present-day definition of dissociative disorders in the American Psychiatric Association's *Diagnostic and Statistical Manual of Mental Disorders, Fifth Edition, Text Revision* (DSM-5-TR) is "a disruption of and/or discontinuity in the normal integration of consciousness, memory, identity, emotion, perception, body representation, motor control, and behavior. Dissociative symptoms can potentially disrupt every area of psychological functioning."[9] In essence, dissociative phenomena entail a disconnection from mainstream consciousness of significant areas of such mental functions as memory and identity; in extreme cases, there is a fragmentation of central consciousness. They are understood to originate from the need to keep overwhelming experiences with insupportable associated affects and meanings separated off, or encapsulated, in the mind. This can have not only defensive or protective functions but also adaptive value in that it may enable the person to continue to function in significant areas of their life. Ultimately, these disorders result in significant impairment or distress in work, social, or other major areas of life function.

Key Distinction in the Usage of the Term "Dissociation"

In the sleep medicine context, it is important to distinguish the different meanings of the term "dissociation" as used in psychiatry as opposed to in sleep medicine because this can cause considerable confusion. In psychiatry, "dissociation" refers to a disconnection among mental functions, effected to avoid extreme psychic distress, and is understood as largely psychogenic in origin. For example, in dissociative amnesia, memory of a trauma and a range of related mental contents may become inaccessible to ordinary conscious mental states. In sleep medicine, the term "wake/sleep state dissociation" refers to the fact that the 3 major states of being, wakefulness, non-rapid eye movement (NREM) sleep, and REM sleep, are quite complex and comprised of multiple elements; individual elements of one state may persist into or emerge during one of the other major states. An example would be in narcolepsy where the muscle atonia that normally occurs during REM sleep may arise during wakefulness in the symptom of cataplexy. Wake/sleep state dissociation is understood to be physiologically based, and what is dissociated, individual physiologic elements of the 3 major states of being, is conceptually quite different from the mental functions that are disconnected in dissociation in the psychiatric sense. However, these phenomena may have some overlap or interaction that has not yet been clearly elucidated.

Five types of dissociative disorders are delineated in the DSM-5-TR: dissociative identity disorder, dissociative amnesia, depersonalization/derealization disorder, other specified dissociative disorder, and unspecified dissociative disorder. A brief description of some of these disorders may convey a sense of the type of phenomena encompassed. Dissociative amnesia involves an inability to recall important autobiographical information, usually traumatic or stressful in nature, which is beyond the bounds of ordinary forgetting. The memory impairment can extend widely to related or contiguous groups of memories; in extreme cases, which typically have a sudden onset, there can be a loss of personal identity. The impairment is in principle reversible, in that the memories were originally encoded. Dissociative identity disorder, formerly known as multiple personality disorder, is the most severe of the dissociative disorders. It is characterized by the presence of "2 or more distinct personality states," involving "marked discontinuity in sense of self and sense of agency, accompanied by related alterations in affect, behavior, consciousness, memory, perception, cognition, and/or sensory-motor functioning."[9] The formerly separate category of dissociative fugue, defined as "Apparently purposeful travel or bewildered wandering that is associated with amnesia for identity or for other important autobiographical information,"[9] is now subsumed as a subtype of dissociative amnesia and also understood to frequently occur in the more encompassing disturbance of dissociative identity disorder.

DETAILED DESCRIPTION OF SLEEP-RELATED DISSOCIATIVE DISORDERS

Myriad widely varying types of behaviors and states have been described in dissociative episodes emerging out of the sleep period. This may lead to uncertainty about why these phenomena are classified together, but in fact they share the core underlying mechanism of dissociation, the need to keep psychologically insupportable memories, affects, meanings, and impulses separated off from central consciousness. Reenactments of childhood sexual or physical abuse, accompanied at times by patients' efforts to defend themselves, are frequently emphasized but many other types of behaviors have been seen. Episodes may involve confused wandering; agitated movement, screaming, and running into furniture or crashing through doors; self-injury or self-mutilation such as burning or cutting oneself; violent or homicidal behavior; assumption of a different personality; and regressive behaviors or trance-like, unresponsive states. This parallels the protean nature of manifestations of daytime dissociative disorders. Patients are usually amnestic for the episodes, although at times they may recall a "dream" afterward that seems to reflect what they were

experiencing, or they may recall traumatic childhood experiences that seem associated with the behavioral phenomena of the dissociative episode.

Episodes can occur quite frequently, commonly several times per week to as many as several episodes per night. Although some episodes may last just a few minutes, duration can be lengthy, often lasting for hours. It has been speculated that there may be differences in the nature of dissociative episodes originating during the sleep period from what is seen in daytime episodes but specific data are not available. This possibility has been discussed varyingly in terms of the different neural organization during sleep, or during the specific NREM or REM sleep state preceding the episode, or, from a more psychological perspective, as related to sleep and sleep stages as states when unconscious conflicts and traumatic memories are varyingly mobilized and mental defense mechanisms are diminished.

Demographics and Prevalence

The cases of SRDD that have been reported to date are preponderantly female. Population prevalence is unknown. They appear to be uncommon in the general sleep medicine population. However, in one series of 150 consecutive patients presenting to a sleep disorders center with recurrent sleep-related injury, 8 (5.3%) had SRDDs.[2] In a series of 29 consecutive patients presenting to a sleep and dissociation research center with daytime dissociative disorders, 8 (27.6%) were found to have a SRDD.[10] Accurately determining the population prevalence will entail sophisticated sampling techniques that proportionately include groups with likely higher prevalence rates.

Onset, Ontogeny, and Clinical Course

The ages of onset reported to date have mostly been in the range from adolescence through middle adulthood. There is one published case with age of onset as early as 6 years.[11] The initial emergence of episodes may be gradual or abrupt. The course appears to be chronic, in some cases with increasing frequency of episodes over time. There can be stress-related exacerbations; in some reported instances, the stress has been a major loss.

Etiology, Pathophysiology, and Pathogenesis

A history of psychological trauma is almost universally found in cases of SRDD. The trauma is understood to be a crucial etiologic source of the insupportable affects and impulses that determine the need to utilize dissociative mechanisms. Frequently, the trauma entails childhood sexual or physical abuse, perhaps especially in the more severe cases with dissociative identity disorder. However, this is by no means always the case. In some instances, the childhood trauma is one of loss/abandonment, or emotionally abusive or harsh treatment. In others, the relevant trauma appears to have occurred in adulthood, for example, a sexual assault or a robbery.

In terms of pathophysiology, what is known is limited and preliminary. It is often thought that dissociative disorders in general are based on a loss of integration, or functional disconnection, among different brain regions or neural networks involved in mental activity, and this would be expected to apply to SRDDs as well. There are suggestions that areas of the brain involved in memory and language may be impaired in the aftermath of severe trauma, and that memories of traumatic events are encoded in brain structures (eg, subcortical and paralimbic structures such as the amygdalae) that are more emotion-dominated and less subject to higher-order cognitive control. In addition, in SRDDs there may be particular factors related to the sleep period in which the episodes occur. The neural organization of sleep, or of NREM or REM sleep in specific, may carry over to some degree and be a factor in determining the nature of dissociative episodes arising a few minutes after awakening or during the transition to sleep.

Associated, Predisposing, and Precipitating Factors

Nearly all of the patients reported with SRDDs have also had a daytime dissociative disorder. Often, there is congruence between the behaviors observed in episodes that emerge during the sleep period and those observed in daytime episodes. The presence of multiple additional serious psychiatric disorders is quite common; major depressive disorder, PTSD, borderline personality disorder, and alcohol and substance abuse are among the most frequently reported.

Where childhood trauma is present, a variety of factors may contribute to determining the degree of pathologic outcome that ensues, including the quality of early family/caretaking relationships and the biological vulnerability to major psychiatric disorder.

A SRDD may be precipitated or exacerbated by significant stress, in several reported cases by a major loss or by experiences that evoke memories of the original trauma.

Complications and Consequences

Complications can include repeated injuries to self, either from purposeful acts of self-harm or self-mutilation such as self-cutting or self-burning or from running into furniture, through doors, and so forth. Injury to others may also occur, for example, from assaultive behavior. Hospitalizations are common with the daytime dissociative disorders and co-occurring psychiatric problems. Disruption of relationships, work, and overall life function can be severe in these disorders.

DIAGNOSIS

The 2005 ICSD-2 diagnostic criteria for SRDD require the presence of a dissociative disorder that meets DSM diagnostic criteria and that includes episodes that occur in close conjunction with the sleep period. If, in addition, polysomnographic study documents a dissociative episode(s) emerging "during sustained EEG wakefulness, either in the transition from wakefulness to sleep or after an awakening from NREM or REM sleep," the criteria are satisfied. If an episode is not observed on polysomnography, there must be a compelling history of sleep-related dissociative episodes reported by observers, and this is further supported if the behaviors observed during the sleep period are similar to what is reported in daytime dissociative episodes. Finally, the symptoms cannot be better explained by another medical disorder or circumstance.[12]

The situation is clearest when a dissociative episode is seen arising out of wakefulness on polysomnographic study. Even then, given the wide range of behaviors that can be seen in dissociative episodes and their overlap with phenomena of other disorders, a history of daytime dissociative episodes that are similar to the episodes seen in the laboratory, and perhaps also a history of psychological trauma, can further buttress the overall clinical impression. If an episode of dissociative behavior is not observed on polysomnography, a history that is compelling for an SRDD, particularly if the behaviors are similar to observed daytime dissociative behaviors, becomes crucial. The failure to find polysomnographic evidence of an NREM parasomnia or of REM sleep behavior disorder (RBD), while useful contributory information, is not by itself compelling evidence in establishing the diagnosis of an SRDD. Evidence of these parasomnias, particularly those arising out of NREM sleep, is by no means always seen on 1 or 2 nights of recording in the sleep laboratory. A further complication is that patients may have both an NREM (or REM) parasomnia *and* an SRDD.

Differential Diagnosis

Differential diagnosis consists primarily of other parasomnias that can involve complex behavior arising out of sleep and sleep-related seizures

(Table 1). Polysomnographically, the NREM disorders of arousal—confusional arousals, sleep terrors, and sleepwalking—emerge directly during arousal from NREM sleep, most often delta sleep, in a state that is an admixture of sleep and wakefulness. RBD occurs during REM sleep, with abnormal loss of muscle atonia and excessive motor activity. In contrast, SRDDs occur during well-established, sustained wakefulness, either in the transition to sleep or after an awakening from N1, N2, or REM sleep. The episodes of dissociative behavior tend to be longer lasting than episodes in the NREM disorders of arousal or REM behavior disorder, although sleepwalking can at times be quite prolonged. The nature of the behaviors can often be helpful in distinguishing dissociative episodes from the disorders of arousal and the acting out of dreams that is seen in RBD. The response to treatment with clonazepam may also be informative: NREM disorders of arousal (as

Table 1
Differential diagnosis of sleep-related dissociative disorders

Alternative Diagnosis	Features Supporting Alternative Diagnosis	Features Supporting SRDD
Somnambulism and other NREM disorders of arousal	Occurs during arousal from NREM, usually N3, sleep in hybrid sleep-wake state Usually in first third of night	Occurs during sustained EEG wakefulness Throughout the night
	Short episodes, although somnambulism can occasionally be more lengthy	Episodes can be lengthy, often more than an hour
	Good response to clonazepam	Does not respond or worsens with clonazepam
	Daytime dissociative episodes not characteristically present	Daytime dissociative episodes almost always present
RBD	Occurs during REM sleep, with loss of muscle atonia	Occurs during sustained EEG wakefulness
	Later in the night	Throughout the night
	Brief episodes	Episodes can be lengthy, often more than an hour
	Good response to clonazepam	Does not respond or worsens with clonazepam
	Daytime dissociative episodes not characteristically present	Daytime dissociative episodes almost always present
Sleep-related eating disorder	Occurs during partial arousals from N3 or N2 sleep	Occurs during sustained EEG wakefulness
	Characteristic episodes of eating, often carelessly, can involve peculiar foods	Widely varied behaviors, may reenact past abuse, although occasionally may include eating
	Daytime dissociative episodes not characteristically present	Daytime dissociative episodes almost always present
Nocturnal seizures	Abnormalities on an expanded 16–20 lead EEG montage (May not be seen in Sleep-Related Hypermotor Epilepsy)	Does not characteristically have EEG abnormalities
	Occurs during N1, N2, or transitional sleep	Occurs during sustained EEG wakefulness
	Brief duration	Episodes can be lengthy, often more than an hour
	Stereotyped behavior	Widely varied behaviors, may reenact past abuse
	Good response to anticonvulsant medication	Not known to respond to anticonvulsant medication
	Daytime dissociative episodes not characteristically present	Daytime dissociative episodes almost always present

Note: SRDD and the above disorders in the differential diagnosis are not mutually exclusive; they may at times co-occur.

well as RBD) generally respond well to clonaze-pam, whereas SRDD typically does not improve and often worsens with that medication.

Sleep-related eating disorder, in the "NREM-Related Parasomnias" category, most often oc-curs during partial arousals from NREM sleep but can occur during a more fully awake state, and with EEG wakefulness. However, the very charac-teristic, repetitive episodes of eating behavior usu-ally permit ready distinction from a dissociative disorder.

Nocturnal seizures can often be diagnosed from abnormalities on an expanded 16-to-20 lead EEG montage, although in cases of Nocturnal Frontal Lobe Epilepsy (Sleep-Related Hypermotor Epi-lepsy) scalp EEG may not show electrographic epileptic ictal pattern. The stereotypic quality of the behavior in sleep-related seizures may be helpful in distinguishing them, as may the typically brief duration of seizures compared with dissocia-tive episodes. At times the response to anticonvul-sant treatment can be informative. An additional complication in polysomnographic diagnosis is that some of the reported cases of SRDDs also have documented histories of seizures, that is, both disorders may be present.

SRDD may occasionally present with symptoms suggestive of narcolepsy (daytime sleepiness and at least one reported auxiliary symptom) but these cases do not demonstrate the objective Multiple Sleep Latency Test findings diagnostic for narco-lepsy and instead have clinical histories and sleep laboratory findings supportive of a dissociative disorder.[13]

Additional differential diagnostic considerations include medical disorders and toxic-metabolic states that can result in alterations of conscious-ness, and malingering.

In view of the central importance of identifying dissociative psychological mechanisms, day-time dissociative episodes, and a history of trauma, an in-depth psychiatric/psychological evaluation is an essential part of the diagnostic procedure.

Given the small number of cases that have been observed to date, it is not possible to know for certain that dissociative episodes always emerge out of a period of sustained wakefulness, rather than, for example, after very brief wakefulness or even directly upon awakening from sleep. Addi-tionally, it is possible that there may be hybrid situ-ations, for example, an episode of somnambulism that also has significant dissociative elements, or that begins as somnambulism and evolves into a dissociative episode. The fact that some episodes of sleep-related eating disorder occur during EEG wakefulness is suggestive here. Further clinical

experience is needed to clarify these and other matters.

Formal Status of the Diagnosis

The diagnosis of SRDD does not have formal recognition in any section of the ICSD-3, after be-ing included in the "Other Parasomnias" section of the ICSD-2. (This situation has now been continued in the ICSD-3-TR.) The omission is re-ported to have been based on the following con-siderations: The parasomnias task force for the ICSD-3 was instructed that SRDD was to be viewed as a psychiatric disorder and would need to be shifted as such to the section on Sleep-Related Medical and Neurologic Disorders. How-ever, because the psychiatric nomenclature (DSM-5-TR), which defines and delineates disso-ciative disorders, does not list SRDDs as a distinct sleep disorder, the diagnosis could not be included in that section of the ICSD either.[3]

This has resulted in a very unfortunate situation. SRDD is a significant consideration in the differen-tial diagnosis of any disorder involving complex behavior arising out of sleep, and is in fact listed in the ICSD-3-TR as part of the differential diag-nosis for NREM disorders of arousal, RBD, and nightmare disorder, with brief mention of some distinguishing features. It is a distinct, sleep-related subgroup of the dissociative disorders based on the defining characteristic of episodes occurring during the sleep period. It entails behav-iors and states during the sleep period that are frequently quite similar to those seen in parasom-nias and often presents to sleep disorders centers as suspected somnambulism. These elements indicate a close connection with the parasomnias. Most importantly for the clinician, the absence of a full description of SRDD anywhere in the ICSD-3-TR is detrimental for optimal diagnosis and man-agement of patients.

Important research, too, that can contribute to further refining our understanding of this disorder and its precise relationship to sleep and nature as a sleep disorder, may be hampered by its omis-sion from the sleep disorders nosology. It would be valuable to know, for example, if there is a sub-group of patients with dissociative disorders whose episodes occur preferentially or exclusively during the sleep period, and if so, what factors in these patients and in sleep may account for this. Awakenings from NREM sleep in particular tend to be gradual; it can take some time to attain a fully integrated and functional brain/mind state. It is plausible that this piecemeal attainment of full wakefulness may provide a fertile ground from which dissociative episodes are more likely to emerge. The same may be true of the period of transition to sleep when the full integration of the mind gradually diminishes.

The related question of whether dissociative episodes arising during the sleep period differ in any systematic way from daytime dissociative episodes warrants investigation. It will be important too to clarify the relationship between SRDD and the proposed parasomnia of trauma-associated sleep disorder, given significant overlapping elements such as the presence of trauma and disruptive nocturnal behaviors.[14] A number of additional reasons for the reinclusion of SRDDs in the ICSD, and in the parasomnias section, have been enumerated.[3]

Further Considerations

SRDDs have been characterized as a psychiatric parasomnia. This designation is valuable in emphasizing the direct link to a psychiatric diagnosis that distinguishes this from other parasomnias, but may be too categorical. There is evidence that psychiatric/psychological factors can play a significant role in other parasomnias, particularly NREM parasomnias that entail complex behavior arising out of sleep. High levels of psychopathology have been found in patients with sleep-related injury related to sleepwalking and sleep terrors,[15] and in samples with sleep-related eating disorders.[16,17] Histories of trauma that seem closely related to the specific parasomnia behaviors have been reported in a number of cases of abnormal sleep-related sexual behavior,[18,19] and childhood abuse of different kinds has been observed at elevated levels in sleep-related eating disorder.[20] Furthermore, dissociative psychological tendencies (without frank dissociative disorders) have been observed in patients with sleep-related eating disorders,[17,20] and some episodes of sleep-related eating occur during virtually complete EEG wakefulness. In these NREM parasomnias, factors related to sleep play a much more central role than in SRDDs, but psychiatric/psychological factors may also be significantly involved in some instances.

TREATMENT

Limited information is available about the treatment of SRDDs. In a number of individual cases, there is mention of medications that were tried, usually with partial or no benefit, or psychological or behavioral treatments that were in progress, had been refused or quickly aborted, or had not been effective. There are, however, several cases in which psychological interventions were reported to have been effective. Two of these were child cases: one was a 6-year-old child for whom an intensive,

structured treatment program that included individual therapy, family and group work, and a daily activity program was successful in resolving sleep-related and daytime dissociative episodes[11]; the other was a 10-year-old child whose exclusively sleep-related episodes were reported to have ceased following tailored individual therapy and family counseling.[21] In these instances, the early identification of the disorder, quick institution of intensive therapy, and fact that the patients were children may have been favorable factors.

Experience with daytime dissociative disorders in adults is relevant, and indicates that, especially in more severe cases, treatment is lengthy, challenging, and difficult. Psychotherapy is the central element. As traumatic material emerges, very intense and potentially overwhelming affects, and often destructive and self-destructive impulses, will be evoked. Safety must be assured and hospitalization is frequently required. Developing trust that the therapist has genuine concern and will not be hurtful, abusive, or negligent is a major and difficult task given the patient's history. Intense pulls to reenact traumatic aspects of the patient's key relationships require skillful management. Psychodynamic understanding is essential; it has been combined, in some treatment strategies that have been developed, with other modalities such as hypnosis, cognitive approaches, and medications to attenuate disabling symptoms. Comorbid psychiatric disorders need to be addressed. Given the complexity and difficulty of many of these cases, treatment needs to be carefully, individually tailored. Psychotherapists with expertise and experience in dealing with trauma and dissociative

---

Box 1
Management of sleep-related dissociative disorders: key elements

- Thorough psychological/psychiatric evaluation as part of the initial workup

- Psychotherapy with a therapist skilled in working with trauma and dissociative disorders, using psychodynamic principles along with cognitive and other elements as needed

- Psychiatric management with a psychiatrist skilled in the use of medications for dissociative disorders (may be the same practitioner as the therapist)

- Additional treatment modalities, for example, family treatment, group therapy, milieu therapy, and inpatient treatment used as indicated

- Address sleep/wake-related issues that may be a factor in the dissociative episodes

disorders and psychiatrists skillful in the use of medications for those disorders should be involved.

It is possible that specific aspects of treatment derived from the association of SRDDs with the sleep period may be developed. A recent report described a patient with daytime and nocturnal dissociative episodes and excessive daytime sleepiness who responded to treatment with modafinil with remission of both the dissociative episodes and the daytime sleepiness.[22] Experience with other parasomnias suggests that it may be helpful to treat any coexisting sleep disorders such as obstructive sleep apnea or periodic limb movements of sleep that cause arousals and may potentiate dissociative episodes. Key principles in the management of SRDDs are summarized in **Box 1**.

SUMMARY

SRDDs are of considerable importance to the sleep clinician. Patients with these conditions present to the sleep clinic and require careful diagnosis and management; they are also a key element in the differential diagnosis of parasomnias involving complex behavior arising out of sleep. In SRDD, phenomena of the psychiatrically defined dissociative disorders emerge during the sleep period. They occur during sustained wakefulness, either in the transition to sleep or following an awakening from N1, N2, or REM sleep. A wide range of behaviors have been observed during episodes, including reenactment of childhood abuse, confused wandering, agitated, frightened activity, self-injury, and violence. Daytime dissociative episodes are almost universally present, as is a background of trauma; there is typically major coexisting psychopathology. Patients are predominantly female. Episodes tend to occur frequently, to be lengthy (often more than an hour), and the course appears to be chronic. Diagnosis is based on both clinical history and polysomnography; differential diagnosis primarily involves other parasomnias and nocturnal seizures. There are at present unsettled differences about the proper status of this diagnosis. Limited information is available about treatment; in a few reported cases, psychological interventions have proven effective.

CLINICS CARE POINTS

- It is essential for the sleep clinician to be familiar with SRDDs. Patients with these conditions present to the sleep clinic where they require careful investigation, accurate diagnosis, and informed referral for treatment. They are also a key element in the differential diagnosis of parasomnias involving complex behavior arising out of sleep.

- A core concept in understanding SRDDs is the psychological mechanism of dissociation, in which mental contents and functions, such as substantial areas of memory, are separated off from central consciousness in order to avoid overwhelming experiences with insupportable affects and meanings. The presenting behaviors and states during episodes may be widely varied but they have in common that underlying mechanism. This usage of the term "dissociation" is quite different from the sleep medicine concept of "wake/sleep state dissociation," in which physiologic elements of 1 of the 3 major states of being, wakefulness, NREM sleep, and REM sleep, persist into or emerge during one of the other major states.

- Referral to clinicians skilled in psychotherapy and medication management in patients with histories of trauma and dissociation is strongly indicated.

DISCLOSURE

The author has no commercial or financial conflicts of interest or funding sources to disclose.

REFERENCES

1. Rice E, Fisher C. Fugue states in sleep and wakefulness: a psychophysiological study. J Nerv Ment Dis 1976;163(2):79–87.
2. Schenck CH, Milner DM, Hurwitz TD, et al. Dissociative disorders presenting as somnambulism: polysomnographic, video and clinical documentation (8 cases). Dissociation 1989;2(4):194–204.
3. Schenck CH, Cramer Bornemann M, Kaplish N, et al. Sleep-related (psychogenic) dissociative disorders as parasomnias associated with a psychiatric disorder: update on reported cases. J Clin Sleep Med 2021;17(4):803–10.
4. Lopez R, Lefevre L, Barateau L, et al. A series of 8 cases of sleep-related psychogenic dissociative disorders and proposed updated diagnostic criteria. J Clin Sleep Med 2022;18(2):563–73.
5. American Academy of Sleep Medicine. International classification of sleep disorders. Diagnostic and coding manual. 2nd edition. Westchester, IL: American Academy of Sleep Medicine; 2005.
6. American Academy of Sleep Medicine. International classification of sleep disorders. 3rd edition. Darien, IL: American Academy of Sleep Medicine; 2014.

7. American Academy of Sleep Medicine. *International classification of sleep disorders*. 3rd edition. Darien, IL: American Academy of Sleep Medicine; 2023. text revision.

8. Loewenstein RJ, Frewen P, Lewis-Fernandez R. Dissociative disorders. In: Sadock BJ, Sadock VA, Ruiz P, editors. Kaplan & Sadock's comprehensive textbook of psychiatry. 10th edition. Philadelphia: Wolters Kluwer; 2017. p. 4272–464.

9. American Psychiatric Association. Diagnostic and statistical manual of mental disorders. 5th edition. Washington, DC: American Psychiatric Publishing; 2022. text revision.

10. Agargun MY, Kara H, Ozer OA, et al. Characteristics of patients with nocturnal dissociative disorders. Sleep Hypn 2001;3(4):131–4.

11. Calamaro CJ, Mason TBA. Sleep-related dissociative disorder in a 6-year-old girl. Behav Sleep Med 2008;6:147–57.

12. American Academy of Sleep Medicine. Sleep related dissociative disorders. In: American Academy of Sleep Medicine. International classification of sleep disorders. Diagnostic and coding manual. 2nd edition. Westchester, IL: American Academy of Sleep Medicine; 2005. p. 159–61.

13. Schenck CH, Mahowald MW. Somatoform conversion disorder mimicking narcolepsy in 8 patients with nocturnal and diurnal dissociative disorders. Sleep Research 1993;22:260.

14. Mysliwiec V, Brock MS, Creamer JL, et al. Trauma associated sleep disorder: a parasomnia induced by trauma. Sleep Med Rev 2018;37:94–104.

15. Schenck CH, Milner DM, Hurwitz TD, et al. A polysomnographic and clinical report on sleep-related injury in 100 adult patients. Am J Psychiatr 1989;146(9):1166–73.

16. Schenck CH, Hurwitz TD, Bundlie SR, et al. Sleep-related eating disorders: polysomnographic correlates of a heterogeneous syndrome distinct from daytime eating disorders. Sleep 1991;14(5):419–31.

17. Winkelman JW, Herzog DB, Fava M. The prevalence of sleep-related eating disorder in psychiatric and non-psychiatric populations. Psychol Med 1999;29: 1461–6.

18. Guilleminault C, Moscovitch A, Yuen K, et al. Atypical sexual behavior during sleep. Psychosom Med 2002;64:328–36.

19. Bejot Y, Juenet N, Garrouty R, et al. Sexsomnia: an uncommon variety of parasomnia. Clin Neurol Neurosurg 2010;112:72–5.

20. Schenck CH, Hurwitz TD, O'Connor KA, et al. Additional categories of sleep-related eating disorders and the current status of treatment. Sleep 1993; 16(5):457–66.

21. Molaie M, Deutsch GK. Psychogenic events presenting as parasomnia. Sleep 1997;20(6):402–5.

22. Fiszman A, Figueira I, Pinna C, et al. Efficacy of Modafinil for dissociative identity disorder with hypersomnia. Sleep Hypn 2020;22(1):1–7.

Sleep-Related Urologic Dysfunction

Rosalia Silvestri, MD

KEYWORDS

• Enuresis • Nocturia • Urinary urge incontinence • Sleep

KEY POINTS

- Sleep enuresis is classified by the ICSD-3-TR as a parasomnia in the context of sleep-related urologic dysfunction and may be characterized as primary or secondary, monosymptomatic or nonmonosymptomatic.
- Nocturia is part of the same parasomnia and indicates an excessive number of voids occurring during the sleep period.
- Nocturnal urinary urge incontinence refers to urinary urgency occurring at night that wakes the sleeping subject who is unable to reach the toilet in time to void their bladder.

INTRODUCTION

Before the most recent revision of the International Classification of Sleep Disorders (ICSD-3),[1] sleep enuresis (SE) was classified under "other parasomnias," indicating sleep-related undesirable events or experiences originating during sleep, unrelated to a specific distribution during rapid eye movement (REM) or non-rapid eye movement (NREM) sleep. It was, in fact, construed as a failure to awaken from sleep in response to a physiologic voiding stimulus. The latest classification (The International Classification of Sleep Disorders - Third Edition - Text Revision [ICSD-3-TR]),[2] instead, lists SE as one of 3 disorders comprising sleep-related urologic dysfunction; the others being nocturia, nocturnal voluntary voiding because of awakening from sleep, and nocturnal urinary urge incontinence (UUI), the unsuccessful waking from sleep to oblige voiding urgency but failing to reach the toilet in time (**Table 1**).

This novel taxonomy follows a recent consensus report by the International Continence Society on the current terminology for nocturia and nocturnal lower urinary tract function.[3] The latter clinically based terminology report updated all relevant definitions from research since the first nocturia standardization document, published in 2002.

For the sake of clarity, the 3 syndromic entities that comprise sleep-related urologic dysfunction will be described separately.

SLEEP ENURESIS

Nocturnal or night bed-wetting, SE's first reference dates back to the Ebers papyrus of 1550 BC.[4] Early reports described enuretic episodes as "dream equivalents,"[5] until Broughton[6] interpreted enuresis as a disorder of arousal, that is, an NREM parasomnia occurring during N3.

However, later polysomnographic evidence did not confirm this link to slow-wave sleep.

Initially, this disorder was distinguished into its more severe form, primary SE, characterized by a lack of nocturnal continence, and its milder form, secondary SE, when bed-wetting episodes manifest after a dry period of at least 6 months in subjects aged older than 5 years.[7] More recently,[2] attention is called to the frequency of nocturnal episodes, less or more than 4/wk, and whether the condition seems to be monosymptomatic or nonmonosymptomatic, that is, linked to other urinary tract symptoms.

SE occurs in up to 20% of 5-year-olds[2] with a spontaneous remitting rate of 15% per year.[8] The male-to-female ratio is 3:1 in children, whereas

Sleep Medicine Center, UOSD of Neurophysiopathology and Movement Disorders, Department of Clinical and Experimental Medicine, University of Messina, Messina, Italy
E-mail address: rsilvestri@unime.it

Sleep Med Clin 19 (2024) 169–176
https://doi.org/10.1016/j.jsmc.2023.10.009

Table 1
Sleep-related urologic dysfunction according to the ICSD-3-TR

Sleep-Related Urologic Dysfunction		
SE	**Nocturia**	**Nocturnal UUI**
Recurrent involuntary voiding during sleep	Urination arising from and followed by sleep	Urinary urgency and leakage after awakening from sleep
At least 1/mo	Three or more episodes/night	Minimal frequency: 1/wk
Age >5 y	Age >5 y	
At least 3 mo duration		

From Medicine AAoS. *International Classification of Sleep Disorders*. Third Edition, Text Revision ed. 2023.

the disorder is reported in 2% to 3% of older adults, primarily in women.[2]

Besides co-occurrence with neurodevelopmental and sleep disorders in children, genetic studies strongly support hereditary factors showing a complex heterogeneity due to a significant interaction with environmental factors. Linkage studies disclosed markers on chromosomes 6, 8, 12, 13, and 22 with different phenotypes.[9,10]

SE prevalence of 77% has been found in children with both parents with enuresis and 44% with only one parent affected.[11]

Rs6313 polymorphism in the 5-hydroxytryptamine receptor 2A gene has been associated with polysymptomatic SE, suggesting that serotonin may influence the polysymptomatic form of this heterogeneous disorder.[12]

Butler and Holland[13] hypothesize that the cause of voiding dysfunction involves 3 possible mechanisms: excessive urine production during sleep, nocturnal bladder overactivity, and difficulty arousing from sleep. Difficulty arousing from sleep seems to play a significant role in children with SE. In fact, young patients with enuresis are often described as difficult to arouse deep-sleepers by their parents; hence, SE has been long interpreted as a maturational sleep delay, confirmed by a higher arousal threshold compared with healthy controls.[14,15]

Sleep studies, including those with simultaneous cystography during polysomnography, have shown an overall reduction in N3 and REM, besides a pathologically increased arousal index.[2] Of note, these sleep structure alterations are similar during nights when SE occurs and when it does not.[16]

Both sleep-disordered breathing (SDB; in up to 47% of children)[17] and a high periodic limb movement index[18] are common findings in SE, the latter correlating with treatment resistance. In this context, autonomic alterations have been recorded preceding an enuretic event: both tachycardia and higher mean arterial pressure have been observed

in children with SE indifferently during wet or dry nights.[19] Autonomic studies also suggest parasympathetic nervous system hyperactivity in children with SE.[20]

SDB seems to prevail in female children suffering from SE, who exhibit greater excessive daytime sleepiness (EDS) and behavioral problems compared with the control population.[21]

As for urinary overproduction at night exceeding the maximum daytime functional capacity, research has shown that children with enuresis do not suffer from arginine vasopressor (AVP) deficiency but rather from a central AVP receptor level defect.[22]

Besides primary abnormalities of this type, excessive urine production coupled with the inability to concentrate the urine may be secondary to several medical conditions, including diabetes insipidus or mellitus, sickle cell disease, and iatrogenic conditions linked to agents such as diuretics and caffeine. Moreover, urinary tract infections may be as common in children as in adults. In contrast, conditions such as neurogenic bladder, dementia, and other neurologic pathologic conditions are more often reported in adult and elderly patients with enuresis.

Risk and precipitating factors for children often include personal and parental anxiety and posttraumatic stress.[23,24] Furthermore, bullied children are more likely to develop enuresis, negatively affecting their self-esteem and social life (sleepovers, camping, and so forth).[25] SE is also overexpressed in mental retardation, attention deficit hyperactivity disorder (ADHD),[26] and autism spectrum disorder (ASD).[27] Maternal factors include age younger than 20 years at the child's birth, smoking, and prematurity.[28]

Differential diagnosis in children should include evaluating possible urinary tract infections, especially when daytime symptoms or abnormalities in the micturition process or urinary flow are present. A sleep study is indicated in the presence of snoring, EDS, adenoid and tonsil hypertrophy, and ADHD to rule out or treat obstructive sleep apnea (OSA) or when nocturnal epileptic seizures are suspected.

Radiological and cystoscopic evaluation, when normal, may be complemented by urodynamic studies to detect detrusor or sphincter problems.[29]

Urodynamic studies have revealed that up to 73% of adults with SE suffer from bladder dysfunction.[30] Overactive bladder and poor voiding due to detrusor underactivity contribute to the pathogenesis of SE in women.[31]

SE management includes pharmacologic and nonpharmacologic treatment depending on patients' age and cause. In children aged older than 6 years, behavioral techniques must be tried first, including fluid restriction, retention control exercises, wetness alarms, biofeedback, and psychotherapy.

The bell-and-pad alarm therapy involves an alarm activated by urination to awaken the child and allow them to do most of the voiding properly in the toilet. This method proved more efficient than drug therapy and assures higher rates of sustained continence.[32,33] Treatment lasts approximately 2 to 3 months, or until the subject has accomplished 14 consecutive dry nights,[34] with a cumulative relapse rate of 30%.[35]

Psychotherapy is indicated only in cases of posttraumatic stress, whereas encouraging results have been obtained using electroacupuncture with a successful rate of 65% in children with monosymptomatic enuresis.[36] Another study using acupuncture to treat 50 children and adolescents suffering from persistent primary SE reported impressive results, with a 76% and 92% cure rate at the 6-month and 1-year follow-up, respectively.[37]

Sleep architecture parameters in children with severe OSA may predict the success of adenotonsillectomy. In fact, children with both severe OSA (apnea-hypopnea index >10) and a prolonged N2 stage are 3.4 times more likely to have a postoperative resolution of SE.[38]

Among experimental treatments, both parasacral transcutaneous electrical nerve stimulation for overly active bladders[39] and functional magnetic stimulation for children with cortical arousal dysfunction[40,41] have obtained partial success.

Medications used for SE treatment thus far include antidepressants, antidiuretics, antispasmodics, and prostaglandin synthesis inhibitors.

Among tricyclic antidepressants, imipramine 25 mg (50–75 mg in older children) 1 or 2 hours before bedtime acts as an alpha-adrenergic stimulant of the renal proximal tubules[42] but is scantly efficient and presents a significant relapse rate.[43] Reboxetine has been used as an alternative[44]

but an extensive review on the use of tricyclic-related drugs to treat SE concluded against its use due to the small and transient effect size, in addition to significant side effects.[43]

Desmopressin (10-40 mcg intranasally or 200-600 mcg orally) is currently the primary antidiuretic prescribed for SE. Unfortunately, it has a short-lasting efficacy despite almost no side effects. The relapse rate is very high on drug discontinuation.[45,46] However, this treatment may be positively combined with alarm therapy and anticholinergic drugs.

A retrospective observational study of ADHD and ASD children with enuresis treated with desmopressin and anticholinergic therapy (34) showed a favorable trend.[47]

Studies with diuretic and antispasmodic drugs (oxybutynin and tolterodine) showed limited efficacy alone but combination therapy research has shown that desmopressin plus tolterodine performs better than desmopressin plus oxybutynin in the treatment of children with primary SE.[48]

NOCTURIA

Nocturia is defined as the need for patients to wake at night one or more times for voiding. Each episode is voluntary, unlike SE, and must be preceded and followed by a sleep period.

Three or 4 voids per night are defined as pathologic. The disorder is more prevalent in the adult and elderly population, with increasing frequency with age (2%–3% in the 20s, nearly 20% in the 70s).[2] Nocturia may lead to sleep deprivation, exhaustion, impaired daytime activities, and cognitive dysfunction. It is, however, underreported and underdiagnosed with inefficient management due to the failure of an etiologic assessment.

Etiologic factors include nocturnal and global polyuria, bladder storage problems, and sleep disorders, among the most common factors.[49]

Nocturnal polyuria is defined as nocturnal urinary overproduction (more than 20% of the total 24-hour urine volume in subjects aged 25–65 years, more than 33% in patients aged older than 65 years). The increased nighttime urine production is usually accompanied by a proportional daytime reduction in hourly urine volume, resulting in a normal 24-hour total urine production.

The hourly urinary production is regulated by AVP released from the posterior pituitary gland in response to hypernatremia or low blood pressure to inhibit urine production. In contrast, atrial natriuretic peptide (ANP) increases renal excretion of sodium and water, acting as a diuretic.[50]

Nocturnal polyuria is a frequent cause of nocturia in elderly patients; this could be linked to several factors, including excessive alcohol or caffeine intake, congestive heart failure with elevated plasma levels of ANP, OSA, peripheral edema, and lower extremity venous insufficiency.

Global polyuria, instead, refers to a urinary overproduction throughout the day, resulting in an increased output of more than 40 mL/kg/24 h. It is always associated with either primary or secondary polydipsia due to diabetes mellitus or insipidus, drug effects, renal insufficiency, or low estrogen levels in women.[49] When polyuria is not the cause of nocturia, bladder storage problems due to reduced bladder capacity or detrusor overactivity need to be ruled out.

Finally, sleep disorders believed to contribute to or even cause nocturia refer mainly to OSA, which may induce nocturia via augmented ANP production. In fact, nocturia occurs in nearly 50% of patients with OSA, and its prevalence increases with increasing OSA severity (57.2%, 64.3%, and 76.9% in mild, moderate, and severe OSA, respectively).[51] Moreover, restless legs syndrome (RLS) alone or combined with OSA may aggravate sleep dysfunction and nocturia.[2] Screening for OSA and other sleep disorders may enable early treatment and reduce cardio and cerebrovascular consequences.

Other contributing factors to nocturia include peripheral edema, a large amount of fluid intake at bedtime, liver failure, depression, Parkinson disease due to reduced sympathetic tone, and, last but not least, normal pregnancy.

Men and women are equally exposed to the risk of nocturia, appraised as 50% after the age of 60 years. Young women (pregnancy effect) are more prone to nocturia, whereas older men aged older than 70 years have an increased risk compared with their female counterparts.[52] Obesity is an independent risk factor, doubling or tripling the incidence of nocturia in both genders.[50]

Patients should be encouraged by their doctors to keep night diaries about their voiding frequencies.

All contributing medical conditions and medications should be carefully assessed and ruled out. The presence of lower urinary tract symptoms may indicate the need for further urologic assessment with the aid of instrumental procedures, including flowmetry, cystoscopy, urodynamics, and laboratory evaluations (glucose, renal function, urinalysis, and so forth), besides physical examination.

Patients with nocturia are exposed to an increased risk of nocturnal falls and fractures, as recently investigated.[53] In fact, nocturia is associated with an excess relative risk of 20% for falls and an excess relative risk of 32% for fractures compared with people without nocturia after adjusting for age, gender, and various comorbidities.

Data from the National Health and Nutrition Examination Survey[54] indicate a significant association of nocturia with all-cause mortality and cardiovascular disease mortality in both men and women. In a subgroup analysis, nocturia was associated with cardiovascular disease mortality in patients with diabetes, hypertension, dyslipidemia, or cardiovascular disease at baseline.

Treatment should be offered to all patients with significant symptoms, aiming toward a 50% reduction of nocturia frequency or no more than 1 to 2 voiding episodes per night because complete cessation of nocturia may not be feasible.

Initial treatment should simply limit evening fluid intake, reduce salt and proteins, promote daytime physical activities, and reduce time spent in bed. Moreover, absorbent pads and mattress covers could help protect the bed.

Behavioral and pelvic floor muscle training in postmenopausal women has significantly reduced nocturia episodes.[55] Sleep hygiene techniques to reduce superficial and fragmented sleep via sleep restriction therapy could potentially consolidate the sleep period. Continuous positive airway pressure (CPAP), if OSA has been detected, has proven significantly effective in reducing nocturia from 2.6 to 0.7 voids per night.[56]

Before considering a medical approach, it should be noted that age-related increases in the 24-hour diuresis rate, sodium clearance, and free water clearance are not specific to subjects experiencing nocturia but rather represent a widespread age-related change. This information should drive both behavioral and pharmacologic interventions. In fact, especially in patients aged older than 65 years, impaired circadian rhythmicity of AVP or decreased renal responsivity to water clearance may constitute the substrate of increased nocturnal voiding episodes.[57]

Finally, pharmacologic therapy for nocturia[50] includes the following:

- *Diuretic therapy timing adjustments* in patients with hypertension or patients with congestive heart failure
- *Alpha-blockers* to reduce detrusor instability and overactivity (doxazosin, terazosin)
- *Anticholinergics* to increase bladder capacity
- *Topical vaginal estrogen* in postmenopausal women
- *Botox bladder injections* in very severe cases
- *Desmopressin* for patients with nocturnal polyuria.

Desmopressin, however, should not be used in patients with chronic heart failure or chronic kidney disease. Desmopressin nasal spray has fewer side effects and has proven effective at different dosages to reduce nocturia episodes, starting with a 0.83 mcg dose.[58]

Other remedies of uncertain value include slow-release melatonin, nonsteroidal anti-inflammatory drugs to decrease glomerular filtration rate, and 5-alpha-reductase inhibitors (finasteride and dutasteride) to treat benign prostatic hyperplasia in men.[50]

Posterior tibial nerve stimulation has been used to improve bladder storage and reduce voiding via pudendal and pelvic sympathetic nerve stimulation.[59]

Combination therapy of medications and behavioral techniques has thus far granted encouraging results with respect to drug therapy alone. Still, it does not seem to be more efficient than behavioral therapy alone (**Table 2**).[60]

NOCTURNAL URINARY URGE INCONTINENCE

UUI is defined as incontinence after awakening from sleep with the inability to reach the bathroom before micturition occurs.[2] Hence, the patient awakens with the urge to void but leakage occurs on their way to the toilet, and they experience wake enuresis as partial or complete involuntary voiding.

UUI is an established risk factor for diurnal and nocturnal falls; it affects nearly 2.1% of all community-dwelling older adults, placing them at risk for hip fractures.[2] Several causes may account for UUI, most of which are in common with nocturia: polyuria, urinary tract pathologic condition, irritable bladder, prostatism, and neurologic disorders such as dementia, Parkinson disease, and neurogenic bladder. Often, in these patients, it is almost impossible to disentangle the contributive role of polyuria, reduced bladder capacity, and neurogenic bladder.

UUI complications include urinary tract infections, decubitus ulcers, insomnia, and sepsis.

Available treatment options include mostly anticholinergics, as discussed above. However, especially in older residents, adverse drug effects include worsening cognitive status and benign prostatic hyperplasia, besides dry mouth and drowsiness.[61]

UUI patients dissatisfied with anticholinergic drug therapy experienced improved treatment outcomes by adding a self-administered behavioral intervention, including pelvic floor muscle training and tailored behavioral techniques to their drug regimen.[62]

Catheterization may be intermittently used. Prostate surgery is indicated in the case of severe obstructive pathologic condition but results are mixed also due to the presence of a central component associated with executive dysfunction.

DISCUSSION

Voiding dysfunction mechanisms and causes are not yet fully disclosed because they may implicate genetic predisposition and overlapping of their 3 main components: urine overproduction, storage capacity, and impaired arousal.

Voiding dysfunction, although very common at different ages, is often overlooked and rarely thoroughly diagnosed. Instead, empirical treatments are often offered without specific consideration for the patient's general health status and pharmacologic history. A vast psychological and social burden ensues from voiding dysfunction, affecting patients as well as caregivers. Sanitary costs are also consistent; nocturia alone costs an estimated US$61 billion to Americans each year due to lost productivity and sick leave, primarily because of preventable falls, fractures, and associated injuries and an estimated annual cost of lost work productivity due to nocturia of € 29 billion in the EU-15.[63]

Frequent complications are seen in the elderly in community-dwelling populations and include sepsis, insomnia, renal dysfunction, fractures, and increased cardiovascular and cerebrovascular mortality.

The role of sleep and sleep disorders needs further elucidation, including the contribution of

Table 2	
Sleep-related urologic dysfunction therapy	
Behavioral Interventions	**Pharmacologic Treatment**
Reduction of fluid intake later in the daytime	Tricyclic antidepressants (children)
Retention control exercises	Desmopressin (nasal/oral)
Alarm devices (SE in children)	Anticholinergic drugs
Acupuncture	Alpha blockers
Transcutaneous parasacral electrical nerve stimulation	Topical vaginal estrogens
Sleep consolidation (medical and CPAP)	Botox bladder injections
Pelvic floor muscle training	Diuretic therapy time adjustment

insomnia and OSA. Simultaneous night recordings of urodynamic and sleep parameters may cast light on proximal triggers and causative mechanisms.

Alleviation of symptoms and potential complications should be the ultimate goal of the dedicated clinician dealing with this pathologic condition.

SUMMARY

SE, nocturia, and UUI represent the multiple concurrent aspects of the newly categorized sleep-related urologic dysfunction. This sleep disorder is included in the parasomnias section of the ICSD-3-TR[2] referring to involuntary events and experiences occurring during any sleep phase and disturbing patients' sleep depth and continuity. Sleep fragmentation and mechanisms referring to hypoxia and negative pressure breathing are also included among the possible causes of voiding dysfunction, especially of primary and secondary SE and polyuria.

The epidemiology of sleep-related voiding dysfunctions spans a vast age spectrum from childhood to seniority and implies idiopathic genetic mechanisms as well as secondary medical causes involving the control of fluid excretion, brain, heart, renal, and bladder pathologic condition.

This article aims to review the principal mechanisms leading to sleep-related urologic dysfunction and indicate the best diagnostic procedures and available treatment options, both medical and behavioral, tailored according to the patient's age and comorbid conditions.

CLINICS CARE POINTS

- SE, nocturia, and UUI have sleep as well as daytime impact and consequences despite being often underrecognized and undertreated.
- Sleep-related urologic dysfunction severely affects patients' sleep and health, with potentially lethal consequences for the elderly.
- A careful medical/pharmacologic history, physical examination, laboratory work, and adequate instrumental procedures should be promoted by the primary care physician (PCP) and sleep specialist in patients reporting nocturnal voiding symptoms.
- Treatment should be established early and tailored to individual needs and comorbidities, avoiding dangerous adverse drug effects that may threaten the patient's life quality and security.

ACKNOWLEDGMENTS

The author greatly acknowledges the assistance of Maria Caterina Di Perri, MS for her valuable contribution in compiling this article.

DISCLOSURE

Rosalia Silvestri has no conflicts of interest to disclose.

REFERENCES

1. American Academy of Sleep Medicine. In: International classification of sleep disorders. 3rd edition. Darien, IL: American Academy of Sleep Medicine; 2014.
2. American Academy of Sleep Medicine. International classification of sleep disorders. 3rd edition, text revision. Darien, IL: American Academy of Sleep Medicine; 2023.
3. Hashim H, Blanker MH, Drake MJ, et al. International continence society (ICS) report on the terminology for nocturia and nocturnal lower urinary tract function. Neurourol Urodyn 2019;38(2):499–508.
4. Glicklich LB. An historical account of enuresis. Pediatrics 1951;8(6):859–76.
5. Pierce CM, Whitman RM, Maas JW, et al. Enuresis and dreaming. Experimental studies. Arch Gen Psychiatry 1961;4:166–70.
6. Broughton RJ. Sleep disorders: disorders of arousal? Enuresis, somnambulism, and nightmares occur in confusional states of arousal, not in "dreaming sleep". Science 1968;159(3819):1070–8.
7. American Academy of Sleep Medicine. The International Classification of Sleep Disorders: Diagnostic and Coding Manual. 2nd edition. Westchester, IL: American Academy of Sleep Medicine; 2005. p. 162–4.
8. Forsythe WI, Redmond A. Enuresis and spontaneous cure rate. Study of 1129 enuretis. Arch Dis Child. Apr 1974;49(4):259–63.
9. Jorgensen CS, Horsdal HT, Rajagopal VM, et al. Identification of genetic loci associated with nocturnal enuresis: a genome-wide association study. Lancet Child Adolesc Health 2021;5(3):201–9.
10. von Gontard A, Schaumburg H, Hollmann E, et al. The genetics of enuresis: a review. J Urol 2001; 166(6):2438–43.
11. Bakwin H. The Genetics of Enuresis. In: Kolvin I, Mac Keith RCI, Meadow SR, editors. Bladder control and enuresis. London: William Heinemann; 1973. p. 73–7.
12. Wei CC, Wan L, Lin WY, et al. Rs 6313 polymorphism in 5-hydroxytryptamine receptor 2A gene association with polysymptomatic primary nocturnal enuresis. J Clin Lab Anal 2010;24(6):371–5.
13. Butler RJ, Holland P. The three systems: a conceptual way of understanding nocturnal enuresis. Scand J Urol Nephrol 2000;34(4):270–7.

14. Alexopoulos EI, Kostadima E, Pagonari I, et al. Association between primary nocturnal enuresis and habitual snoring in children. Urology 2006;68(2):406–9.

15. Ersu R, Arman AR, Save D, et al. Prevalence of snoring and symptoms of sleep-disordered breathing in primary school children in istanbul. Chest 2004; 126(1):19–24.

16. Soster LA, Alves RC, Fagundes SN, et al. Non-REM sleep instability in children with primary monosymptomatic sleep enuresis. J Clin Sleep Med 2017; 13(10):1163–70.

17. Alexopoulos EI, Malakasioti G, Varlami V, et al. Nocturnal enuresis is associated with moderate-to-severe obstructive sleep apnea in children with snoring. Pediatr Res 2014;76(6):555–9.

18. Dhondt K, Baert E, Van Herzeele C, et al. Sleep fragmentation and increased periodic limb movements are more common in children with nocturnal enuresis. Acta Paediatr 2014;103(6):e268–72.

19. Bader G, Neveus T, Kruse S, et al. Sleep of primary enuretic children and controls. Sleep 2002;25(5): 579–83.

20. Yakinci C, Mungen B, Durmaz Y, et al. Autonomic nervous system functions in children with nocturnal enuresis. Brain Dev 1997;19(7):485–7.

21. Stone J, Malone PS, Atwill D, et al. Symptoms of sleep-disordered breathing in children with nocturnal enuresis. J Pediatr Urol 2008;4(3):197–202.

22. Eggert P. What's new in enuresis? Acta Paediatr Taiwan 2002;43(1):6–9.

23. Akan S, Urkmez A, Yildirim C, et al. Late-onset secondary nocturnal enuresis in adolescents associated with post-traumatic stress disorder developed after a traffic accident. Arch Ital Urol Androl 2015; 87(3):250–1.

24. Eidlitz-Markus T, Shuper A, Amir J. Secondary enuresis: post-traumatic stress disorder in children after car accidents. Isr Med Assoc J 2000;2(2): 135–7.

25. Williams K, Chambers M, Logan S, et al. Association of common health symptoms with bullying in primary school children. BMJ 1996;313(7048):17–9.

26. Shreeram S, He JP, Kalaydjian A, et al. Prevalence of enuresis and its association with attention-deficit/hyperactivity disorder among U.S. children: results from a nationally representative study. J Am Acad Child Adolesc Psychiatry 2009;48(1):35–41.

27. von Gontard A, Hussong J, Yang SS, et al. Neurodevelopmental disorders and incontinence in children and adolescents: attention-deficit/hyperactivity disorder, autism spectrum disorder, and intellectual disability-A consensus document of the International Children's Continence Society. Neurourol Urodyn 2022;41(1):102–14.

28. Rona RJ, Li L, Chinn S. Determinants of nocturnal enuresis in England and scotland in the '90s. Dev Med Child Neurol 1997;39(10):677–81.

29. Parekh DJ, Pope JCt, Adams MC, et al. The use of radiography, urodynamic studies and cystoscopy in the evaluation of voiding dysfunction. J Urol 2001;165(1):215–8.

30. Yeung CK, Sreedhar B, Sihoe JD, et al. Differences in characteristics of nocturnal enuresis between children and adolescents: a critical appraisal from a large epidemiological study. BJU Int 2006;97(5): 1069–73.

31. Song QX, Li J, Gu Y, et al. The clinical features and predictive factors of nocturnal enuresis in adult women. Front Med 2021;8:744214.

32. Monda JM, Husmann DA. Primary nocturnal enuresis: a comparison among observation, imipramine, desmopressin acetate and bed-wetting alarm systems. J Urol 1995;154(2 Pt 2):745–8.

33. Oredsson AF, Jorgensen TM. Changes in nocturnal bladder capacity during treatment with the bell and pad for monosymptomatic nocturnal enuresis. J Urol 1998;160(1):166–9.

34. Alqannad EM, Alharbi AS, Almansour RA, et al. Alarm therapy in the treatment of enuresis in children: types and efficacy review. Cureus 2021; 13(8):e17358.

35. Gim CS, Lillystone D, Caldwell PH. Efficacy of the bell and pad alarm therapy for nocturnal enuresis. J Paediatr Child Health Jul-Aug 2009;45(7–8):405–8.

36. Bjorkstrom G, Hellstrom AL, Andersson S. Electroacupuncture in the treatment of children with monosymptomatic nocturnal enuresis. Scand J Urol Nephrol 2000;34(1):21–6.

37. El Koumi MA, Ahmed SA, Salama AM. Acupuncture efficacy in the treatment of persistent primary nocturnal enuresis. Arab J Nephrol Transplant 2013;6(3):173–6.

38. Thottam PJ, Kovacevic L, Madgy DN, et al. Sleep architecture parameters that predict postoperative resolution of nocturnal enuresis in children with obstructive sleep apnea. Ann Otol Rhinol Laryngol 2013;122(11):690–4.

39. Tugtepe H, Thomas DT, Ergun R, et al. The effectiveness of transcutaneous electrical neural stimulation therapy in patients with urinary incontinence resistant to initial medical treatment or biofeedback. J Pediatr Urol 2015;11(3):137 e1–e5.

40. But I, Varda NM. Functional magnetic stimulation: a new method for the treatment of girls with primary nocturnal enuresis? J Pediatr Urol 2006;2(5):415–8.

41. Xiang B, Biji S, Liu JX, et al. Functional brainstem changes in response to bladder function alteration elicited by surgical reduction in bladder capacity: a functional magnetic resonance imaging study. J Urol 2010;184(5):2186–91.

42. Hunsballe JM, Rittig S, Pedersen EB, et al. Single dose imipramine reduces nocturnal urine output in patients with nocturnal enuresis and nocturnal polyuria. J Urol 1997;158(3 Pt 1):830–6.

43. Caldwell PH, Sureshkumar P, Wong WC. Tricyclic and related drugs for nocturnal enuresis in children. Cochrane Database Syst Rev 2016;2016(1): CD002117.

44. Lundmark E, Stenberg A, Hagglof B, et al. Reboxetine in therapy-resistant enuresis: a randomized placebo-controlled study. J Pediatr Urol 2016; 12(6):397 e1–e397 e5.

45. Moffatt ME, Harlos S, Kirshen AJ, et al. Desmopressin acetate and nocturnal enuresis: how much do we know? Pediatrics 1993;92(3):420–5.

46. Skoog SJ, Stokes A, Turner KL. Oral desmopressin: a randomized double-blind placebo controlled study of effectiveness in children with primary nocturnal enuresis. J Urol 1997;158(3 Pt 2):1035–40.

47. Gor RA, Fuhrer J, Schober JM. A retrospective observational study of enuresis, daytime voiding symptoms, and response to medical therapy in children with attention deficit hyperactivity disorder and autism spectrum disorder. J Pediatr Urol 2012;8(3):314–7.

48. Azarfar A, Esmaeili M, Naseri M, et al. Comparison of combined treatment with desmopressin plus oxybutynin and desmopressin plus tolterodine in treatment of children with primary nocturnal enuresis. J Renal Inj Prev 2015;4(3):80–6.

49. Nguyen LN, Randhawa H, Nadeau G, et al. Canadian urological association best practice report: diagnosis and management of nocturia. Can Urol Assoc J 2022;16(7):E336–49.

50. Leslie SW, Sajjad H, Singh S, Nocturia. [Updated 2023 Mar 11]. In: StatPearls [Internet]. Treasure Island (FL): StatPearls Publishing; 2023 Jan-. Available at: https://www.ncbi.nlm.nih.gov/books/NBK518987/.

51. Oztura I, Kaynak D, Kaynak HC. Nocturia in sleep-disordered breathing. Sleep Med 2006;7(4):362–7.

52. Bosch JL, Weiss JP. The prevalence and causes of nocturia. J Urol 2010;184(2):440–6.

53. Pesonen JS, Vernooij RWM, Cartwright R, et al. The impact of nocturia on falls and fractures: a systematic review and meta-analysis. J Urol 2020;203(4): 674–83.

54. Moon S, Kim YJ, Chung HS, et al. The relationship between nocturia and mortality: data from the national health and nutrition examination Survey. Int Neurourol J 2022;26(2):144–52.

55. Wu C, Newman D, Schwartz TA, et al. Effects of unsupervised behavioral and pelvic floor muscle training programs on nocturia, urinary urgency, and urinary frequency in postmenopausal women: secondary analysis of a randomized, two-arm, parallel design, superiority trial (TULIP study). Maturitas 2021;146:42–8.

56. Wang T, Huang W, Zong H, et al. The efficacy of continuous positive airway pressure therapy on nocturia in patients with obstructive sleep apnea: a systematic review and meta-analysis. Int Neurourol J 2015;19(3):178–84.

57. Monaghan TF, Bliwise DL, Denys MA, et al. Phenotyping nocturnal polyuria: circadian and age-related variations in diuresis rate, free water clearance and sodium clearance. Age Ageing 2020;49(3):439–45.

58. Kaminetsky J, Fein S, Dmochowski R, et al. Efficacy and safety of SER120 nasal spray in patients with nocturia: pooled analysis of 2 randomized, double-blind, placebo controlled, phase 3 trials. J Urol 2018;200(3):604–11.

59. McPhail C, Carey R, Nambiar S, et al. The investigation of percutaneous tibial nerve stimulation (PTNS) as a minimally invasive, non-surgical, non-hormonal treatment for overactive bladder symptoms. J Clin Med 2023;12(10). https://doi.org/10.3390/jcm12103490.

60. Burgio KL, Kraus SR, Johnson TM 2nd, et al. Effectiveness of combined behavioral and drug therapy for overactive bladder symptoms in men: a randomized clinical trial. JAMA Intern Med 2020;180(3): 411–9.

61. Demaagd GA, Davenport TC. Management of urinary incontinence. P t 2012;37(6):345–361h.

62. Wyman JF, Klutke C, Burgio K, et al. Effects of combined behavioral intervention and tolterodine on patient-reported outcomes. Can J Urol 2010;17(4): 5283–90.

63. Holm-Larsen T. The economic impact of nocturia. Neurourol Urodyn 2014;33(Suppl 1):S10–4.

Parasomnias During the COVID-19 Pandemic

Felice Di Laudo, MD[a], Greta Mainieri, MD[a,b], Federica Provini, MD, PhD[a,b],*

KEYWORDS

- COVID-19 • Pandemic • Sleep disorders • Parasomnias • Lockdown • Healthcare workers
- Telemedicine

KEY POINTS

- Acute SARS-CoV2 infection and chronic disease in long-COVID patients have a massive impact on sleep, worsening pre-existing sleep disorders or triggering a new onset of sleep disorders, both directly due to the infection itself and indirectly due to increase of stress and anxiety symptoms.
- The allostatic load is the exaggerated and abnormal activity of brain areas that orchestrate the "stress response", and the pandemic is a factor that increases the allostatic load, which may be closely related to sleep in a bidirectional way: when sleep dysregulation is present, stress reactivity is increased and, on the other hand, stressors lead to sleep problems.
- Lockdown and quarantine, that is, the measures imposed to tackle COVID-19 diffusion worldwide, increased the rates of sleep disturbances, in particular insomnia, but also NREM and REM parasomnias.
- Children and healthcare workers were populations at particular risk of developing sleep disturbances, in particular parasomnias, during the COVID-19 pandemic. Due to the global reduction of sleep lab attendance after COVID-19 outbreak, parasomnias were investigated only by administering questionnaires.
- Sleep studies with adequate preparation, telemedicine and home videos may overcome the issue of massive reduction in performing sleep studies during future exceptional situations as the pandemic was in these years.

BACKGROUND

Parasomnias are undesirable physical events or experiences that occur during entry into sleep, within sleep, or during arousal from sleep. Parasomnias may occur during non-rapid eye movement sleep (NREM), rapid eye movement sleep (REM), or during transitions to and from sleep.[1] Many parasomnias are the result of mixed states with the concomitant presence of multiple state-determining biomarkers. According to the recent view of sleep as a "complex local phenomenon", different states of consciousness, such as wakefulness, NREM sleep and REM sleep, can concurrently result in these "altered", but not necessarily pathologic,[2] states.

Non-rapid Eye Movement Parasomnias: Predisposing Factors and Precipitants

NREM sleep parasomnias are motor manifestations characterized by the occurrence of incomplete awakenings from NREM sleep; confusional arousals, sleep terrors, and sleepwalking are the 3 main clinical entities, currently grouped under the name of "disorders of arousal" (DoA).[1] The lifetime prevalence of DoA is around 7%, and it is higher in childhood than in adults.[3] Although the exact pathophysiological mechanisms are not still

[a] Department of Biomedical and NeuroMotor Sciences (DiBiNeM), University of Bologna, Via Massarenti, 9, Pad. 11, Bologna 40138, Italy; [b] IRCCS Istituto delle Scienze Neurologiche di Bologna, Via Altura, 3, Bologna 40139, Italy
* Corresponding author. IRCCS Istituto delle Scienze Neurologiche di Bologna, Bellaria Hospital, Bologna 40139, Italy.
E-mail address: federica.provini@unibo.it

Sleep Med Clin 19 (2024) 177–187
https://doi.org/10.1016/j.jsmc.2023.10.012
1556-407X/24/© 2023 Elsevier Inc. All rights reserved.

fully elucidated, the proposed "3-Ps model" for DoA pathophysiology identifies predisposing, priming, and precipitating factors: on a predisposed genetic background,[4] different priming factors could provoke DoA episodes, especially when possible precipitating factors are present (**Fig. 1**).[5] A "4th P" has been suggested, when the persistence of unresolved causes may lead to the perpetuation of DoA in adulthood.[6] DoA occur in the first third of the night, when the amount of slow wave sleep (SWS) is greater, so factors that deepen SWS or increase SWS fragmentation are related to the occurrence of DoA episodes.[7–13]

Rapid Eye Movement Parasomnias

REM parasomnias include 3 main clinical entities: recurrent isolated sleep paralysis, nightmare disorder, and REM sleep behavior disorder (RBD). Sleep paralysis is characterized by an inability to perform voluntary movements at sleep onset or on waking from sleep that may last seconds to minutes and usually resolves spontaneously or by sensorial stimulations.[1] Anxiety is usually a core feature of sleep paralysis and may be associated with auditory, visual, or tactile hallucinations, or the sense of a presence in the room. Predisposing factors are sleep deprivation and irregular sleep-wake schedules, while some studies reported mental stress as a precipitating factor.[14]

Nightmare disorder is characterized by recurrent, highly dysphoric dreams that generally occur during REM sleep and often result in awakening. Nightmares are very common in children, most frequently involving anxiety, fear, or terror (frequently undistinguished from confusional arousals or sleep terrors) but also anger, rage, embarrassment, and disgust.[1] Associations with psychopathology have been identified, as well as with the clinical use of antidepressants, antihypertensives, dopamine-receptor agonists, GABAergic drugs, acetylcholine, and histamine.[15]

RBD is characterized by loss of the physiologic muscle atonia and by abnormal motor behaviors emerging during REM sleep that may cause injury to the patients and/or to their bedpartners. RBD usually manifests as an attempted enactment of unpleasant, action-filled, and violent dreams in which the individual is being confronted, attacked, or chased by unfamiliar people or animals: the dream action often corresponds closely to the observed sleep behaviors.[1] RBD can emerge acutely with drug withdrawal or toxic-metabolic states or can be triggered by antidepressant/other medications.[16] Chronic RBD can be associated with medical or neurologic disorders, mostly α-synucleinopathies.[16]

RBD is defined as "isolated" when it occurs in the absence of any other medical condition.[16]

Coronavirus Disease-2019 Outbreak

In December 2019, the Chinese Center for Disease Control and Prevention reported a cluster of pneumonia cases with unknown cause, observed in the Chinese city of Wuhan. The first complete viral genome sequence (January 2020) was eventually named "2019 novel coronavirus (2019-nCoV/SARS-CoV-2)". The virus caused the coronavirus disease 2019 (COVID-19) and spread rapidly worldwide with its symptoms ranging from fully asymptomatic to severe disease and death. In March 2020, the World Health Organization (WHO) declared COVID-19 a pandemic. It has infected 769,806,130 patients globally, causing 6,955,497 deaths as of August 16, 2023.[17] Before the production and

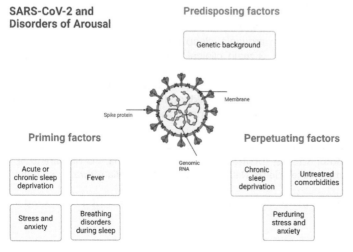

SARS-CoV-2 and Disorders of Arousal

Predisposing factors

Genetic background

Membrane

Spike protein

Genomic RNA

Priming factors

| Acute or chronic sleep deprivation | Fever |

| Stress and anxiety | Breathing disorders during sleep |

Perpetuating factors

| Chronic sleep deprivation | Untreatred comorbidities |

| Perduring stress and anxiety |

Fig. 1. Disorders of Arousal in SARS-CoV-2 infection.

marketing of vaccines, the only measures to manage the spread of the virus were social distancing, wearing masks, frequent hand hygiene, and quarantines. After the first vaccine was approved by the Food and Drug Administration and European Medicines Agency in December 2020, a proportion of 13,499,865,692 SARS-CoV-2 vaccine doses have been administered as of August 20, 2023.[17] In the meantime, a high number of variants appeared and, even though at the time of this writing COVID-19 is not a public health emergency of international concern anymore, it is still a dangerous infectious disease, especially for frail patients. During the COVID-19 pandemic, and particularly during spring 2020, most countries worldwide imposed restrictions on the free circulation of people to contrast SARS-CoV2 spreading, including lockdown and quarantine. "Lockdown" is a state or period in which movement within or access to an area is restricted in the interests of public safety or health. "Quarantine", instead, is a specific period of time in which a person positive to COVID-19, or that may have had contact with a positive one, must stay or be kept away from others in order to prevent the spread of the disease. In the following 2 years, restrictions have been imposed in countries or regions where virus spreading was more aggressive, while other countries chose various options on how to face the health emergency (**Box 1**).

DISCUSSION
Impact of Coronavirus Disease-2019 Pandemic on Sleep

Both directly (through the infection itself) and indirectly (through the changes in daily routine and the psychological impact during lockdown and quarantines), COVID-19 had a massive impact on sleep. A meta-analysis of 250 studies comprising about half-million participants revealed that during the COVID-19 pandemic the pooled estimated prevalence of sleep disturbances (including poor sleep quality and insomnia) was 40%.[18] Patients infected with COVID-19 appeared the most affected by sleep disturbances, but also other populations, particularly children and healthcare workers (HWs), experienced sleep disturbances independently of viral infection, due to the exceptional living conditions imposed during lockdown and quarantine. Sleep dysfunction due to COVID-19 pandemic is a multi-faceted condition, including insomnia, disrupted sleep continuity, changes in sleep-wake cycle, and decreased sleep quality: the colloquial terms "coronasomnia" or "COVID-somnia" have been proposed to encompass all these symptoms.[19] The COVID-19 outbreak has been considered one of the most

---

Box 1
Clinical vignette

A 35 y.o. woman with positive family history for Disorders of Arousals (brother and mother) affected by sleepwalking and confusional arousals since she was 8 y.o., experienced COVID-19 infection in May 2021. During her first episode of sleepwalking the patient left her bed and ran in her house rising the shutters and getting injured. After that she experienced only two or three episodes of sleepwalking until she was 35 y.o. Since the adolescence the patient reported 6 to 7 confusional arousals per year, appearing especially related to social alcohol assumption and sleep deprivation.

In the beginning of May 2021, the patient presented symptoms related to an upper respiratory infection: firstly, cough and sore throat; then, after 2 days, fever up to 38°C and mild headache. At that time, she lived with her partner, both resulted positive to COVID-19 antigenic test and, as indicated by Italian normative, began the quarantine. She threated her symptoms with Paracetamole and after 4 days she was completely asymptomatic, while only after 14 days she had a negative COVID-19 test. During the first week of quarantine, she experienced confusional arousals once or twice per night, witnessed by her partner as she could open her eyes, look around confusedly, even manipulate objects near the bed. After COVID-19 symptoms remission, she gradually decreased the number of confusional arousals, up to one per month. We gave her general advice, such as to protect the room where she slept, in order to avoid possible traumatism, to maintain regular sleep patterns and an adequate number of hours of sleep per night, to avoid factors that can trigger the episodes (alcohol intake before going to bed, sleep deprivation, sleeping in a noisy/bright room).

---

stressful periods of recent years, due to its wide impact on economics, healthcare, sociality, and everyday routine worldwide. The brain adapts to orchestrate an anticipatory "stress response" to threats, in order to keep the "internal milieu" stable: this active process of adaptation has been named "allostasis". The repeated activation of allostatic mechanisms leads to a chronically elevated and dysregulated brain activity named "allostatic load".[20] The occurrence of repeated challenges, failure to adjust to these repeated challenges, failure to shut off the response after the challenge is ceased, and failure to mount an adequate response are 4 conditions that lead to allostatic load.[21] The pandemic impact and prolonged duration are an example of allostatic load, which may lead to COVID-19 effects over time. Allostatic load and sleep may be closely related; when sleep dysregulation is present, stress reactivity is increased, and, on the other hand, stressors lead to sleep problems due to, for example, dysregulation of the hypothalamic-pituitary-adrenal axis.[22] Thus, this vicious cycle may increase an individual's vulnerability to the detrimental effects of stress, with a significant impact on health and quality of life.[23] During the pandemic, HWs were a population particularly affected by pandemic-related sleep dysfunction, because of the higher stress exposure than in the general population due to the higher potential for contracting the virus, being exposed to COVID-19 positive patients or, more in general, to a large volume of patients in addition to increased working shifts.[24] During the early stages of the COVID-19 outbreak the percentage of HWs with Pittsburg Sleep Quality Index of more than 5 (a higher score indicates a lower sleep quality) increased from 61.9% to 69.3%.[25] Insomnia was the most frequent reported symptom (23.6%–68.3%) and the incidence of comorbid moderate to severe sleep apnea in insomnia reached 38.5%, indicating a high comorbidity rate of sleep apnea and insomnia attributable to stress.[26,27] Depression and anxiety,[25] worries about the COVID-19 outbreak,[28] or being worried about being infected[29], and pre-existing psychological diseases or sleep medication[28] are the psychological factors associated with sleep disturbances in HWs. Other factors related to higher rate of sleep disturbances in HW were female sex,[30] age in the fifth decade (particularly 41–45 years),[31] carrying the burden of caring for the elderly or children[32] and being unmarried.[31] There are many possible factors that may explain this higher incidence of sleep disturbances in HW, including of course an increase in working hours.[31] Then, as previously reported, being a shift worker increased insomnia rate and the risk of COVID-19 infection.[32,33]

Among frontline HWs (FHW) who are engaged in the direct diagnosis, treatment, and care of COVID-19 patients, doctors experienced less sleep disturbances than nurses, as previously reported during the SARS outbreak, probably because nurses had more frequent shift works and more direct contacts with COVID-19 patients than doctors, although this may vary in different clinical settings.[34,35]

Acute and Chronic Effects of COVID-19 Infection on Sleep

In the past 2 years, many scientific works have shown a strong relationship between SARS-CoV2 infection and sleep disorders, especially in patients with more severe COVID-19 symptoms or even hospitalized and recently discharged patients, who can be adopted as a model of acute effect of COVID-19 on sleep.[24] In fact, both a new onset and worsening of previously reported sleep disorders (particularly insomnia and parasomnias) were experienced in COVID-19 patients. Up until now, the responsible mechanisms of this association are still unclear. However, different hypotheses have been suggested such as the interference with specific neuronal pathways, the activation of a neuroinflammation process, indirectly the use of medications, experiencing more stress and anxiety, or all of them in different combinations (**Fig. 2**). Adding further complexity to the issue, patients with pre-existing sleep disorders experienced slower recovery from the viral infection and worse outcomes from the disease, suggesting that the relationship between COVID-19 and sleep disorder might be bi-directional.[36] It is still unclear what degree of sleep dysfunction in patients hospitalized for COVID-19 is specific to the viral illness or to other hospital-related factors. In hospitalized COVID-19 patients, the prevalence of sleep disturbance ranges from 33.3% to 84.7% among different studies; in particular, insomnia, both terminal and initial, may be severe up to the necessity of pre-

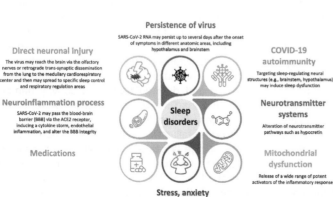

Persistence of virus
SARS-CoV-2 RNA may persist up to several days after the onset of symptoms in different anatomic areas, including hypothalamus and brainstem

Direct neuronal injury
The virus may reach the brain via the olfactory nerves or retrograde trans-synaptic dissemination from the lung to the medullary cardiorespiratory center and then may spread to specific sleep control and respiratory regulation areas

Neuroinflammation process
SARS-CoV-2 may pass the blood-brain barrier (BBB) via the ACE2 receptor, inducing a cytokine storm, endothelial inflammation, and alter the BBB integrity

Medications

Sleep disorders

COVID-19 autoimmunity
Targeting sleep-regulating neural structures (e.g., brainstem, hypothalamus) may induce sleep dysfunction

Neurotransmitter systems
Alteration of neurotransmitter pathways such as hypocretin

Mitochondrial dysfunction
Release of a wide range of potent activators of the inflammatory response

Stress, anxiety

Fig. 2. Different mechanisms for sleep disruption in Covid-19.

scribing drug treatments.[37] Sleep disturbances appeared immediately after admission in half of hospitalized COVID-19 patients, without any sex difference and, furthermore, the frequency of sleep symptoms doubled from day 2 to day 7,[38] indicating that they experienced maybe more that an acute psychological response to the disease. The prolonged hospitalization may have acted as a repeated challenge for the allostatic process of these patients, and this dysfunctional activation, that is, the allostatic load, may have worsened sleep disturbances. A more severe clinical course during COVID-19 infection was experienced by patients having concurrent sleep disturbances. Among patients with COVID-19 symptoms, the risk of severe infection was found to be 6-fold to 8-fold higher in the presence of decreased sleep status and reduced sleep hours in the week prior to the diagnosis.[39] A Chinese cohort of 165 patients showed poor sleepers had lower absolute lymphocyte count and increased neutrophil-to-lymphocyte ratio compared to good sleepers, and 12% of poor sleepers required intensive care unit care while none of the good sleepers did.[40] Sleep disturbances were 1 of the most common symptoms experienced also during post-COVID-19 conditions (ie, COVID-19 symptoms appearing or continuing after 3 months from the clinical onset of COVID-19 and lasting for at least 2 months), interestingly affecting 10% to 20% of COVID-19 patients, together with fatigue, shortness of breath, cognitive dysfunction, memory disturbances and muscle pain or spasm, according to WHO.[41,42] Different pathophysiological hypotheses have been proposed to explain the relationship between sleep disturbances and persisting COVID-19 infection, but there is still little evidence on the precise mechanism involving sleep disturbances (see **Fig. 2**). The persistence of the virus in hypothalamus and brainstem[43] may lead to a disruption of the sleep-wake cycle resulting in insomnia or poor quality of sleep[44]; other hypotheses include post-COVID-19 autoimmunity,[45] alterations of neurotransmitter systems[46], or mitochondrial dysfunction.[47] Finally, inflammation can modify sleep by increasing NREM sleep and decreasing REM sleep, and vice versa; sleep disturbances have been shown to lead to increased neuroinflammation and blood-brain barrier disruption.[48,49]

The Effects of Lockdown on Sleep: Focus on Parasomnias

Many studies explored the effects of lockdown and/or quarantine periods on sleep. In the early phase of the lockdown, the prevalence of difficulty initiating or maintaining sleep was reported at

around 24% and was associated with older age, sex female, reduction in income, having elderly dependents, alcohol use, depression, and higher rates of anxiety depressive symptoms and stress.[50,51] Investigating people who shifted to remote work during lockdown, which was labeled "smart working" in Italy, showed that although the percentage of subjects not reaching at least 7 hours of sleep per night in weekdays decreased from 61.01% to 35.01% in the smart-working group,[52] smart-working subjects experienced a delay in their chronotype. In particular, this effect was encountered in younger participants, due to the effect of electronic devices[53] and (imposed) free-running conditions on human sleep-wake cycle.[52] Interestingly, where some pre-pandemic good sleepers experienced worse sleep during the lockdown measures, some patients with pre-pandemic insomnia paradoxically experienced a meaningful improvement in sleep quality. This finding appeared related to the individual different emotional attitude toward the lockdown, which influenced the perceived sleep quality.[54]

Sleep disturbances during the pandemic were reported across all age ranges of younger children,[55] including infants,[56] toddlers[57], and school-age youth.[58] In a population of young children aged 6 months to 4 years,[59] the lockdown reduced the number and duration of naps and increased the length of nocturnal sleep, with no impact on the total duration of sleep over 24 hours; furthermore, children experienced more difficulties in initiating and maintaining sleep and an increased frequency of parasomnias. Similar results were shown among children aged 4 to 6 years,[60] when compared with pre-pandemic findings, they had later bedtimes and wake times, longer nocturnal but shorter nap duration. The use of screens with consequent exposure to bright light was associated with poorer mental health and greater perceived stress, as well as sleep disturbance.[61] In addition, in children's wake-sleep schedules, the reduction of outdoor and physical activity, and the increase of stress and anxiety are the main suggested reasons causing sleep disruption during the pandemic.[62,63] On the other hand, teens and young adults were reported sleeping more and having fewer sleep issues during the pandemic,[64] probably because of the online school schedule that let them wake up later in the morning, following the physiologic delay in sleep-wake circadian rhythmicity typical of adolescence.

Coronavirus Disease-2019 and Parasomnias

COVID-19 pandemic conditions might have had an impact on both REM and NREM parasomnias, even if there is little evidence in literature regarding

Table 1
Investigation parasomnias during COVID-19 pandemic

PARASOMNIAS During COVID-19	Investigated Presence	Frequency	Methods of Evaluation	Studied Population	Subjects (Number)
NREM					
Confusional Arousals	NO	-	-	-	-
Sleepwalking	YES	Increased	QUESTIONNAIRES	Healthy children/adolescents; Children with Autism Spectrum Disorder and Attention Deficit and Hyperactivity Disorder; Healthcare workers	4820
Sleep Terrors	YES	Increased	QUESTIONNAIRES		
Sleep Related Eating Disorders	NO	-	-	-	-
REM					
REM Sleep Behavior Disorder (RBD)	YES (REM sleep without atonia with no application of RBD diagnostic criteria)	Increased	VIDEO-POLYSOMNOGRAPHY	Patients with suspected sleep disorder after COVID-19 infection	11
Dream Enactment with no application of RBD diagnostic criteria	YES	Increased	QUESTIONNAIRES	General population	21.870
Recurrent Isolated Sleep Paralysis	NO	-	-	-	-
Nightmare Disorder (ND)	YES (Nightmares without ND diagnostic criteria)	Increased	QUESTIONNAIRES	Patients after COVID-19 infection; General population	2262
OTHER					
Exploiding Head Syndrome	NO	-	-	-	-
Sleep Related Hallucinations	YES	Increased	QUESTIONNAIRES	Narcolepsy type 1 patients	50
Sleep Enuresis	NO	-	-	-	-

this specific topic. The lack of scientific papers on parasomnias during the COVID-19 pandemic might be a consequence of the overall reduction of hospital or outpatient attendances for non-essential medical complaints during the pandemic, leading to fewer parasomnia diagnoses and lack of follow-up information. Data on parasomnias during the COVID-19 pandemic were mainly obtained by subjective questionnaires.

In a study on 544 COVID-19 patients during the pandemic,[65] nightmare frequency was significantly higher in the COVID-19 participants than in controls with a linear correlation between high COVID-19 disease severity and a higher number of reported nightmares. Moreover, having post-traumatic stress disorder (PTSD) and anxiety symptoms was associated with greater nightmare frequency. A cross-sectional web study on 19,355 participants[66] showed higher dream recall frequency during the pandemic than before. Female gender, younger age, nightmares, sleep talking, sleep maintenance problems, and symptoms of RBD and PTSD were associated with high dream recall frequency. A large-scale international online survey on 26,539 subjects[67] found that dream enactment behaviors (DEBs) were 2 to 4 times higher in the general population during the COVID-19 pandemic than in previous studies. DEBs were associated with male sex, smoking, alcohol consumption, olfactory impairment, depression and anxiety symptoms, OSA symptoms, and PTSD symptoms. DEBs are 1 core symptom of RBD, and this result may hint at a possible increase in the occurrence of isolated RBD in COVID-19 patients. However, DEBs may be linked to other sleep disorders, and these data need for confirmatory polysomnographic studies. In a study[68] on 11 patients with suspected sleep disorder after acute COVID-19, 4 patients (36%) presented REM sleep without atonia at video-polysomnography, while none of them had RBD complaint in their past clinical history.

One study on the impact of COVID-19 on sleep in adult HWs[33] showed a higher frequency of parasomnias including nightmares, sleepwalking, and sleep terrors, compared to non-HWs; being a shift worker was found as an independent risk factor for developing parasomnias. It is well known[8] how rotational shift workers have a higher risk of experiencing parasomnias due to circadian rhythm misalignment and sleep deprivation that may increase sleep pressure.

In pediatric patients with Autism Spectrum Disorder and Attention-deficit/Hyperactivity disorder, sleep and psychological disturbances were investigated with questionnaires during lockdown: difficulties in falling asleep, hypnic jerks, rhythmic movement disorder, night awakenings, restless sleep, sleepwalking, and daytime sleepiness were increased compared to pre-pandemic conditions (see **Fig. 1**).[69]

Management of Parasomnias During Coronavirus Disease-2019

One important point is to treat SARS-CoV2 infection following current guidelines, because the virus may trigger parasomnias due to its associated symptoms, such as fever or respiratory distress.

The general mainstays of parasomnia's treatment (both NREM and REM) remain valid also in patients with SARS-CoV2 infection. In particular for DoA it is necessary to recommend regular sleep-wake routine, quiet and dark bedroom environment, avoidance of sleep deprivation, or of excessive alcohol intake; for RBD, it is recommended to reduce the height of the bed, place a mattress on the floor adjacent to the bed, place pillows or other soft items between the patient and the headboard, and remove any bedside object or furniture that could cause injuries.[70–73]

Pharmacologic options for DoA are Clonazepam (0.5–2 mg at bedtime), low doses of antidepressants, and extended-release Melatonin (2-12 mg at bedtime).[74] Clonazepam is the first drug choice in patients with RBD, while extended-release Melatonin could be used in patients with associated sleep breathing disorders, neurodegenerative diseases, and elderly patients.[73,75] In Nightmare Disorder, Prazosin is recommended especially when nightmares are associated to PTSD.[76]

Non-pharmacological interventions include psychotherapy and Cognitive Behavioral Therapy (CBT).[76] A beneficial role of CBT in contrasting the lockdown-induced changes has been documented in a study on 12 patients attending a group CBT program for NREM parasomnias in the UK.[77] This program was specifically designed to target comorbid insomnia, anxiety, stress, and other psychological aspects, priming and precipitating factors.[76] Despite the negative psychosocial and lifestyle changes during lockdown, which could have a negative impact on sleep and affect parasomnia phenotypes, the 12-patient cohort remained overall clinically stable during follow-up.

SUMMARY

In this article, we discussed the impact of the COVID-19 pandemic on sleep disturbances and the limited available evidence on NREM and REM parasomnias (**Table 1**). This probably reflects the great difficulties in the activities of many sleep laboratories around the world created by the COVID-19 pandemic. Due to the impact of sleep disorders on quality of life and development of comorbidities, it is important to perform polysomnography studies to establish definitive diagnoses: appropriate precautions and safe protocols are needed to guarantee safety for both the patient and the staff.[78] In addition, telemedicine as well as home-made videos in the assessment of sleep disorders and particularly in parasomnias may offer useful alternatives to reduce hospital inflow and improve the clinical management of patients.[79–81]

CLINICS CARE POINTS

- Sleep disorders and COVID-19 may have a bidirectional pathophysiological relationship: both acute SARS-CoV2 infection and chronic "long-COVID" may trigger the occurrence of new-onset sleep disturbances while pre-existing sleep disorders may worsen the clinical course of the viral disease.

- Other aspects of the pandemic, such as lockdown for general population and quarantine for COVID-19 patients and contacts, may independently cause sleep disturbances, mainly due to the increase of stress and anxiety symptoms and the sudden changes in sleep-wake habits.

- During the COVID-19 pandemic, the most frequent reported sleep disorder was insomnia. Some authors described higher rates of NREM and REM parasomnias, often investigated only by means of questionnaires and with conflicting results in the literature.

- Healthcare workers are at particular risk of developing sleep disturbances and COVID-19 pandemic resulted in higher rates of insomnia and parasomnias in this population, due to increased stress and anxiety and increased load of work and shift working schedules. Recognizing this risk could markedly improve healthcare workers quality of life.

- The management of the patient with sleep disorder was a major challenge during the COVID-19 pandemic; however, performing PSG studies with adequate attention to hygiene and use of personal protective equipment, the growing diffusion of telemedicine and home-made infrared videos may overcome the issues of the current pandemic and may prove as useful tools for future challenges.

DISCLOSURES

The authors have nothing to disclose.

REFERENCES

1. American Academy of Sleep Medicine. International Classification of sleep disorders. 3rd edition. Darien (IL): American Academy of Sleep Medicine; 2023. text revision.
2. Sodré ME, Wießner I, Irfan M, Schenck CH, Mota-Rolim SA. Awake or sleeping? Maybe both. A review of sleep-related dissociative states. J Clin Med 2023;12(12):3876.
3. Stallman HM, Kohler M. Prevalence of sleepwalking: a systematic review and meta-analysis. PLoS One 2016;11(11):e0164769.
4. Petit D, Pennestri MH, Paquet J, et al. Childhood sleepwalking and sleep terrors: a longitudinal study of prevalence and familial aggregation. JAMA Pediatr 2015;169(7):653–8.
5. Pressman MR. Factors that predispose, prime and precipitate NREM parasomnias in adults: clinical and forensic implications. Sleep Medicine Rev 2007;11(1):5–33.
6. Mainieri G, Loddo G, Provini F. Disorders of arousal: a Chronobiological Perspective. Clocks and Sleep 2021;3(1):53–65.
7. Pilon M, Montplaisir J, Zadra A. Precipitating factors of somnambulism Impact of sleep deprivation and forced arousals. Neurology 2008;70(24):2284–90.
8. Bjorvatn B, Magerøy N, Moen BE, et al. Parasomnias are more frequent in shift workers than in day workers. Chronobiol Int 2015;32(10):1352–8.
9. Larsen CH, Dooley J, Gordon K. Fever-associated confusional arousal. Eur J Pediatr 2004;163(11):696–7.
10. Lopez R, Jaussent I, Dauvilliers Y. Pain in sleepwalking: a clinical Enigma. Sleep 2015;38(11):1693–8.
11. Juszczak GR, Swiergiel AH. Serotonergic hypothesis of sleepwalking. Med Hypotheses 2005;64(1):28–32.
12. Giuliano L, Fantuzzo D, Mainieri G, et al. Adult-onset sleepwalking secondary to Hyperthyroidism: Polygraphic evidence. J Clin Sleep Med 2018;14(2):285–7.
13. Eid B, Bou Saleh M, Melki I, et al. Evaluation of chronotype among children and associations with BMI, sleep, anxiety, and depression. Front Neurol 2020;11:416.
14. Tomoka T, Kazuhiko F, Sasaki Y, et al. Factors related to the occurrence of isolated sleep paralysis elicited during a multi-phasic sleep-wake schedule. Sleep 2002;25(1):89–96.
15. Pagel JF, Helfter P. Drug induced nightmares - an etiology based review. Hum Psychopharmacol 2003;18(1):59–67.

16. Stefani A, Trenkwalder C, Arnulf I, et al. Isolated rapid eye movement sleep behaviour disorder: clinical and research implications. J Neurol Neurosurg Psychiatry 2023;94(7):581–2.

17. WHO COVID-19 Dashboard. Geneva: World Health Organization, 2020. Available online: https://covid19.who.int/(last cited: 20 August 2023).

18. Jahrami HA, Alhaj OA, Humood AM, et al. Sleep disturbances during the COVID-19 pandemic: a systematic review, meta-analysis, and meta-regression. Sleep Med Rev 2022;62:101591.

19. Bhat S, Chokroverty S. Sleep disorders and COVID-19. Sleep Med 2022;91:253–61.

20. Cortelli P, Pierangeli G, Montagna P. Is migraine a disease? Neurol Sci 2010;31(Suppl 1):S29–31.

21. McEwen BS. Protective and damaging effects of stress mediators. N Engl J Med 1998;338(3):171–9.

22. van Dalfsen JH, Markus CR. The influence of sleep on human hypothalamic-pituitary-adrenal (HPA) axis reactivity: a systematic review. Sleep Med Rev 2018;39: 187–94.

23. Christensen DS, Zachariae R, Amidi A, et al. Sleep and allostatic load: a systematic review and meta-analysis. Sleep Med Rev 2022;64:101650.

24. Lin YN, Liu ZR, Li SQ, et al. Burden of sleep disturbance during COVID-19 pandemic: a systematic review. Nat Sci Sleep 2021;13:933–66.

25. Zhao X, Zhang T, Li B, et al. Job-related factors associated with changes in sleep quality among healthcare workers screening for 2019 novel coronavirus infection: a longitudinal study. Sleep Med 2020;75:21–6.

26. Zhou Y, Wang W, Sun Y, et al. The prevalence and risk factors of psychological disturbances of frontline medical staff in China under the COVID-19 epidemic: Workload should be concerned. J Affect Disord 2020;277:510–4.

27. Zhuo K, Gao C, Wang X, et al. Stress and sleep: a survey based on wearable sleep trackers among medical and nursing staff in Wuhan during the COVID-19 pandemic. Gen Psychiatr 2020;33(3): e100260.

28. Zhan Y, Liu Y, Liu H, et al. Factors associated with insomnia among Chinese front-line nurses fighting against COVID-19 in Wuhan: a cross-sectional survey. J Nurs Manag 2020;28(7):1525–35.

29. Zhang C, Yang L, Liu S, et al. Survey of insomnia and related social psychological factors among medical staff involved in the 2019 novel coronavirus disease outbreak. Front Psychiatry 2020;11:306.

30. Şahin MK, Aker S, Şahin G, et al. Prevalence of depression, anxiety, distress and insomnia and related factors in healthcare workers during COVID-19 pandemic in Turkey. J Community Health 2020;45(6):1168–77.

31. Jain A, Singariya G, Kamal M, et al. COVID-19 pandemic: psychological impact on anaesthesiologists. Indian J Anaesth 2020;64(9):774–83.

32. Wang W, Song W, Xia Z, et al. Sleep disturbance and psychological profiles of medical staff and non-medical staff during the early outbreak of COVID-19 in Hubei Province, China. Front Psychiatry 2020;11:733.

33. Herrero San Martin A, Parra Serrano J, Diaz Cambriles T, et al. Sleep characteristics in health workers exposed to the COVID-19 pandemic. Sleep Med 2020;75:388–94.

34. Lim RK, Wambier CG, Goren A. Are night shift workers at an increased risk for COVID-19? Med Hypotheses 2020;144:110147.

35. Phua DH, Tang HK, Tham KY. Coping responses of emergency physicians and nurses to the 2003 severe acute respiratory syndrome outbreak. Acad Emerg Med 2005;12(4):322–8.

36. Maas MB, Kim M, Malkani RG, et al. Obstructive sleep apnea and risk of COVID-19 infection, hospitalization and respiratory failure. Sleep Breath 2021;25(2):1155–7.

37. Yue L, Wang J, Ju M, et al. How psychiatrists coordinate treatment for COVID-19: a retrospective study and experience from China. Gen Psychiatr 2020; 33(4):e100272.

38. Liguori C, Pierantozzi M, Spanetta M, et al. Subjective neurological symptoms frequently occur in patients with SARS-CoV2 infection. Brain Behav Immun 2020;88:11–6.

39. Huang B, Niu Y, Zhao W, et al. Reduced sleep in the week prior to diagnosis of COVID-19 is associated with the severity of COVID-19. Nat Sci Sleep 2020; 12:999–1007.

40. Zhang J, Xu D, Xie B, et al. Poor-sleep is associated with slow recovery from lymphopenia and an increased need for ICU care in hospitalized patients with COVID-19: a retrospective cohort study. Brain Behav Immun 2020;88:50–8.

41. Soriano JB, Murthy S, Marshall JC, et al. WHO clinical case definition working group on post-COVID-19 condition. A clinical case definition of post COVID-19 condition by a Delphi consensus. Lancet Infect Dis 2022;22(4):e102–7.

42. Davis HE, Assaf GS, McCorkell L, et al. Characterizing long COVID in an international cohort: 7 months of symptoms and their impact. EClinicalMedicine 2021;38:101019.

43. Stein SR, Ramelli SC, Grazioli A, et al. SARS-CoV-2 infection and persistence in the human body and brain at autopsy. Nature 2022;612(7941):758–63.

44. Gupta R, Pandi-Perumal SR. SARS-CoV-2 infection: paving way for sleep disorders in long term. Sleep Vigil 2021;5(1):1–2.

45. Rojas M, Rodríguez Y, Acosta-Ampudia Y, et al. Autoimmunity is a hallmark of post-COVID syndrome. J Transl Med 2022;20(1):129.

46. Iranzo A. Sleep and neurological autoimmune diseases. Neuropsychopharmacology 2020;45(1): 129–40.

47. de Boer E, Petrache I, Goldstein NM, et al. Decreased fatty acid oxidation and altered lactate production during exercise in patients with post-acute COVID-19 syndrome. Am J Respir Crit Care Med 2022;205(1):126–9.

48. Schultheiß C, Willscher E, Paschold L, et al. The IL-1β, IL-6, and TNF cytokine triad is associated with post-acute sequelae of COVID-19. Cell Rep Med 2022;3(6):100663.

49. Semyachkina-Glushkovskaya O, Mamedova A, Vinnik V, et al. Brain mechanisms of COVID-19-sleep disorders. Int J Mol Sci 2021;22(13):6917.

50. Dal Santo F, Gonzàlez-Blanco L, Rodrìguez-Revuelta J, et al. Early impact of the COVID-19 outbreak on sleep in a large Spanish sample. Behav Sleep Med 2022;20(3):100–15.

51. Marelli S, Castelnuovo A, Somma A, et al. Impact of COVID-19 lockdown on sleep quality in university students and administration staff. J Neurol 2021;268(1):8–15.

52. Leone MJ, Sigman M, Golombek DA. Effects of lockdown on human sleep and chronotype during the COVID-19 pandemic. Curr Biol 2020;30(16):R930–1.

53. Bhat S, Pinto-Zipp G, Upadhyay H, et al. "To sleep, perchance to tweet": in-bed electronic social media use and its associations with insomnia, daytime sleepiness, mood, and sleep duration in adults. Sleep Health 2018;4(2):166–73.

54. Kocevska D, Blanken TF, Van Someren EJW, et al. Sleep quality during the COVID-19 pandemic: not one size fits all. Sleep Med 2020;76:86–8.

55. Bacaro V, Chiabudini M, Buonanno C, et al. Sleep characteristics in Italian children during home confinement due to COVID-19 outbreak. Clin Neuropsychiatry 2021;18(1):13–27.

56. Kahn M, Barnett N, Glazer A, et al. Infant sleep during COVID-19: longitudinal analysis of infants of US mothers in home confinement versus working as usual. Sleep Health 2021;7(1):19–23.

57. Markovic A, Mühlematter C, Beaugrand M, et al. Severe effects of the COVID-19 confinement on young children's sleep: a longitudinal study identifying risk and protective factors. J Sleep Res 2021;30(5):e13314.

58. Cellini N, Di Giorgio E, Mioni G, et al. Sleep and psychological difficulties in Italian school-age children during COVID-19 lockdown. J Pediatr Psychol 2021;46(2):153–67.

59. Lecuelle F, Leslie W, Huguelet S, et al. Did the COVID-19 lockdown really have no impact on young children's sleep? J Clin Sleep Med 2020;16(12):2021.

60. Liu Z, Tang H, Jin Q, et al. Sleep of preschoolers during the coronavirus disease 2019 (COVID-19) outbreak. J Sleep Res 2021;30(1):e13142.

61. Nagata JM, Abdel Magid HS, Pettee Gabriel K. Screen time for children and adolescents during the coronavirus disease 2019 pandemic. Obesity 2020;28(9):1582–3.

62. Okely AD, Kariippanon KE, Guan H, et al. Global effect of COVID-19 pandemic on physical activity, sedentary behaviour and sleep among 3- to 5-year-old children: a longitudinal study of 14 countries. BMC Publ Health 2021;21(1):940.

63. El Refay AS, Hashem SA, Mostafa HH, et al. Sleep quality and anxiety symptoms in Egyptian children and adolescents during COVID-19 pandemic lockdown. Bull Natl Res Cent 2021;45(1):134.

64. Bruni O, Malorgio E, Doria M, et al. Changes in sleep patterns and disturbances in children and adolescents in Italy during the Covid-19 outbreak. Sleep Med 2022;91:166–74.

65. Scarpelli S, Nadorff MR, Bjorvatn B, et al. Nightmares in people with COVID-19: did coronavirus infect our dreams? Nat Sci Sleep 2022;14:93–108.

66. Fränkl E, Scarpelli S, Nadorff MR, et al. How our dreams changed during the COVID-19 pandemic: effects and correlates of dream recall frequency - a multinational study on 19,355 adults. Nat Sci Sleep 2021;13:1573–91.

67. Liu Y, Partinen E, Chan NY, et al. Dream-enactment behaviours during the COVID-19 pandemic: an international COVID-19 sleep study. J Sleep Res 2023;32(1):e13613.

68. Heidbreder A, Sonnweber T, Stefani A, et al. Video-polysomnographic findings after acute COVID-19: REM sleep without atonia as sign of CNS pathology? Sleep Med 2021;80:92–5.

69. Bruni O, Breda M, Ferri R, et al. Changes in sleep patterns and disorders in children and adolescents with attention deficit hyperactivity disorders and autism spectrum disorders during the covid-19 lockdown. Brain Sci 2021;11(9):1139.

70. Siclari F, Khatami R, Urbaniok F, et al. Violence in sleep. Brain 2010;133(Pt 12):3494–509.

71. Drakatos P, Marples L, Muza R, et al. NREM parasomnias: a treatment approach based upon a retrospective case series of 512 patients. Sleep Med 2019;53:181–8 [published correction appears in Sleep Med. 2020 Jan;65:186].

72. Attarian H. Treatment options for parasomnias. Neurol Clin 2010;28(4):1089–106.

73. Dauvilliers Y, Schenck CH, Postuma RB, et al. REM sleep behaviour disorder. Nat Rev Dis Primers 2018;4(1):19.

74. Proserpio P, Terzaghi M, Manni R, et al. Drugs used in parasomnia. Sleep Med Clin 2022;17(3):367–78.

75. Howell M, Avidan AY, Foldvary-Schaefer N, et al. Management of REM sleep behavior disorder: an American Academy of Sleep Medicine systematic review, meta-analysis, and GRADE assessment. J Clin Sleep Med 2023;19(4):769–810.

76. Aurora RN, Zak RS, Auerbach SH, et al. Best practice guide for the treatment of nightmare disorder in adults. J Clin Sleep Med 2010;6(4):389–401.

77. O'Regan D, Nesbitt A, Biabani N, et al. A novel group cognitive behavioral therapy approach to adult non-rapid eye movement parasomnias. Front Psychiatry 2021;12:679272.

78. Laroche M, Biabani N, Drakatos P, et al. Group cognitive behavioural therapy for non-rapid eye movement parasomnias: long-term outcomes and impact of COVID-19 lockdown. Brain Sci 2023; 13(2):347.

79. Cilea R, Guaraldi P, Barletta G, et al. Performing sleep studies after the COVID-19 outbreak: practical suggestions from Bologna's sleep unit. Sleep Med 2021;77:45–50.

80. Shamim-Uzzaman QA, Bae CJ, Ehsan Z, et al. The use of telemedicine for the diagnosis and treatment of sleep disorders: an American Academy of Sleep Medicine update. J Clin Sleep Med 2021;17(5): 1103–7.

81. Lopez R, Barateau L, Chenini S, et al. Home nocturnal infrared video to record non-rapid eye movement sleep parasomnias. J Sleep Res 2023; 32(2):e13732.

Forensic Implications of the Parasomnias

Brian Holoyda, MD, MPH, MBA[a,b,c,d,]*

KEYWORDS

- Parasomnia • Sexsomnia • Sleep-related violence • Sexual behavior in sleep • Paraphilias
- Paraphilic disorders • Malingering

KEY POINTS

- Sleep-related violence (SRV) and sexual behavior in sleep (SBS) can occur in various sleep disorders, including confusional arousal, non-rapid eye movement parasomnias, rapid eye movement behavior disorder, and nocturnal frontal epilepsy.
- SRV and SBS can result in injury, sexual assault, or death of bed partners or other individuals, resulting in criminal charges and request for forensic assessment.
- Forensic experts evaluating alleged SRV and SBS may be asked to clarify a defendant's diagnosis and assess his or her criminal responsibility and risk of violence.

INTRODUCTION

Parasomnias are undesirable physical events or experiences that occur at the onset of sleep, during sleep, or on arousal from sleep. Non-rapid eye movement (NREM) parasomnias are often benign, whereas rapid eye movement (REM) parasomnias are usually more aggressive because the individual reacts to distressing dream imagery. NREM and REM parasomnias, along with rare conditions such as nocturnal frontal lobe epilepsy, have been implicated in interpersonal aggression toward bed partners or others, also known as sleep-related violence (SRV). Increasingly, parasomnias are also recognized as a cause of sexual behavior in sleep (SBS). Due to adverse outcomes to bed partners and others including injury, sexual abuse, and death, individuals who engage in SRV or SBS may be charged with violating criminal statutes. In such cases, the defendant's attorney or the court may request an expert assessment to clarify an individual's diagnosis. Relevant forensic questions may include the effect of the defendant's alleged parasomnia on criminal responsibility, the risk of future SRV or SBS, and the risk of future physical and sexual violence when awake. This article reviews the available literature on SRV and SBS, identifies forensic issues relevant to the diagnosis of a parasomnia in the forensic context, and delineates additional considerations related to criminal responsibility and violence risk assessment that expert evaluators assessing alleged SRV and SBS may face.

OVERVIEW OF SLEEP-RELATED VIOLENCE AND SEXUAL BEHAVIOR IN SLEEP

SRV may occur in the context of NREM parasomnias, REM parasomnias, and nocturnal seizures and includes acts of aggression toward oneself, one's bed partner, other people, animals, and inanimate objects.[1] NREM parasomnias are often benign and include sleepwalking, confusional arousals, and night terrors but they may sometimes result in physical aggression, including striking, kicking, pulling hair, or use of a weapon. Individuals with NREM parasomnias may be unresponsive and difficult to arouse or become combative with attempts to interact with or restrain them. They typically do not remember their actions

a Contra Costa County Detention Health Services, Martinez, CA, USA; b Department of Psychiatry and Behavioral Medicine; c Martinez Detention Facility, 1000 Ward Street, Martinez, CA 94553, USA; d Forensic Psychiatrist, Denver, CO, USA
* Martinez Detention Facility, 1000 Ward Street, Martinez, CA 94553.
E-mail address: holoyda@gmail.com

Sleep Med Clin 19 (2024) 189–198
https://doi.org/10.1016/j.jsmc.2023.10.010
1556-407X/24/© 2023 Elsevier Inc. All rights reserved.

following the parasomnia episode.[2] Patients with REM behavior disorder (RBD), however, present with dream enactment behaviors resulting from violent or frightening dreams including kicking, punching, running, and yelling. RBD is most often encountered in older men without a history of violence and often serves as a prognostic indicator of alpha-synucleinopathies. REM parasomnias are more common in the second half of the night and individuals typically remember their dream content when awakened from the episode.[3] Finally, SRV may occur in seizure disorders, such as sleep-related epilepsy. Individuals with such conditions may exhibit brief, vigorous, or ballistic behaviors such as screaming, flipping over, or thrashing of limbs, although movements are nondirected and lack a purposeful appearance.[4]

The first epidemiologic survey of SRV, conducted in the United Kingdom, found that approximately 2.1% of a sample between the ages of 15 and 100 years reported currently engaging in SRV. Those who reported SRV were more likely to experience sleep talking, bruxism, hypnic jerks, and hypnagogic hallucinations and to have substance use and mental health problems.[5] The next epidemiologic study of SRV included nearly 20,000 subjects interviewed from 6 European countries, of whom 1.6% reported current SRV.[6] The prevalence of SRV did not differ between men and women except in the United Kingdom, where more men than women reported SRV. Subjects aged 34 years or younger had a higher prevalence of SRV. SRV varied in frequency, with more than half of respondents reporting SRV 1 night per month, a quarter reporting SRV several nights per week, and the remainder reporting SRV at an intermediate frequency. Notably, three-quarters of subjects indicated that they experienced vivid dreams at the time of the SRV, including dreams of being attacked by a person or animal or attempting to protect a loved one from harm, whereas only 10% noted no dreaming associated with SRV. Such a description suggests that REM parasomnias are more common than NREM parasomnias because most patients with NREM parasomnias do not recall associated dream imagery. Additional symptoms of parasomnias were more common in the SRV group, with 72.8% reporting at least 1 symptom compared with 34.3% in the non-SRV group. Hypnagogic hallucinations were the most reported symptom (55.0% vs 24.6%) but SRV subjects were 9 times more likely to endorse sleepwalking and sleep terrors than non-SRV subjects. Nearly one-third (31.4%) of SRV subjects indicated they had hurt themselves or someone else during SRV regardless of frequency with injuries including bruises (42.9%), nose bleeds (25.5%), fractures

(21.6%), abrasions (15.7%), pulled hair (23.5%), and head contusions (13.7%).

There are various aspects of an individual's history that may support a finding of SRV. SRV due to an NREM parasomnia typically occurs during the first third or half of the sleep period during which there is a greater proportion of NREM sleep. Individuals reporting SRV are significantly more likely to have family members with SRV, sleep terrors, and sleepwalking. Mood disorders and physical illness are also significantly associated with SRV.[6] Early research suggested that factors such as psychological distress and substance abuse are more common in individuals with SRV,[5,7] whereas Ohayon and Schenk's large-scale epidemiologic survey did not find stress or tobacco, alcohol, caffeine, illicit drug, or psychotropic medication use to be significantly related to SRV.[6] Individuals with SRV tend to report difficulty initiating sleep and breathing pauses during sleep but sleep–wake schedules and sleep duration that are similar to those without SRV.

There is much less known about SBS. In 1997, Fedoroff and colleagues first described parasomnia-related sexual behavior in a case series evaluating the motivations of men who sexually assaulted sleeping victims.[8] Shapiro and colleagues later coined the term "sexsomnia,"[9] which entered the lexica of the Diagnostic and Statistical Manual of Mental Disorders, Fifth Edition (DSM-5) in 2013[10] and the International Classification of Sleep Disorders, Third Edition (ICSD-3) in 2014.[11] SBS includes sexual acts that one may perform during wakefulness, such as masturbation, sexual vocalizations, fondling, and anal, oral, or vaginal penetration, as well as spontaneous orgasm.[12] Schenck reports that the 2 most common causes of SBS in clinical populations are NREM parasomnias, including confusional arousals and sleepwalking, and obstructive sleep apnea.[13] He also identifies nocturnal seizures and treatment with pramipexole in Parkinson's disease and selective serotonin reuptake inhibitors (SSRIs) as potential causes. Although documented cases of SBS are relatively sparse compared to SRV, it is potentially more common than SRV. In a cross-sectional analysis of 1000 adult Norwegians, Bjorvatn and colleagues found a lifetime and current prevalence of SBS of 7.1% and 2.7%, respectively.[14] In contrast, lifetime and current prevalence of SRV causing self-injury were 4.3% and 2.7%, respectively, and lifetime and current prevalence of SRV causing injury to others were 3.85% and 0.4%, respectively.

Sexsomnia has been linked to priming factors such as alcohol and other drug use, psychotropic medication, sleep deprivation, circadian rhythm disruption, fatigue, psychological stress, and other sleep disorders including obstructive sleep apnea, periodic limb movements, restless legs syndrome, and bruxism.[15–17] Most individuals with sexsomnia have a history of prior or current nonsexual NREM parasomnia. Most individuals have a history of or currently experience sleepwalking, sleep talking, or sleep terrors. Only 11.1% to 35.3% of subjects in research studies report no prior or current nonsexual NREM parasomnias.[18,19] Similar to other NREM parasomnias, most instances of sexsomnia occur during the initial third of the night. Bed partners report that individuals who engage in SBS tend to be more direct and aggressive and less focused on the partner. They note that SBS may include sexual activities that are atypical for the individual[19] and that the episodes are often brief, abruptly initiated, and short, lasting less than 30 minutes.[12] Consistent with other NREM parasomnias, most people report complete amnesia for sexsomnia,[13] whereas a minority demonstrate patchy or full recall, particularly if the bed partner initiated the sexual activity.[19] Individuals do not often attempt to conceal their actions and are typically upset when they become aware of them.[12]

The relationship of alcohol ingestion to the priming of NREM parasomnias is a topic of considerable academic debate.[20–22] In a survey of 39 patients with slow wave sleep disorders, 11 of 12 of those endorsing regular alcohol consumption reported that alcohol intake increased their parasomnia behaviors.[23] Alternatively, Pressman describes how the neurophysiology of alcohol's γ-aminobutyric acid type A (GABA-A) inhibitory activity opposes the known decrease in GABA-A inhibition observed in sleepwalking.[24] Alcohol intoxication can disrupt sleep architecture and alcoholic blackouts can mimic parasomnia behaviors, making it crucial to properly assess subjects' alcohol intake. Due to the lack of validated scientific evidence, the recently published *International Classification of Sleep Disorders, Third Edition, Text Revision* (ICSD-3-TR)[25] no longer lists alcohol as a trigger for sleepwalking. The ICSD-3-TR states that parasomnias should not be entertained or diagnosed in the setting of acute alcohol intoxication or when the observed behavior is better explained by alcohol intoxication or illicit drug use.

SLEEP-RELATED VIOLENCE AND SEXUAL BEHAVIOR IN SLEEP IN COURT

SRV and SBS can lead to physical injury, sexual abuse, and death. It is not surprising, then, that individuals who engage in SRV and SBS may face legal consequences for their behavior. In 2014, Ingravallo and colleagues published the first systematic review of medico-legal cases stemming from SRV and SBS.[1] The authors identified 9 cases of SRV and 9 cases of SBS published between the years 1985 and 2011. All 9 of the SRV cases stemmed from a single sleep-related incident. The 9 defendants were all males between the ages of 14 to 42 years. Four of them reported ongoing sleep disturbance, 4 reported a history of parasomnias, and 3 reported a history of SRV. Behaviors were varied and included stabbing one's cousin to death; shooting one's wife; driving 23 km to the house of a wife's parents and beating and stabbing a mother-in-law to death; strangling one's wife while dreaming about being chased by armed Japanese soldiers; and throwing one's son out of a third-floor window. There were 10 victims, 6 of whom were female and 7 of whom were adults. Five defendants faced a charge of murder, 3 faced a charge of attempted murder, and 1 faced charges of both murder and attempted murder. Six defendants put forth defenses of sleepwalking; of these, 2 were acquitted, 2 were convicted, and 2 had their cases dropped or deserted. Other diagnoses included night terrors in 2 defendants who were acquitted and obstructive sleep apnea in 1 defendant who was convicted. Defendants received evaluations of varying depth with components including psychiatric evaluation, neurologic evaluation, electroencephalogram (EEG), head computed tomography (CT), and video-polysomnography (v-PSG).

In Ingravallo and colleagues' review of 9 medico-legal cases of SBS, all but 1 stemmed from a single incident.[1] As in the cases of SRV described above, all defendants were males. The range of ages was similar to the cases of SRV, as well. Six defendants had a clinical history of sleepwalking, sleepwalking with other parasomnias, or snoring. The reported behaviors included drinking a beer while naked in a major urban thoroughfare; fondling breasts; digital penetration of a vagina; and oral, anal, and vaginal penetration of a woman sleeping in a room separate from that of the defendant. Aside from the case involving a man walking nude on a road, all cases had a single female victim. Charges were varied and included sexual assault, sexual battery, rape, sexual misconduct, repeated sexual fondling, and indecent exposure. Five defendants put forth defenses of sleepwalking and 1 a defense of sexsomnia, whereas 3 defendants did not have an explicit defense. Experts diagnosed sleepwalking in 3 cases, NREM parasomnia in 3 cases, nocturnal complex seizure in 1 case, "parasomnic behavior" in 1 case, and parasomnia overlap disorder involving sleepwalking, SBS, and REM sleep behavior disorder in 1 case. Eight of 9 defendants received an acquittal, whereas the outcome of 1 defendant's case was unknown. Forensic evaluations ranged in depth as in the SRV cases.

In 2015, Organ and Fedoroff published an analysis of 10 cases of sexsomnia from Canada occurring between 1966 and 2013.[26] Similar to Ingravallo and colleagues' systematic review,[1] all defendants were males and had female victims. Only 4 subjects had known prior parasomnias. The authors noted that alcohol was a "priming factor" in 8 of the 10 cases. Four defendants received outright acquittals, whereas 4 were found guilty due to "lack of supporting evidence." In 1 case, a defendant was found not criminally responsible on account of a mental disorder before receiving an absolute discharge from a government psychiatric facility. The outcome of 1 case was pending at the time of publication.

In 1 final case series of SBS, Mohebbi and colleagues reviewed 8 American cases from 2004 to 2012 in which a defendant presented a sleep disorder as a defense for repeated sexually inappropriate behavior.[27] Consistent with the previously described case series, all 8 defendants were males. In contrast, however, all cases involved minor female victims, except 1 case that involved 2 minor male victims. All victims knew the defendant. Most defense experts diagnosed the defendant with an NREM parasomnia such as sleepwalking, sleep terrors, and sexsomnia. Despite this, the defendant was found guilty in 7 of 8 cases; in the remaining case, an appellate court reversed and remanded the verdict of guilt due to the exclusion of an expert's testimony on sexsomnia.

The published medico-legal case series of SRV and SBS are limited in scope and do not account for all cases in which SRV and SBS have been presented in court. Regardless, differences in the outcomes of the cases suggest potential trends in how legal decision-makers view these phenomena. For example, it is notable that all defendants received an acquittal in the cases of SBS reviewed by Ingravallo and colleagues,[1] whereas there were no known acquittals in the series presented by Mohebbi and colleagues.[27] It is possible that the legal decision-makers in cases involving recurrent sexual abuse of children are less likely to find in favor of a defendant, regardless of the amount and quality of supporting evidence that the individual has a parasomnia. Also notable is the variation in the degree of interpersonal aggression involved in cases of SRV and SBS. All the cases of SRV presented by Ingravallo and colleagues[1] involved charges of homicide or attempted homicide, rather than less-violent behaviors such as striking, kicking, or hair-pulling. In contrast, cases of SBS included behaviors ranging from standing naked in public to repeated sexual assault, consistent with the variability in sexually inappropriate behavior.

THE FORENSIC EVALUATION OF PARASOMNIAS

With the growing recognition of SRV and SBS and sexsomnia's recent inclusion in the DSM and ICSD, there has been an increasing interest in the forensic evaluation of parasomnias. Some authors have attempted to delineate some guidelines for the evaluation of alleged parasomnias in the forensic context,[1,28,29] although there is no clear consensus on what constitutes an adequate assessment. In fact, some experts opine that the evidence base of SRV and SBS is too limited to support the proposal for international guidelines on the forensic evaluation of SRV and SBS and instead recommend the prioritization of further research into sleep behaviors.[30] This is a legitimate concern; however, defendants and their attorneys may increasingly view a defense of SRV and SBS as worthy of consideration, prompting forensic evaluation and the production of expert opinion. Experts asked to evaluate such claims would therefore benefit from some evidence-based recommendations to assist in conducting such assessments.

Research on Forensic Referrals for Sleep-Related Violence and Sexual Behavior in Sleep

In 2019, Bornemann and colleagues published a review of 351 referrals to a forensic sleep medicine center during 11 years.[31] Of those, only 110 (31%) were found to be "possibly sleep-related" and accepted for rendering an opinion by a forensic sleep medicine expert. The 241 other cases were rejected because they were believed to be related to a medical condition, a psychiatric condition, alcohol intoxication, or illicit drug use. The most common referrals related to sexual assault (n = 52), murder (n = 18), and driving under the influence of drug or alcohol (n = 7). Seventy-seven cases involved a parasomnia, including 46 sexsomnia cases. In cases of parasomnia, most perpetrators were men (n = 69, 90%) and most victims were women (n = 62, 81%). In the 46 cases of sexsomnia, all perpetrators were men and most victims were women (n = 43, 93%). Other causes for SRV and SBS included zolpidem side effects (n = 17), sleep deprivation (n = 7), obstructive sleep apnea (n = 6), and insomnia (n = 2). Notably, the authors did not report any cases of malingering or feigned parasomnia in their review.

Diagnostic Considerations

One of the primary tasks of a forensic evaluator in cases of SRV and SBS is to determine if the individual suffers from a parasomnia or other sleep disorder. As the diagnosis of RBD and nocturnal seizure disorders is more straightforward and less forensically fraught than the diagnosis of NREM parasomnias, this section will focus on NREM parasomnias. **Table 1** summarizes relevant elements of the forensic evaluation of SRV and SBS. An in-depth clinical history is necessary and includes a sleep history, psychiatric history, neurologic history, substance use history, family history of sleep disorders, sexual history, and violence history. Descriptions of the SRV events should be consistent with common clinical findings of NREM parasomnias (see Text **Box 1**). Sleep comorbidities, shift work, psychological stress, fatigue, and psychotropic medication use are also relevant areas of inquiry. It is necessary to obtain collateral information from victims, current or prior bed partners, or family members who may be aware of a history of behaviors consistent with a parasomnia.[28] **Table 2** summarizes findings that suggest an explanation other than an NREM parasomnia for SRV.

The value of v-PSG in forensic evaluations of SRV and SBS is debatable for multiple reasons.

Video-polysomnography may not capture an episode of NREM parasomnia-related behaviors,[18] which is particularly true in studies of SBS.[19] In fact, there have been few reported cases of SBS occurring in the laboratory setting at all.[32] A failure to identify evidence of an NREM parasomnia in v-PSG, therefore, does not rule out the possibility that an individual has one. However, v-PSG may provide evidence of other sleep disorders that could trigger or contribute to episodes of SRV or SBS, such as sleep apnea, periodic limb movements, among others. From a legal perspective, however, there may be little utility in obtaining v-PSG. Even if an individual demonstrates evidence of an NREM parasomnia in the laboratory, such a finding does not mean that he or she was asleep at the time of the alleged offense.[33] Experts have noted that, "there is absolutely no after-the-fact polysomnography finding that could possibly have any relevance as to whether the accused was sleepwalking at the time of the event in question."[34] Expert evaluators should therefore consider the potential evidentiary benefit of v-PSG when deciding whether to obtain one in the forensic context.

Table 1
Components of the forensic evaluation of alleged sleep-related violence and sexual behavior in sleep

Component of Evaluation	Factors to Consider
Sleep history	• Description of alleged parasomnia-related behaviors based on collateral data from bed partner/family member observer. • Childhood history of an NREM parasomnia • Previous known history of parasomnias, SRV, and SBS • History of other comorbid sleep disorders (untreated obstructive sleep apnea, insomnia, circadian rhythm disorders, periodic limb movements, and so forth) • Identification of potential parasomnia triggers, including fatigue, and illicit substance use, psychotropic medication use, shift work, and cross-time zone travel
Other relevant history	• Psychiatric history (including treatment with psychotropic serotonergic medications) • Substance use history • Neurologic history • Family history of sleep disorders • Sexual history (for cases of SBS) • Violence and legal history
Collateral information	• Collateral report of parasomnia-related behaviors (from family members or prior or current bed partners) • Relationship between victim and defendant, including a history of violence or abuse
Neurologic evaluations	• EEG • CT head or MRI brain (if concern for an organic lesion) • v-PSG (weigh the evidentiary benefit beforehand)
Psychophysiological evaluations (in cases of SBS)	• VRT assessment of sexual interests • PPG to assess sexual arousal disorder

<table>
<tr><td>

Box 1
Expected features of sleep-related violence due to non-rapid eye movement parasomnia

- A history of similar episodes
- Some interaction with the environment
- Usually brief duration
- Without apparent motivation
- Victim is someone who just happened to be present
- Horror or confusion on return of consciousness
- No efforts to escape, conceal the act, or evade responsibility
- Occurs at least 1 h after sleep onset or on awakening
- Not better explained by another mental disorder, medical condition, medication, or substance use

Adapted from Cramer-Bornemann, M. A., Mahowald, M. W. (2017). Sleep Forensics: Criminal Culpability for Sleep-Related Violence. In Kryger, M., Roth, T., Dement, W. C. (Eds.), Principles and Practice of Sleep Medicine, 6th Edition. Amsterdam, NE: Elsevier.

</td></tr>
</table>

Malingering

Because a parasomnia defense can lead to acquittal or a finding of not criminally responsible, defendants may increasingly attempt to feign a history of SRV or SBS to evade criminal responsibility for their acts. Apart from observing a defendant pretending to engage in violent or sexual behavior while undergoing v-PSG, there are no objective measures by which to identify malingered parasomnias. Forensic experts must rely on collateral information and clinical history to identify inconsistencies or other evidence of feigning in a defendant's narrative.[28] **Table 3** summarizes some potential indicators of feigned parasomnia. Efforts to hide evidence of one's alleged SRV or SBS are inconsistent with genuine

NREM parasomnias because most individuals lack awareness of their behaviors unless informed by others. Examples include threatening a victim, wearing a condom, and removing clothing or linens from the location of the act. Failing to take steps to avoid repeat acts of SRV and SBS after becoming aware of one's behavior is also concerning. One might expect a conscientious adult to seek out medical attention or otherwise prevent contact with potential victims after learning that he has perpetrated SRV or SBS. Rational preventive behaviors would include locking bedroom doors, storing potential weapons securely, and sleeping in separate rooms. This is likely one reason why all the defendants in Mohebbi and colleagues' case series[27] were convicted of sex offenses: repeated sexual abuse of children in the absence of efforts to reduce one's own risk suggests alternative motives for the behavior. Additional warning signs for feigned parasomnias include recall of the incident and new-onset SRV or SBS as the sole presenting parasomnia-related behavior.

Psychosexual Evaluation of Sexual Behavior in Sleep

In cases of alleged SBS, a forensic psychiatrist with expertise in psychosexual evaluation is crucial to identify the presence of atypical sexual interests, or paraphilias, or other psychological motivations that may play a role in sexual behavior.[28] A thorough psychosexual evaluation often includes a clinical interview, the review of collateral records, the interview of collateral informants, and objective testing of sexual interests and sexual arousal. In the clinical interview, the evaluator will obtain a detailed sexual history assessing childhood exposure to sexual stimuli and activity, pornography exposure and use, masturbatory practices, sexual acts with others, and a review of potential paraphilic fantasies and interests. Perhaps not surprisingly, individuals undergoing evaluation following SBS who wish to present a sexsomnia defense may not be forthcoming about atypical or problematic sexual

Table 2
Findings indicative of sleep-related violence not due to non-rapid eye movement parasomnia

Finding	Potential Explanation for SRV
Alcohol intoxication before sleep	Alcohol-induced blackout; alcohol intoxication state
Illicit drug use before sleep	Other intoxication state
Zolpidem use before sleep	Zolpidem-induced parasomnia
Dream imagery recall	RBD
Efforts to conceal the act or evade responsibility	Malingering (**Table 3**)

Table 3
Potential indicators of feigned sleep-related violence and sexual behavior in sleep

Element	Explanation
Attempts to conceal one's behavior	Threatening a victim or hiding evidence indicates that the defendant is aware of the behavior and attempting to evade responsibility for it
Recurrent SRV and SBS after being notified of violent or sexual acts in sleep	A failure to take steps to reduce one's risk of engaging in SRV or SBS after being informed of the behavior suggests either a disregard for potential victims or feigned parasomnia
Full recall of episodes of SRV and SBS	Individuals typically lack memory of the events that occur in NREM parasomnias or have memory of dream imagery in REM parasomnias
SRV or SBS as sole parasomnia-related behavior in new-onset parasomnia	Most individuals who engage in SRV or SBS have other co-occurring parasomnias. New-onset SRV or SBS without additional parasomnia symptoms should raise one's suspicion for malingering

Adapted from Holoyda et al., 2021.[28]

interests, so the use of collateral records and informants and objective measures can be useful. Software that assesses visual reaction time (VRT) and penile plethysmography (PPG) can provide evidence of atypical sexual interest and arousal, respectively.[35]

An expert conducting a forensic evaluation of SBS should always consider paraphilias in the differential diagnosis. For example, a case involving child victims necessitates an evaluation for possible pedophilic disorder. Legal records and collateral informants may provide evidence of pedophilic interest, for example, use of child sexual exploitation materials or a history of grooming behavior. Alternatively, a scenario characterized by particularly violent or brutal sexual behavior should raise suspicion for sexual sadism disorder. Former bed partners may note that the individual has a history of aggressive and injurious sexual behavior. As previously noted, some bed partners of individuals with SBS report more direct, less partner-focused, and sometimes atypical sexual activity.[19] The forensic expert should therefore attempt to identify numerous sources of evidence indicative of a paraphilic disorder before making such a diagnosis. Diagnosing a paraphilic disorder based solely on the reported SBS would be inappropriate.

Violence Risk Assessment and the Relationship of Sleep-Related Violence and Sexual Behavior in Sleep to Waking Behavior

The relationship between SRV and an individual's risk of violence in waking life is unknown.[28] There are no studies assessing the violence histories of individuals with known or alleged SRV. It is unclear if standardized violence risk assessments such as the Violence Risk Appraisal Guide-Revised or the History-Clinical-Risk Version 3 are relevant in the evaluation of individuals with a history of SRV and criminal sanction for such behavior. The relationship between SBS and waking sexuality is similarly mysterious. It is unclear if an individual's waking sexual orientation and sexual interests remain constant during SBS. If an adult man is accused of engaging in SBS with another man or prepubescent children, it is unclear if such behavior suggests an underlying homosexual orientation or pedophilic interest, respectively. Such questions are particularly relevant for treating clinicians and forensic experts involved in developing risk management strategies for individuals with SRV and SBS. If SRV and SBS are phenomena truly independent from a person's behavior in waking life, then treatment of the underlying parasomnia or other sleep disorders should reduce the risk of a recurrence of violence and sexually violent behavior. Whether this is the case remains unclear. Of course, an individual may theoretically have a parasomnia co-occurring with a paraphilic disorder. Determining that a defendant's inappropriate sexual behavior is secondary to a parasomnia rather than a paraphilic interest when the purported SBS is consistent with one's paraphilic interest would be particularly challenging. There should be substantial evidence supporting a finding of SBS before proffering such an opinion.

Criminal Responsibility

The most relevant forensic question in cases of SRV and SBS is the defendant's criminal responsibility.

To commit a crime, an individual must have *mens rea* (guilty mind) and perpetrate an *actus reus* (guilty act). In addition, some criminal statutes establish the degree of intent that an individual must possess at the time of the offense to be convicted. Levels of intent in criminal law include purposely, knowingly, recklessly, and negligently. In cases involving SRV and SBS related to a parasomnia, an individual may be completely unaware of his or her behavior and, therefore, lack *mens rea* and fail to develop any degree of intent to commit a crime. Theoretically, individuals with a known history of SRV and SBS who fail to take steps to protect bed partners or others in the vicinity and engage in SRV or SBS could be accused of a reckless or negligent criminal intent, either consciously disregarding the risk of sexual abuse or failing to be aware of the risk, respectively.[36] A parasomnia defense provides a defendant the opportunity to negate his or her *mens rea* at the time of an offense through an insanity plea or to demonstrate that he or she lacked the capacity to develop the requisite criminal intent for the crime. It is the parasomnia's effect on criminal responsibility that renders it potentially attractive to would-be malingerers. Forensic assessments of criminal responsibility for SRV and SBS therefore require cautious formulation of a diagnosis, evaluation of alternative explanations for the alleged behavior, and consideration of malingering.

After a finding of current mental illness and dangerousness, individuals who are found not guilty by reason of insanity (NGRI) are typically remanded to a forensic psychiatric hospital setting and remain there until they are no longer dangerous to the community. As noted above, there is no research on the risk of waking violence posed by individuals who engage in genuine SRV and SBS. It is therefore unclear what purpose treatment in an inpatient forensic hospital setting might serve. Forensic evaluators tasked with evaluating individuals found NGRI based on a parasomnia may have to develop a risk mitigation plan for those returning to the community.[28] Risk mitigation strategies may include mandated outpatient sleep medicine treatment, avoidance of triggers for parasomnias, treatment of the parasomnia and co-occurring sleep and psychiatric disorders, and restrictions on sleeping arrangements with bed partners and other individuals in the home environment. Legal decision-makers may experience fear or worry about conditionally releasing an individual found NGRI for SRV or SBS, in which case the forensic expert may provide education about parasomnias and the limited research regarding the risk for violence posed by individuals with parasomnias.

SUMMARY

Although more research is necessary to better understand SRV and SBS, defendants, attorneys, and legal decision-makers increasingly seek forensic assessment of alleged SRV and SBS in criminal cases. Conducting an adequate forensic assessment of alleged SRV and SBS requires an understanding of sleep medicine and forensic psychiatry. Malingering, criminal responsibility, and psychosexual considerations are all potentially relevant in such cases. Despite a limited evidence base, forensic experts may serve an important role in educating attorneys, juries, and judges about parasomnias and associated SRV and SBS.

CLINICS CARE POINTS

- The role of v-PSG in the forensic evaluation of alleged parasomnia is questionable. Attorneys and experts should carefully consider the evidentiary benefit of obtaining v-PSG for a defendant before doing so.

- The forensic evaluation of alleged sexsomnia requires a psychosexual evaluation conducted by a forensic psychiatrist to rule out the presence of a rational alternative motive for the act, such as a paraphilic sexual interest.

- Defendants found not criminally responsible based on a parasomnia diagnosis may be mandated to treatment at a forensic psychiatric hospital or in the community. Forensic evaluators and clinicians must identify and develop a risk management strategy to reduce the likelihood of future SRV and SBS.

ACKNOWLEDGMENTS

Dr B. Holoyda would like to thank Basil B. Holoyda, M.D. of Neurology Associates in Macon, GA for reviewing this article and providing constructive feedback.

DISCLOSURES

The author has no financial or other disclosures to make regarding this article.

REFERENCES

1. Ingravallo F, Poli F, Gilmore EV, et al. Sleep-related violence and sexual behavior in sleep: a systematic review of medical-legal case reports. J Clin Sleep Med 2014;10(8):927–35.

2. Castelnovo A, Lopez R, Proserpio P, et al. NREM sleep parasomnias as disorders of sleep-state dissociation. Nat Rev Neurol 2018;14(8):470–81.

3. St. Louis EK, Boeve BF. REM sleep behavior disorder: diagnosis, clinical implications, and future directions. Mayo Clin Proc 2017;92(11):1723–36.

4. Nobili L, Proserpio P, Combi R, et al. Nocturnal frontal lobe epilepsy. Curr Neurol Neurosci Rep 2014;14: 424. https://doi.org/10.1007/s11910-013-0424-6.

5. Ohayon MM, Caulet M, Priest RG. Violent behavior during sleep. J Clin Psychiatry 1997;58(8):369–76.

6. Ohayon MM, Schenck CH. Violent behavior during sleep: prevalence, comorbidity and consequences. Sleep Med 2010;11(9):941–6.

7. Moldofsky H, Gilbert R, Lue FA, et al. Sleep-related violence. Sleep 1995;18(9):731–9.

8. Fedoroff JP, B A, Woods V, et al. A case-controlled study of men who sexually assault sleeping victims. In: Shapiro C, Smith AM, editors. Forensic aspects of sleep. Chichester, UK: John Wiley & Sons; 1997.

9. Shapiro CM, Trajanovic NN, Fedoroff JP. Sexsomnia–a new parasomnia? Can J Psychiatry 2003; 48(5):311–7.

10. American Psychiatric Association. Diagnostic and statistical manual of mental disorders. Fifth Edition. Washington, DC: American Psychiatric Association; 2013.

11. American Academy of Sleep Medicine. International classification of sleep disorders. Third Edition. Darien, IL: American Academy of Sleep Medicine; 2014.

12. Trajanovic NN, Shapiro CM. Sexsomnias. In: Thorpy MJ, editor. The parasomnias and other sleep-related movement disorders. Cambridge, UK: Cambridge University Press; 2010. p. 70–80. https://doi.org/10.1111/j.1365-2869.2008.00693.x.

13. Schenck CH. Update on sexsomnia, sleep related sexual seizures, and forensic implications. NeuroQuantology 2015;13(4):518–41.

14. Bjorvatn B, Gronli J, Pallesen S. Prevalence of different parasomnias in the general population. Sleep Med 2010;11(10):1031–4.

15. Drakatos P, Marples L, Muza R, et al. Video polysomnographic findings in non-rapid eye movement parasomnia. J Sleep Res 2019;28(2):e12772.

16. Martynowicz H, Smardz J, Wieczorek T, et al. The Co-occurrence of sexsomnia, sleep bruxism and other sleep disorders. J Clin Med 2018;7(9). https://doi.org/10.3390/jcm7090233.

17. Muza R, Lawrence M, Drakatos P. The reality of sexsomnia. Curr Opin Pulm Med 2016;22(6):576–82.

18. Banerjee D. Sleepwalking and sleeptalking. In: DR M, editor. Sleep medicine. Melbourne, Australia: IP Communications; 2017.

19. Dubessy AL, Leu-Semenescu S, Attali V, et al. Sexsomnia: a specialized non-REM parasomnia? Sleep 2017;40(2). https://doi.org/10.1093/sleep/zsw043.

20. Ebrahim I, Fenwick P. Letter to the Editor re: Pressman et al. Alcohol-induced sleepwalking or confusional arousal as a defense to criminal behavior: a review of scientific evidence, methods and forensic considerations. J Sleep Res (2007) 16, 182-212. J Sleep Res 2008;17:470–2.

21. Pressman MR, Mahowald MW, Schenck CH, et al. No scientific evidence that alcohol causes sleepwalking. J Sleep Res 2008;17:473–4.

22. Pressman MR, Mahowald MW, Schenck CH, Borenmann MC, et al. Alcohol, sleepwalking and violence: lack of reliable scientific evidence. Brain 2013;136:e229.

23. Maschauer EM, Gabryelska A, Morrison I, et al. Alcohol as a trigger affecting symptom severity and frequency of slow wave sleep disorders. J Clin Sleep Med 2017;13(9):1111.

24. Pressman MR. The neurophysiological and neurochemical effects of alcohol on the brain are inconsistent with current evidence based models of sleepwalking. Sleep Med Rev 2019;43:92–5.

25. American Academy of Sleep Medicine. International classification of sleep disorders. Third Edition, Text Revision. Darien, IL: American Academy of Sleep Medicine; 2023.

26. Organ A, Fedoroff JP. Sexsomnia: sleep sex research and its legal implications. Curr Psychiatry Rep 2015;17(5):34.

27. Mohebbi A, Holoyda BJ, Newman WJ. Sexsomnia as a defense in repeated sex crimes. J Am Acad Psychiatry Law 2018;46(1):78–85.

28. Holoyda BJ, Sorrentino RM, Mohebbi A, et al. Forensic evaluation of sexsomnia. J Am Acad Psychiatry Law 2021;49(2):202–10.

29. Cramer-Bornemann MA, Mahowald MW. Sleep forensics. criminal culpability for sleep-related violence. In: Kryger M, Roth T, Dement WC, editors. Principles and practice of sleep medicine. 6th edition. Amsterdam, NE: Elsevier; 2017.

30. Rumbold J, Morrison I, Riha RL. Calls for an international consensus on sleep-related violence and sexual behavior in sleep are premature. J Clin Sleep Med 2014;10(11):1253.

31. Bornemann MAC, Schenck CH, Mahowald MW. A review of sleep-related violence: the demographics of sleep forensic referrals to a single center. Chest 2019;155(5):1059–66.

32. Yeh SB, Schenck CH. Sexsomnia: a case of sleep masturbation documented by video-polysomnography in a young adult male with sleepwalking. Sleep Sci 2016;9(2):65–8.

33. Bornemann MAC. Sexsomnia: a medicolegal case-based approach in analyzing potential sleep-related abnormal sexual behaviors. In: Kothare SV IA, editor. Parasomnias: clinical characteristics and treatment. New York, NY: Springer; 2013. p. 431–61.

34. Mahowald MW, Schenck CH, Cramer-Bornemann M. Finally–sleep science for the courtroom. Sleep Med Rev 2007;11(1):1–3.

35. Holoyda BJ, Newman WJ. Recidivism risk assessment for adult sexual offenders. Curr Psychiatry Rep 2016;18(2):17.

36. American Law Institute. (1985), Model penal code : official draft and explanatory notes : complete text of Model penal code as adopted at the 1962 Annual Meeting of the American Law Institute at Washington, DC, May 24, 1962. The Institute; Philadelphia, PA.

Educational Resources to Support Patients with Parasomnias

Courtney D. Molina, BS[a], Adreanne Rivera, BS[b], Alon Y. Avidan, MD, MPH[a],*

KEYWORDS

- Parasomnia • REM sleep behavior disorder • Dream enactment behavior • Alpha-synucleinopathy
- Parkinson disease • Neurodegeneration

KEY POINTS

- This article lists credible and accessible online resources about parasomnias (ie, sleepwalking, night terrors, and rapid eye movement sleep behavior disorder [RBD0]) for both patients and health-care providers.
- Educational resources focused on these abnormal behaviors can empower patients to take an active role in managing their conditions in partnership with their clinicians.
- An extensive "Frequently Asked Questions (FAQ) About RBD" is also featured in this article as a tool to help clinicians and patients better identify and manage RBD, as well as understand the relationship between RBD and the alpha-synucleinopathies (Parkinson disease, Lewy Body Dementia, and multiple system atrophy).

INTRODUCTION

People suffering from parasomnias are continuously searching for credible information about their conditions even before they are seen by sleep clinicians.

Websites on parasomnias seem to be focused on common disorders of arousal (sleepwalking and sleep terrors) and are specific to parents in search of information whereas websites specifically on rapid eye movement (REM) parasomnias address REM sleep behavior disorder (RBD) extensively. Due to the risk of people with dream enactment behavior (DEB) who are searching for resources first learning about the potential connection between RBD and neurologic conditions through the web, it is crucial that websites highlight the critical need to be seen by a sleep clinician for confirmation of diagnosis. The resources on the Internet can provide this information accurately and remind patients that a clinician must address diagnosis and management. Patient education and accessibility to clinically validated resources can affect patients' ability to advocate for themselves, most especially in a clinical setting. Several websites focused on sleep and parasomnias can empower patients with the knowledge to take an active role in managing their conditions, collaborating with their clinicians in clinical management, enrolling in registries, and joining newsletters sponsored by these resources.

The resources listed below are examples of websites that are both credible and accurate in disseminating accurate and helpful information for patients.

GENERAL SLEEP EDUCATION WEBSITES
American Academy of Sleep Medicine Sleep Education

This website, developed by the American Academy of Sleep Medicine (AASM), provides an extensive overview of sleep medicine topics for patients and

[a] Department of Neurology, UCLA, David Geffen School of Medicine at UCLA, 710 Westwood Boulevard, RNRC, C153, Mail Code 176919, Los Angeles, CA 90095-1769, USA; [b] UCLA Clinical Translational Science Institute, 10911 Weyburn Avenue 3rd Road Floor, Los Angeles, CA 90095, USA
* Corresponding author
E-mail address: avidan@mednet.ucla.edu

Sleep Med Clin 19 (2024) 199–210
https://doi.org/10.1016/j.jsmc.2023.12.002

clinicians alike[1](https://sleepeducation.org). Articles address healthy sleep habits, sleep disorders, sleep studies and tests, treatment paradigms, and a sleep product guide. They may be embedded with helpful companion videos, or printable infographics. A unique section lists AASM Health Advisories in succinct, easy-to-read summaries discussing a variety of topics such as "Healthy sleep during a pandemic" and "Melatonin use in children and adolescents." Certain topics for advocacy are also made available, listing sleep initiatives, current legislation, and AASM campaigns. A printable peer review summary of minority health and sleep is also a helpful tool.

Project Sleep

Project Sleep is a 501(c) (3) nonprofit organization that educates people on the intersection of crucial sleep-related topics—sleep health and sleep hygiene, sleep disorders, and sleep equity—founded by narcolepsy patient and advocate, Julie Flygare JD.[2] (https://project-sleep.com/) This website gives a broad overview of sleep-related topics in a variety of easy-to-read articles, infographics, videos, links to research opportunities, and a companion podcast. Common sleep disorders described include narcolepsy, insomnia, obstructive sleep apnea, RBD, and restless legs syndrome. An interactive self-assessment can be completed using the Sleep Disorders Symptom Checklist-25.[30] Additionally, an annual application is put out every winter for Rising Voices, a summer program to train people with various sleep disorders in public speaking to develop the next generation of patient advocates. Notably, Project Sleep provides links to the AASM's website, endorsing formal consultation with a board-certified sleep specialist for serious concerns of a sleep disorder, with the caveat that all health journeys typically start with one's primary care physician.

National Sleep Foundation

The National Sleep Foundation is a nonprofit organization founded in 1990, to share educational materials, research opportunities, and campaigns to improve the public's sleep health[3] (https://www.thensf.org). Tools such as the Sleep Health Index and Sleep in America Poll gather more insight into the public's sentiments toward sleep and how that may affect other areas of health including mental health. Sleep Health Topics include articles about sleep apnea, insomnia, excessive sleepiness, and narcolepsy; however, they do not delve beyond the most common sleep disorders and discuss parasomnias.

Sleep Foundation

Having previously been affiliated with the National Sleep Foundation, the Sleep Foundation website broke off into its own separate entity in 2019, sharing free articles revolving around sleep hygiene, sleep disorders, sleep news, and product reviews[4] (https://www.sleepfoundation.org/). Overviews of sleep disorders are broad, listing relevant publications and related articles, adhering to their policy of providing up to date, medically accurate sources. Resources are palatable for audiences without a prior background in sleep medicine, detailing significant topics of interest for the general public, such as the difference between home sleep apnea and in-laboratory sleep tests, the pros and cons of melatonin and magnesium supplementation, and relaxation techniques.

UpToDate

Although a comprehensive source of the causes, differential diagnoses, assessments, and treatments of numerous conditions, UpToDate is of greater benefit for practitioners than the general public (and requires a subscription to gain access to all resources[5] (https://www.uptodate.com/). However, some educational materials can be printed or included in after-visit summaries to be shared with patients. The most extensive educational materials are for RBD, offering 2 handouts—"The Basics" and "Beyond the Basics"—providing a summary of RBD at an easy-to-read (5th grade) level and an in-depth version with some medical jargon (12th grade reading level). Patient education for the other parasomnias is more limited with a focus on children—"Patient education: Sleepwalking in children (The Basics)" and "Patient education: Night terrors, confusional arousals, and nightmares in children (The Basics)." Despite a higher incidence rate of these parasomnias in pediatric populations—which often resolve by adulthood—it would be remiss to overlook the importance of educational materials concerning the clinical presentations of these parasomnias in adult populations as well.

Parasomnias and Disruptive Sleep Disorders from Cleveland Clinic

This site provides a concise, medically reviewed summary of the parasomnias, grouping them by non-REM or REM-type.[6] (https://my.clevelandclinic.org/health) Links to in-depth articles are available for some parasomnias—somnambulism, sleep-related eating disorder, nightmares, RBD, and exploding head syndrome—providing additional helpful information on the topic. Because this site is part of the Cleveland Clinic's Health Library, articles with a broader overview of sleep and sleep disorders may also be of utility for persons with a limited knowledge of sleep medicine.

Sleep Medicine: Patient and Family Education from Seattle Children's Hospital

This helpful website lists many patient education resources discussing a variety of topics in pediatric sleep medicine, including what to expect at a sleep medicine appointment, general tips, and condition-specific handouts. PDFs are available in both English and Spanish[7] (https://www.seattlechildrens.org/clinics/sleep-medicine/).

Mayo Clinic, Navigate to "Department" Search for Sleep

The Mayo Clinic's Center for Sleep Medicine website provides an extensive list of the sleep disorders treated at their clinic[8] (https://www.mayoclinic.org). However, only the more common disorders link to an in-depth guide, including nightmares, night terrors, RBD, and sleepwalking. Of note, parasomnias is listed as a separate entity, although the above disorders fall under the umbrella of "Parasomnias." Each article provides an easy-to-read overview of the disorder's symptoms, causes, and methods for diagnosis and treatment.

European Sleep Research Society

This website, which is affiliated with the Journal of Sleep Research, provides resources for sleep medicine researchers and clinicians with emphasis on supportive aides for those early in their career[9] (ESRS.eu). Most helpful to the general specialist, the European Sleep Research Society has a catalog of free webinars concerning various sleep-related topics as well as a free online course on the fundamentals of sleep. However, their curriculum seems more geared toward topics such as sleep apnea, insomnia, sleep deprivation, and circadian rhythm disorders, and lack mention of the parasomnias.

American Academy of Sleep Medicine

The AASM's website caters to specialists in the field of sleep medicine, setting practice standards, promoting research, and disseminating information about healthy sleep[10] (https://aasm.org). Several AASM patient guides are available for download covering diagnosis and testing for sleep apnea, insomnia, hypersomnia but fail to discuss other common sleep disorders such as the

parasomnias. Guides are made available in both English and Spanish. Additionally, provider fact sheets are available for download, including one for the identification of RBD.

Associated Professional Sleep Societies, LLC

This website represents a joint endeavor by the AASM and Sleep Research Society for the annual SLEEP meeting[11] (https://www.sleepmeeting.org). Since its inauguration in 1986, this conference has been a leading proponent for presentation of cutting edge research, informational sessions, networking, and career development opportunities for clinicians and researchers in the field of sleep medicine. Recordings of select sessions are available online for purchase for attendees and nonattendees alike.

RAPID EYE MOVEMENT SLEEP BEHAVIOR DISORDER
North American Prodromal Synucleinopathy Consortium

- Website
  - Homepage link: https://www.naps-rbd.org;[12] (https://www.naps-rbd.org/)
  - This website is entirely dedicated to RBD, serving dual-purpose: (1) to provide information for those who are concerned about DEMs or have recently been diagnosed with RBD as well as (2) information for healthcare providers who might be responsible for the diagnosis and management of patients with this condition. As of now, resources include short videos and research citations but promise to continually expand their educational materials. Notably, the website also features a sign-up for the NAPS Consortium Registry for future research studies.
- North American Prodromal Synucleinopathy (NAPS) remedy (RBD education delivery)
  - REMEDY (REM Sleep Behavior Disorder Education Delivery) link: https://www.naps-rbd.org/education **Fig. 1**, "RBD Educational Brochure" is an example of an educational resource that can be provided to patients to improve parasomnias and RBD education (**Fig. 1**) but may help improve recognition of RBD based on the Mayo Sleep Questionnaire. The brochure also helps direct prospective patients to the NAPS Educational Website for Specific RBD educational resources and register to receive key resources (see **Fig 2**).
  - REMEDY serves as an education resources portal and is designed to provide patients, loved ones, physicians, researchers, and other interested parties with information

N⋀PS CONSORTIUM
For REM Sleep Behavior Disorder

Parasomnias

- Parasomnia is a sleep disorder consisting of abnormal and undesirable behaviors that occur during sleep.

REM Sleep Behavior Disorder (RBD)

- RBD involves loss of muscle paralysis during dream sleep. This protective effect, which usually prevents us from acting out our dreams, is lost, leading to abnormal vocalizations and behaviors.
- Some of these behaviors can result in sleep disruption and injury when people with RBD act on their dreams
- RBD Requires a Sleep Medicine Consultation with a Sleep Clinician and a Sleep Study Confirmation

Important Facts About RBD

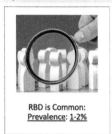
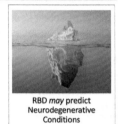

RBD is Common: Prevalence: 1-2%

RBD *may* predict Neurodegenerative Conditions

For more information about RBD and and NAPS, please visit: https://www.naps-rbd.org

Visit Our Website   Data Request Form

Contact Us
Website: naps-rbd.org
Email: info@naps-rbd.org

Fig. 1. RBD patient brochure (naps consortium).[31]

N⋀PS CONSORTIUM
For REM Sleep Behavior Disorder

"Have you ever been told, or suspected yourself, that you seem to 'act out your dreams' while asleep (for example, punching, flailing your arms in the air, making running movements, etc.)?"

If you answered "yes"," you may need to be evaluated for a condition known as REM Sleep Behavior Disorder (RBD)

The North American Prodromal Synucleinopathy (NAPS) Consortium on RBD:

- Promotes education for individuals living with RBD, as well as partners and family of people diagnosed with RBD, and those wanting to learn more about RBD.
- Provides support, clinical care, discovery, community engagement, and educational support.
- Allows patients and health care partners to join the REM Sleep Behavior Disorder Registry to identify potential research participants, but also assist care teams providing care to people with RBD, and to study RBD therapy and outcomes.

THOSE LIVING WITH RBD   LEARN MORE ABOUT RBD   HEALTHCARE PROFESSIONALS

Fig. 2. The North American Prodromal Synucleinopathy (NAPS) consortium on RBD.

about RBD, clinical studies, research opportunities, and other important information (https://www.naps-rbd.org/education).

- ○ All information shared in this portal has been reviewed and validated by sleep physicians in the NAPS Consortium Team. This portal is also being continually maintained and kept up-to-date by sleep physicians in the NAPS Consortium Team.
- ○ This portal contains resources including the following:
  - Educational videos addressing frequently asked questions by patients such as defining RBD, RBD management, history of RBD, and the RBD diagnosis process (https://www.naps-rbd.org/videos).
  - Links to past webinars held by sleep physicians.
  - Links to reputable and credible scientific articles that expand on RBD's link to neurodegenerative disease, RBD's clinical features and case series, RBD's current

treatments, and clinical trial planning (https://www.naps-rbd.org/education).
- • NAPS YouTube Channel (**Fig. 3**)
  - ○ Link: https://www.youtube.com/@naps consortiumforremsleepb7898
  - ○ The NAPS YouTube Channel is managed by the NAPS Consortium REO (Research Education Outreach) Team. The YouTube Channel has content focusing on the following:
    - Patient education
    - NAPS Consortium research updates
    - Patient testimonies
    - Recordings of patient webinars hosted by sleep physicians
- • NAPS Social Media
  - ○ The NAPS social media platforms are managed by the NAPS Consortium REO (Research Education Outreach) Team. The content shared in the NAPS social media platforms has been reviewed and approved by sleep physicians in the NAPS Consortium Team and has the following areas of focus:

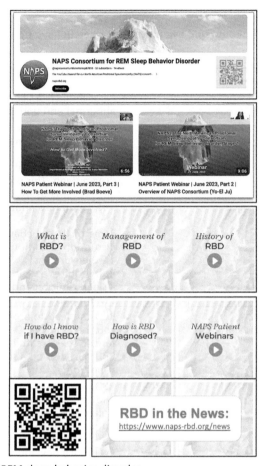

Fig. 3. NAPS consortium for REM sleep behavior disorder.

- Share new research publications related to RBD and sleep medicine. Summarize the importance of each new research publication and translate it into layman's term. The purpose is to help patients stay up-to-date with scientific discoveries and advancements in sleep medicine as well as make these articles more easily accessible to patients.
- Clinical research study recruitment
- Education for patients, industry partners, and sleep medicine physicians
- Promotion of recent and upcoming events related to sleep medicine (including conferences or webinars)
  - The frequency of new posts are 2 to 3 times a week on each platform.
  - Links:
    - Facebook: https://www.facebook.com/NAPSConsortium/
    - Instagram: https://www.instagram.com/napsconsortium/
    - Twitter: https://twitter.com/napsconsortium

  - A list of "Frequently Asked Questions (FAQ) About RBD" is provided below to help clinicians communicate educational information about RBD (**Table 1**).

DIALOGUE SPECIFIC TO NEUROPROTECTIVE MEASURES

The alpha-synucleinopathies, including Parkinson disease, have a prodromal period in which the neurodegeneration has commenced but are not yet clinically significant enough for official diagnosis. Common symptoms that may indicate the prodromal period include anosmia, constipation, depression, motor impairment, orthostatic hypotension, and iRBD.[23] However, of these symptoms, RBD has the highest predictive value with between 50% and 80% of patients with RBD phenoconverting to Parkinson disease within the decade after receiving their diagnosis—and manifestation of these symptoms is nevertheless after significant degeneration has already occurred.[17,19,20,23,26] As noted in RBD

Table 1
Frequently asked questions about rapid eye movement sleep behavior disorder

Question	Discussion
What is RBD and what causes it?	
What is a parasomnia?	• Parasomnia is a sleep disorder consisting of abnormal and undesirable behaviors that occur during sleep[13]
What is RBD?	• RBD is a type of parasomnia that occurs during REM sleep[13,14] • RBD involves loss of muscle paralysis during dream sleep. This protective effect, which usually prevents us from acting out our dreams, is lost, leading to abnormal vocalizations and behaviors[13–15] • Some of these behaviors can result in sleep disruption and injury when people with RBD act on their dreams[13–15] • RBD requires a sleep medicine consultation with a sleep clinician and a sleep study confirmation[13,14,16]
Why is it important to know that you have RBD and treat it?	• RBD can lead to accidental injury to yourself or your bed partner. Due to these risks, it is important to seek treatment[13,14] • RBD may also be a sign of a future neurologic condition[13–15,17,18]
What causes RBD?	• RBD presents in 2 forms: isolated (idiopathic) and symptomatic (secondary)[14,18] • Isolated or idiopathic RBD (iRBD) refers to evolution that is spontaneous without an underlying cause. Many people with iRBD will eventually develop a neurodegenerative condition—specifically, Parkinson disease, Lewy body dementia, or multiple system atrophy, which are collectively referred to alpha-synucleinopathies. These neurologic conditions manifest when an abnormal misfolding of a normal protein (synuclein) accumulates inside nerve cells (neurons) causing them to degenerate[14,17–20] • Symptomatic or secondary RBD manifests due to an underlying cause, such as an alpha-synucleinopathy[14,18,20] • People who take certain antidepressants can develop RBD. This is called drug-induced RBD. Recent research indicates that 50% of patients develop RBD because of medications (serotonergic antidepressant "SSRIs")[15,20]
Can certain medications "cause" RBD?	• Medication/drug-induced RBD can be characterized by DEB coinciding with the initiation of certain medications but particularly serotonergic antidepressants such as selective serotonin reuptake inhibitors (SSRIs) and serotonin and norepinephrine reuptake inhibitors[15,21] • Although a patient with long-term use of SSRIs may be recently diagnosed with RBD, carefully reviewing when the DEB manifested may point to whether the behaviors are attributed to SSRI's or are of another cause.
	(continued on next page)

Table 1
(continued)

Question	Discussion
	• After proper consultation with a patient's primary care provider (PCP) or mental health provider, the patient may discontinue the SSRIs or switch from SSRIs to another antidepressant class such as bupropion if it is safe to do so. If the DEBs persist, it is clinically probable that the RBD is of another cause, and its management would continue as normal[21]
Can RBD be caused by chemical exposure?	• Due to the limited information revolving around RBD and its risk for phenoconversion to the alpha-synucleinopathies, many RBD studies are collecting baseline information such as patients' occupations, lifestyle factors, and environmental hazards to assess for any correlations[18] • Positive correlations include pesticide exposure (a common risk factor for Parkinson disease), carbon dioxide (CO_2) poisoning (of which, is known to induce parkinsonism), and cigarette smoking[22,23]
Diagnosis	
How do you know that you have RBD?	• If you answer "Yes" to the following question, then it is important to be evaluated for RBD: "Have you ever been told, or suspected yourself, that you seem to 'act out your dreams' while asleep (eg, punching, flailing your arms in the air, making running movements, and so forth)?"[5]
How is RBD diagnosed?	• RBD is diagnosed after a careful consultation by a sleep physician or a specialist with training in evaluating and managing parasomnias • It requires the presence of repeated episodes of abnormal behaviors at night (DEBs) and a verification by an in-laboratory sleep study (nocturnal polysomnogram) of the muscle tone during REM sleep (referred to as REM sleep without atonia [RSWA])[13,14,16,24] • People who experience repetitive DEB and RSWA may be diagnosed with RBD but the diagnosis must be established after a careful review of the clinical history by a trained clinician[13,14,16]
What are the diagnostic tools to confirm diagnosis?	• The diagnosis of RBD is based on the interview with a specialist in Sleep Medicine and a subsequent overnight sleep study in the sleep laboratory[14,16]
Can you diagnose RBD without a sleep study or use a wearable device to diagnose it?	• You cannot diagnose RBD without a confirmatory polysomnography (sleep study)[1,13,24] • The current AASM diagnostic criteria include both a history of DEBs and REM sleep without muscle atonia—that is, the absence of muscle paralysis during REM sleep—which can only be assessed by the use of an electromyography (EMG) during the REM stage of sleep

(continued on next page)

Table 1
(continued)

Question	Discussion
	• Wearables, such as Fitbit© or Apple Watch©, do not currently possess the capabilities to assess muscle tone and therefore cannot be used to diagnose RBD. However, future endeavors to incorporate wearables technology into the diagnostic toolkit add another avenue for patients and clinicians to pursue diagnosis that is both simple and cost effective
What is known about the negative predictive value in the absence of RSWA from a single PSG in individuals who have previously experienced dream enactment episodes at home?	• Sleep studies that fail to capture RSWA most commonly fail to capture an adequate amount of REM sleep, if any, for evaluation • We consider the polysomnography (PSG) to be a snapshot of a person's sleep; however, it does not paint the full portrait. Therefore, individuals with a history of DEBs are encouraged to take safety measures in their bedroom environment and record any dream enactment episodes. Those that have DEBs more frequently or intensely are encouraged to begin melatonin therapy for "clinically probable" RBD. In the future, another PSG may be used to reassess for RBD
Is there much concern about nonspecialized PSG readers (even at academic institutions) missing RSWA– that is, if RSWA was not noted as a finding in the PSG report, how confident can one be that RSWA was not actually present during the PSG?	• Yes, PSGs must be tailored to assess for RSWA by addition of an EMG to evaluate muscle tone. If RSWA is not mentioned in the PSG report, we cannot be certain that the study included an EMG montage
Management of RBD	
How is RBD managed?	• It is ideal to maintain a safe sleeping environment to prevent potentially injurious nocturnal behaviors (sleeping bag, sleeping on the floor, and removal of sharp objects) • Depending on the frequency and severity of dream enactment episodes, melatonin or benzodiazepines are generally very effective in managing RBD in most patients with the condition[13,21,24] • The most used benzodiazepine is clonazepam[16,21,24] • People with RBD should receive regular follow-up care
I use melatonin at 3 mg but that does not help that much. What should I do next?	• First, look at the formulation of melatonin. Is it a regular formulation or does it say "time-release" or "extended release" melatonin? If the melatonin is not time-release, consider switching formulations • If the melatonin is time-release, increase the dose to 5 mg or two 3 mg tablets, for a total of 6 mg • Of note, in the United States, melatonin is an over-the-counter agent; as such, there is greater variance between formulations. Switching brands may also improve the DEBs due to these potential differences in efficacy[21]

(continued on next page)

Table 1
(continued)

Question	Discussion
Once diagnosed with RBD, is there an optimal approach for evaluating the effectiveness of different treatment options (melatonin, clonazepam, and so forth)? Currently, I am recording my nighttime behaviors using a night camera and reviewing motion events. It is not ideal but currently all I have to go by beyond rating of restfulness on waking	• There is no optimal approach for evaluating the effectiveness of treatment modalities. Especially in the absence of a bed partner to corroborate the presence of dream enactment episodes, recording unusual behaviors via a night camera and keeping a sleep diary are effective ways to track how frequently the DEBs continue and the nature of the episodes
Is there any experience to be shared yet about dual orexinergic receptor antagonist (DORA) as a potential treatment of RBD?	• A recent study using a mouse model found that implementation of DORAs significantly increased total sleep duration and reduced DEBs[25] • Although this study yields promising results, clinical trials have yet to use human subjects[25]
What does it mean if you have RBD:	
How far away are we from predicting phenoconversion?	• Current data are emerging to help provide clinicians with data to help predicting the risk of phenoconversion. Phenoconversion rate is probably lowest in young patients aged <50 y and increases by 1%–2% each decade.[8,14] In older patients aged >65–70 y, phenoconversion is probably highest, at 6% every year from diagnosis[20]
Management of neurologic disease associated with RBD	
What do you see as the most promising current ideas or areas of inquiry in the search for potential interventions to arrest synucleinopathy during the prodromal phase?	• The prodromal phase is marked by any indicators that may suggest the onset of neurodegeneration. Common symptoms include constipation, depression, anosmia (loss of smell), orthostatic hypotension, motor impairment, and iRBD[17,19,20,23] • However, many of these markers are not noticeable until significant degeneration has already occurred (ie: motor impairment is often not noticed until ~50% neuronal loss of the substantia nigra)[23] • Various studies are currently searching for potential biomarkers to identify progression as early as possible[19,23]
Realistically speaking, what does the timeline look like for getting there?	• Although it is an exciting time for us concerning the attention and resources that are focused on RBD and neurodegenerative conditions, we still cannot predict an accurate timeline for arresting synucleinopathy in the prodromal phase. As many advancements are being made, we still have to keep in mind that our research is often a "marathon" and not a "sprint" for solutions
Because RBD patients are the ideal group to involve in neuroprotective treatments, how can the public and family doctors be better prepared to identify RBD symptoms? It took me 5 y to get diagnosed because it was thought to be stress related or just bad dreams	• The visibility of sleep medicine continues to grow—many patients do not even consider sleep to be an expansive opportunity to improve their health until consulting with other providers on their health-care team • We call on our general practitioner and general neurology colleagues to refer patients for a full sleep evaluation, as even "bad dreams" or more

(continued on next page)

Table 1 (continued)	
Question	**Discussion**
	"benign" displays of poor sleep may indicate other sleep disorders such as sleep-disordered breathing or underlying sleep deprivation • Certain organizations committed to the research and treatment of RBD have created tools to better advocate for patients with RBD, including diagnostic criteria for clinicians and patient information guides, videos, or sign-ups for clinical trials for those who suspect or have recently been diagnosed with RBD. Among these are the American Academy of Sleep Medicine (AASM), the Sleep Research Society (SRS). the National Sleep Foundation, and our own NAPS Consortium
What is known about the role of antidepressants on RBD symptoms and progression timeline?	• It is known that some antidepressants may worsen and or exacerbate RBD symptoms.[15] There is an ongoing debate about whether these antidepressants may be a primary causative factor of RBD[15]
Is it possible to "delay" or "prevent" progression to neurodegeneration in people with diagnosis of RBD?	• Because RBD may present a window of opportunity to predict future neurodegenerative conditions, the diagnosis of RBD may offer those at risk to begin specific treatments to mitigate this risk. However, at the time of writing this article (January 2024), no specific therapy is currently available
Patient advocacy	
Are there any support groups for people with RBD?	• Currently, there is no organized network of RBD support groups. This is one of the high priorities of our NAPS Consortium, and we are working on developing this initiative
RBD research	
How do I get involved in NAPS?	All NAPS research sites and their respective institutions have regulations related to participation in clinical research. Interested participants may reach out to NAPS at https://www.naps-rbd.org for further inquiry
	We will continue to follow individuals with RBD who were enrolled in the NAPS study before developing Parkinson disease or other neurologic disorders

manuscrips in this issue, more recent data from the Mayo Clinic highlights that the strongest independent predictor of phenoconversion risk was the patient's age at the time when RBD diagnosis was made with the following observations: Age < 50 years may represent the lowest phenoconversion rates at about 1% per year, 2%/year risk of phenoconversion for 50-60 year age bracket, 4%/year for those 60-70 years of age, and 6%/year for those older than >70 (Alexandres, McCarter, Boeve, et al., 2023. unpublished data). As researchers aim to identify these prodromal markers, subsequent efforts can be made to pinpoint neuroprotective measures to slow or halt the neurodegeneration in its earliest stages. As of now, the best neuroprotective agent is exercise. The literature suggests that regular, intense exercise in midlife significantly reduced the risk of developing Parkinson disease later in life.[27,28] On the whole, exercise is not specified so long as it is vigorous but previous studies have looked at the benefits of cycling, running, dancing, tai chi, yoga, and weight lifting.[27,29] Exercise is also indicated to have general positive effects on patient's living with Parkinson, evoking neuroplasticity of the brain, reducing mild cognitive impairment, counteracting muscle weakness, and improving gait and balance.[24,27–29]

SUMMARY

As the field of sleep medicine continues to expand, more resources are needed to educate the public of common sleep disorders and how to pursue diagnosis by a sleep professional. Although sleep apnea and insomnia are widely regarded as the "bread and butter" of sleep medicine, the limitations to parasomnia educational materials must be addressed, particularly due to the unusual and stress-inducing nature of the behaviors. Many of the parasomnias, such as sleep terrors and somnambulism, often present in child and adolescent populations; however, their lesser-known presentations in older populations may point to other disorders such as untreated sleep-disordered breathing. A diagnosis of RBD also often leaves patients and their loved ones with unease due to both the unsettling nature of the DEBs and its high risk of phenoconversion to the alpha-synucleinopathies. Proper tools are needed to identify and counsel these patients given the serious nature of their disorder, including how to mitigate harm in the bedroom environment, what to look for in the phenoconversion process to an alpha-synucleinopathy, how to empower patient participation in forthcoming clinical trial endeavors, and advocate for strong patient–provider relationships.

FUNDING STATEMENT

This work was funded by National Institutes of Health-National Institute on Aging (NIH-NIA), U19 AG071754, and the Karen Toffler Charitable Trust.

ACKNOWLEDGMENTS

This publication was supported in part by the National Institutes of Health, United States (NIH) grants R34AG056639 (NAPS) and U19-AG071754 (NAPS2). Its contents are solely the reresponsibility of the authors and do not necessarily represent the official views of the NIH. The authors would like to express their sincere appreciation and gratitude to the entire NAPS consortium, the Karen Toffler Charitable Trust (https://tofflertrust.org), and the Education Committee of the North American Prodromal Synucleinopathy Consortium for RBD, Stage 2 (NAPS2, https://www.naps-rbd.org). **Table 1** was developed following previous NAPS RBD Patient Webinars which were supportd by other NAPS investogators, Dr Aleksandar Videnovic, MD, MSc, (Harvard Medical School), Michael Howell, MD (University of Minnesota) and NAPS administative laisons, Jennifer McLeland, PhD and Ms Leah Taylor (Washington University).

DISCLOSURE

Dr Avidan has received consultant fees from Avadel, Merck, Takeda, Idorsia and speaker honoraria from Avadel and Idorsia.

CLINICS CARE POINTS

- Parasomnias are undesirable nocturnal events occurring during sleep or the transition into or out of sleep. The events may occur in nonrapid eye movement (NREM) or rapid eye movement (REM) sleep and consist of abnormal behaviors (eg, sleep-related eating) or dream enactment (eg, REM sleep behavior disorder). While patients are thirsty for education about parasomnias, with a few exceptions, the Internet may not provide consistent educational resources about these diagnoses.

- REM sleep behavior disorder (RBD) is identified by episodes of dream enactment in which the patient is exhibiting behaviors such as punching, kicking, or yelling out while asleep.

- RBD may only be diagnosed after a polysomnography captures epochs of REM sleep without muscle atonia.

- RBD is a high predictive factor for alpha-synucleinopathy neurodegeneration (Parkinson's disease, dementia with Lewy Bodies, multiple system atrophy), termed "phenoconversion.

REFERENCES

1. Home Page – Sleep Education – American Academy of Sleep Medicine. Sleep Education. https://www.sleepeducation.org/.
2. Project Sleep Home Page. Project Sleep. https://project-sleep.com/.
3. National Sleep Foundation. The National Sleep Foundation. https://www.thensf.org/.
4. Better Sleep for a better you. Sleep Foundation. https://www.sleepfoundation.org/.
5. UpToDate: Industry-leading clinical decision support. UpToDate. https://www.uptodate.com/home.

6. Cleveland Clinic Parasomnias: Causes, symptoms, types & management. Cleveland Clinic. https://my.-clevelandclinic.org/health/diseases/12133-para-somnias–disruptive-sleep-disorders.

7. Patient and family education – sleep medicine – seattle children's. Seattle Children's Hospital. https://www.seattlechildrens.org/clinics/sleep-medi-cine/patient-family-resources/.

8. Top-ranked hospital in the nation-Mayo Clinic. Mayo Clinic. https://www.mayoclinic.org/.

9. ESRS. ESRS Home: European Sleep Research Society. ESRS. https://esrs.eu/.

10. American Academy of Sleep Medicine: AASM: Sleep: Medical society. American Academy of Sleep Medicine – Association for Sleep Clinicians and Researchers. https://aasm.org/.

11. Sleep 2023. APSS annual meeting: AASM: SRS. SLEEP meeting. https://www.sleepmeeting.org/.

12. NAPS consortium for REM sleep behavior disorder. NAPS Consortium for REM Sleep Behavior Disorder. https://www.naps-rbd.org/.

13. Boeve BF. REM sleep behavior disorder: updated review of the core features, the REM sleep behavior disorder-neurodegenerative disease association, evolving concepts, controversies, and future directions. Ann N Y Acad Sci 2010;1184:15–54.

14. McCarter SJ, St Louis EK, Boeve BF. REM sleep behavior disorder and REM sleep without atonia as an early manifestation of degenerative neurological disease [published correction appears in Curr Neurol Neurosci Rep. 2012 Apr;12(2):226]. Curr Neurol Neurosci Rep 2012;12(2):182–92.

15. Baltzan M, Yao C, Rizzo D, et al. Dream enactment behavior: review for the clinician. J Clin Sleep Med 2020;16(11):1949–69.

16. Högl B, Stefani A. REM sleep behavior disorder (RBD): update on diagnosis and treatment. Somnologie 2017;21(Suppl 1):1–8.

17. Postuma RB, Gagnon JF, Bertrand JA, et al. Parkinson risk in idiopathic REM sleep behavior disorder: preparing for neuroprotective trials. Neurology 2015;84(11):1104–13.

18. Postuma RB, Montplaisir JY, Pelletier A, et al. Environmental risk factors for REM sleep behavior disorder: a multicenter case-control study. Neurology 2012;79(5):428–34.

19. Berg D, Crotty GF, Keavney JL, et al. Path to Parkinson disease prevention: conclusion and outlook. Neurology 2022;99(7 Suppl 1):76–83.

20. Howell M, Schenck C. Rapid eye movement sleep behavior disorder. UpToDate. https://www.uptodate.com/contents/rapid-eye-movement-sleep-behavior-disorder.

21. Howell M, Avidan AY, Foldvary-Schaefer N, et al. Management of REM sleep behavior disorder: an American academy of sleep medicine clinical practice guideline. J Clin Sleep Med 2023;19(4):759–68.

22. Jacobs ML, Dauvilliers Y, St Louis EK, et al. Risk factor profile in Parkinson's disease subtype with REM sleep behavior disorder. J Parkinsons Dis 2016; 6(1):231–7.

23. Postuma RB, Gagnon JF, Montplaisir J. Clinical prediction of Parkinson's disease: planning for the age of neuroprotection. J Neurol Neurosurg Psychiatr 2010;81(9):1008–13.

24. Lang AE, Espay AJ. Disease modification in Parkinson's disease: current approaches, challenges, and future considerations. Movement Disorders 2018; 33(5):660–77.

25. Kam K, Vetter K, Tejiram RA, et al. Effect of aging and dual orexin receptor antagonist on sleep architecture and Non-REM oscillations including an REM behavior disorder phenotype in the PS19 mouse model of tauopathy. J Neurosci 2023; 43(25):4738–49.

26. Elliott JE, Lim MM, Keil AT, et al. Baseline characteristics of the North American prodromal Synucleinopathy cohort. Ann Clin Transl Neurol 2023;10(4): 520–35.

27. Ahlskog JE. Does vigorous exercise have a neuroprotective effect in Parkinson disease? Neurology 2011;77(3):288–94.

28. Janssen Daalen JM, Schootemeijer S, Richard E, et al. Lifestyle interventions for the prevention of Parkinson disease. Neurology 2022;99(7):42–51.

29. Hou L, Chen W, Liu X, et al. Exercise-induced neuroprotection of the nigrostriatal dopamine system in Parkinson's disease. Front Aging Neurosci 2017;9. https://doi.org/10.3389/fnagi.2017.00358.

30. Klingman KJ, Jungquist CR, Perlis ML. Introducing the sleep disorders symptom checklist-25: A primary care friendly and comprehensive screener for sleep disorders. Sleep Med Res 2017;8(1):17–25.

31. Boeve BF, Molano JR, Ferman TJ, et al. Validation of the Mayo Sleep Questionnaire to screen for REM sleep behavior disorder in a community-based sample. J Clin Sleep Med 2013;9(5):475–80.

Moving?

Make sure your subscription moves with you!

To notify us of your new address, find your **Clinics Account Number** (located on your mailing label above your name), and contact customer service at:

Email: journalscustomerservice-usa@elsevier.com

800-654-2452 (subscribers in the U.S. & Canada)
314-447-8871 (subscribers outside of the U.S. & Canada)

Fax number: 314-447-8029

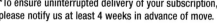

Elsevier Health Sciences Division
Subscription Customer Service
3251 Riverport Lane
Maryland Heights, MO 63043

*To ensure uninterrupted delivery of your subscription, please notify us at least 4 weeks in advance of move.

Printed and bound by CPI Group (UK) Ltd, Croydon, CR0 4YY

03/10/2024

01040365-0005